FETAL HEART MONITORING
Principles and Practices

Fourth Edition

Editors

Audrey Lyndon, RNC, PhD, CNS

Linda Usher Ali, MS, RNC

Contributors

Linda Usher Ali, MS, RNC

Joanne D. Barnes, MS, RNC

Rebecca L. Cypher, MSN, PNNP

Dodi Gauthier, BSN, MEd, RNC

Karen M. Harmon, BSN, MSN, RN, RNC, CNS

G. Eric Knox, MD

Audrey Lyndon, RNC, PhD, CNS

Patricia Robin McCartney, PhD, RNC, F.

Nancy O'Brien-Abel, MN, RNC

Kathleen Rice Simpson, PhD, RNC, FAAI

Catharine M. Treanor, MS, RNC

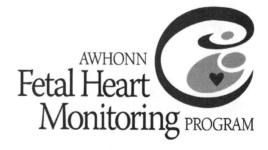

AWHONN
Fetal Heart
Monitoring PROGRAM

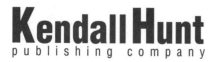

Kendall Hunt
publishing company

Any procedure or practice described in this book should be applied by the health care practitioner only under appropriate supervision in accordance with professional guidelines, and in light of the specific circumstances of each practice situation. The information contained in this book does not define a standard of care, nor is it intended to dictate an exclusive course of management. It presents general methods and techniques of practice that are currently viewed widely as acceptable, based on current research and used by recognized authorities. Proper care of individual patients may depend on many individual factors as well as professional judgment. The information presented here is not designed to define standards of practice for employment, licensure, discipline, legal or other purposes. Variations and innovations that are consistent with law and that demonstrably improve the quality of patient care should be encouraged. Care has been taken to confirm the accuracy of information presented and to describe generally accepted practices. However, the authors, editors, and publisher expressly disclaim any responsibility for errors or omissions or for any consequences resulting from the application of the information in this book and make no warranty, express or implied, with respect to the contents of the book.

The author and publisher have endeavored to ensure that drug selection and dosage set forth in this text are in accordance with current recommendations and practice at the time of publication. However, in view of ongoing changes in government regulations, and the constant flow of information relating to drug therapy and drug reactions, the reader is urged to check the package insert for each drug for any changes in indications and dosage and for added warnings and precautions. This is particularly important when the recommended agent is a new or infrequently used drug. It is the responsibility of the health care provider to ascertain the most current FDA status and guidance on drugs or devices planned for use in their clinical practice.

Requests for permission to use or reproduce material from this book should be directed to permissions@awhonn.org or mailed to: permissions: AWHONN, 2000 L Street, NW, Suite 740, Washington D.C 20036.

Second Printing

Copyright © 1993, 1997, 2003, and 2009 by the Association of Women's Health, Obstetric and Neonatal Nurses (AWHONN), 2000 L Street, N.W., Suite 740, Washington D.C. 20036.

ISBN 978-0-7575-6234-1

Printed in the United States of America
10   9   8   7   6   5   4

CONTENTS

SECTION ONE

Theoretical Basis for Fetal Heart Monitoring

SECTION TWO

Maternal-Fetal Assessment

SECTION THREE

Fetal Monitoring: Diagnosis and Intervention

SECTION FIVE

Advanced Fetal Heart Monitoring Principles and Practices

PREFACE

When it began in 1992, the Association of Women's Health, Obstetric, and Neonatal Nurses (AWHONN) Fetal Heart Monitoring Principles and Practices Workshop (FHMPP) consisted of a single two-day workshop designed to validate the knowledge and skills of registered nurses in the use of fetal heart monitoring technologies. In the intervening years, the course evolved into the AWHONN Fetal Heart Monitoring Program (FHMP) and includes courses and supporting materials addressing the needs of the novice clinician through those appropriate for the expert level clinician The AWHONN FHMP today is a dynamic, comprehensive series of fetal heart monitoring courses and resources designed for use by a multidisciplinary clinical audience including professional nurses, midwives, and physicians. While the purpose of the book is primarily to support the AWHONN FHMP courses, perinatal health care providers may also find it a useful stand-alone practice resource.

This edition of *Fetal Heart Monitoring Principles and Practices* completes the program transition to the National Institutes of Child Health and Development (NICHD) definitions for terms used in describing fetal heart rate findings. This transition was initiated by AWHONN in 2005 based on the recognition that use of standardized terminology among health care providers to communicate fetal heart monitoring information is important to the promotion of patient safety. Use of standardized terminology is consistent with Joint Commission recommendations (Sentinel Event Alert # 30). AWHONN and ACOG both support adoption of a common language for fetal heart monitoring as one step toward improving communication between providers during labor and birth.

The core principles of the FHMP have been retained in this edition. These principles include an emphasis on a physiologic framework for decision making, an evidence-based approach to the care of laboring women and their families, and a commitment to supporting the full range of fetal heart rate assessment technology, including auscultation.

AWHONN participated in the 2008 NICHD Workshop on definitions, interpretation, and research guidelines for electronic fetal monitoring. The three-tiered classification system for EFM patterns fits well with the existing AWHONN Dynamic Physiologic Response Model for interpreting FHR characteristics, and the 2008 classification system and other definition changes are fully integrated into this text.

The 2008 NICHD guidelines for interpretation of EFM tracings also have implications for the interpretation and communication of FHR data obtained by intermittent auscultation. In order to maintain a consistent language for discussion of FHR findings, two categories for interpretation of IA are also presented which are consistent with the three-tiered EFM system. Thus the terms "reassuring" and "nonreassuring" are replaced by Category I (normal) and Category II (indeterminate) for interpretation of auscultation findings, and by Category I (normal), Category II (indeterminate) and Category III (abnormal) for interpretation of electronic fetal monitoring findings in this text. All providers are encouraged to continue the important focus on using a common language for communicating FHR findings. The terms "reassuring" and "nonreassuring" are used in a limited way in the text to discuss interpretation of some types of testing (e.g. biophysical profile results), and are also used in quotation marks when discussing research findings that were originally reported using these terms.

Major changes for the fourth edition include complete transition to the NICHD terminology for describing FHR findings, integration of the physiologic basis for fetal monitoring into a single chapter, increased focus on using the least invasive methods of monitoring as appropriate to maternal-fetal condition, and increased attention to supportive care and the physiologic management of oxytocin and second stage labor as methods of supporting fetal well being. The chapter on fetal cardiac rhythm disturbances has also been extensively reorganized and updated. In keeping with the current language usage in the literature, we have eliminated the distinction between "arrhythmia" and "dysrhythmia" in this edition, and refer to all fetal cardiac rhythm disturbances as arrhythmias.

Note on interpretation of terms used in this textbook: In this text "clinician" refers to professional nurses, midwives, and physicians practicing in accordance with their education and training and within the parameters of their institutional, state, provincial, regional, or other regulatory scope of practice and professional guidelines. The term "midwife" refers to certified nurse midwives and certified midwives in the United States, and registered midwives in Canada.

REVIEWERS

The Association of Women's Health, Obstetric and Neonatal Nurses, the editors, and chapter contributors are indebted to all who shared their time and expertise in reviewing the chapters for this book.

Donna Adelsperger, RN, MEd
Susan Bellebaum, BSN, RNC
Kris Bourgeois, RNC, MS
Deborah A. Cruz, MSN, CRNP
Janet K. Cunningham, MS, RNC
Robin Evans, RN, MSN
Lawrence DeVoe, MD
Dodi Gauthier, BSN, MEd, RNC
Ann C. Holden, RN, BScN, MSc(T), PNC

Helain J. Landy, MD
Susan Ellis-Murphy, BSN, MA, RNC
Linda Goodwin RNC, MEd
Patricia Robin McCartney, RNC, PhD, FAAN
Nancy O'Brien-Abel, MN, RNC
Kathy O'Connell, MN, RN
Denise Palmer, MS, RN, CNS
Mimi Pomerleau, MSN, RNC

Theoretical Basis for Fetal Heart Monitoring

1. Read This Book
2. Take the On-Line Test
3. Earn Continuing Nursing Education Credit

www.awhonn.org/fhm

AWHONN is accredited as a provider of continuing nursing education by the American Nurses Credentialing Center's Commission on Accreditation.

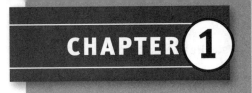

CHAPTER 1

Intrapartum Fetal Monitoring: A Historical Perspective

Patricia Robin McCartney

INTRODUCTION

Fetal heart rate (FHR) assessment is performed in nearly all births, and electronic fetal monitoring is a common obstetric procedure in the United States and Canada today. This introduction to fetal heart monitoring (FHM) education includes an overview of the history of FHR assessment, evidence about FHM practice, development of professional guidelines, standardization of terminology, evolution of FHM education, and use of the nursing process as a framework for applying FHM education to practice. These components provide a historical context and understanding of the state of the science as a basis for the AWHONN Fetal Heart Monitoring Program.

HISTORY OF FETAL HEART RATE SURVEILLANCE

Assessment of the FHR is an indirect measure of fetal oxygenation in antepartum and intrapartum care. This overview highlights the development of techniques to assess the fetus by assessing the FHR and uterine activity (UA) along with adjunct assessment techniques such as ultrasonography, fetal scalp blood sampling, fetal scalp stimulation, acoustic stimulation, pulse oximetry, and computer analysis. This review is based on material from several more comprehensive sources, including Goodlin (1979), Schmidt and McCartney (2000), and Wulf

(1985). Association of Women's Health, Obstetric, and Neonatal Nurses (AWHONN, 2005), Bloom et al. (2006), and Devoe et al. (2006) are the source materials after the year 2000. Key events are summarized in Table 1-1.

Clinicians and researchers seeking ways to prevent fetal death (mortality) and neurologic damage (morbidity) shaped the evolution of FHM techniques. Clinical assessment of the FHR and UA began with unassisted auscultation (examiner's ear on the maternal abdomen) and palpation (examiner's hands on the abdomen) and expanded with the addition of mechanical devices and electronic technology. Contemporary practice is the result of more than a century of development by practitioners dedicated to promoting optimal birth outcomes by identifying and implementing best practices for fetal heart assessment, interpretation, and intervention.

Fetal Heart Rate

Clinical assessment of the FHR began almost 200 years ago, when the Swiss surgeon Mayor in 1818 and the French physician and nobleman Kergaradec (Jean-Alexandre Le Jumeau, Vicomte de Kergaradec) in 1821 reported the presence of fetal heart sounds obtained by auscultation. Mayor used the ear-to-abdomen method, but Kergaradec used a wooden stethoscope and is credited as the first practitioner to recommend assessing fetal heart sounds for diagnostic

Table 1-1	A Chronology of Major Fetal Heart Monitoring Developments
Date	**Development**
1818	Mayor listens to FHR with ear on woman's abdomen.
1821	Kergaradec obtains FHR by stethoscope and relates FHR to fetal life and well-being.
1893	Von Winckel publishes text with auscultation criteria for diagnosing fetal distress.
1906	Cremer uses abdominal and intravaginal leads for fetal ECG.
1917	Hillis describes the head fetoscope.
1958	Hon reports preliminary EFM research.
1961	Saling measures fetal scalp pH.
1964	Callagan adapts Doppler ultrasonography to detect FHR.
1968	Hammacher and Hewlett-Packard market commercial EFM.
1971	International panel approves EFM pattern terminology.
1972	Hon develops the spiral fetal scalp electrode.
1976	Haverkamp reports randomized trial comparing EFM and auscultation.
1977	Read uses acoustical stimulation to assess fetal well-being.
1978	Dawes-Redman criteria for computer analysis of FHR.
1982	Clark uses scalp stimulation to assess fetal well-being.
1985	Manning reports findings on the biophysical profile.
1986	Paine publishes the auscultation acceleration test.
1992	AWHONN introduces a standardized FHR monitoring education program.
1997	NICHD panel recommends standardized EFM definitions.
1999	Thacker and Stroup report meta-analysis of EFM clinical trials.
2000	FDA conditionally approves the fetal pulse oximeter.
2006	U.S. clinical trial of fetal heart ST analysis (STAN) is undertaken.
2006	AWHONN and ACOG standardize FHM language to the 1997 NICHD definitions in educational resources.
2008	NICHD panel recommends standardized categories for interpretation of EFM patterns. AWHONN incorporates interpretation categories into educational resources.

AWHONN, Association of Women's Health, Obstetric and Neonatal Nurses; ECG, electrocardiogram; EFM, electronic fetal monitoring; FDA, U.S. Food and Drug Administration; FHM, fetal heart monitoring; FHMPP, Fetal Heart Monitoring Principles and Practices; FHR, fetal heart rate; NICHD, National Institute of Child Health and Human Development.

purposes. In 1833, Evory Kennedy in Dublin wrote a comprehensive monograph, *Observations on Obstetric Auscultation,* intended to convince doubting colleagues to use Kergaradec's auscultation technique. Kennedy's textbook described the slowness of the FHR return when a contraction "is passing on" and the effects of fetal head and funic compression on the FHR.

During the mid-1800s, a number of investigations using auscultation were reported, including identifying the normal FHR range and correlating FHR with other clinical findings, such as maternal fever, gestational age, fetal weight, fetal sex, and fetal movement. Clinicians debated methods of auscultation (stethoscope vs. ear-to-abdomen), the ideal positioning of the mother (standing vs. supine), and the necessity of exposing the pregnant woman's abdomen during the procedure. Clinicians also investigated physiologic causes for changes in the FHR. In Germany in 1858, Schwartz wrote in a text that the FHR should be counted during labor, both between and during contractions, as a method of assessing fetal well-being. Schwartz related fetal bradycardia to both fetal head compression and decreased placental function caused by the reduction in blood flow during uterine contractions. He was the first to investigate fetal breathing activity. In 1885, Schatz described umbilical cord compression; in 1903, Seitz claimed that FHR decelerations were indicators of fetal oxygenation and described head compression.

In 1849 in the United States, Kilian proposed that finding a FHR of less than 100 beats per minute (bpm) or greater than 180 bpm could identify "fetal distress" that required forceps intervention. Von Winckel in Germany in 1893 formulated specific criteria to identify "fetal distress" as determined by auscultation: tachycardia greater than 160 bpm, bradycardia less than 120 bpm, or irregularity of the FHR. Von Winckel's criteria and auscultation guidelines were followed for the next 75 years (Wulf, 1985).

In the early 1900s, the fetoscope replaced auscultation with the ear or binaural or monaural stethoscope. The head fetoscope was first described in the literature by Hillis (1917) as a metal band over the head attached to a common binaural stethoscope. The original purpose for the device was to enable the obstetrician to listen to second-stage fetal heart tones without using any hands, thus remaining "surgically prepared" for the birth. However, additional benefits were improved assessment from bone conduction and the ability to press the bell of the stethoscope firmly against the abdomen. This device came to be known as the DeLee-Hillis fetoscope to acknowledge both obstetrician inventors.

The use of technology to assess the FHR began with indirect measurement using abdominal devices and direct measurement using fetal devices. Pestalozza in 1891 and Hofbauer and Weiss in 1908 reported use of phonocardiography, a mechanical process using a microphone-like apparatus that amplified and continuously recorded the FHR through the maternal abdominal wall. Many years later, Hammacher in 1962 improved the clarity of the phonocardiographic signal and connected the FHR with the recording of uterine contractions. One hundred years ago, the cardiologist Cremer applied abdominal and vaginal electrodes to obtain a fetal electrocardiogram (ECG) on the fetus of a woman who was not in labor.

In the 1950s, Hon in the United States, Caldeyro-Barcia in Uruguay, and Hammacher in Germany began to report success with electronic monitors that could continuously record indirect abdominal phonocardiography and electrocardiography. In one of the earliest reports, Hon (1958) described using silver electrodes inside light plastic shells on the mother's abdomen and thigh. Hon compared the FHR and patterns of FHR changes with labor variables and neonatal outcomes. Because of poor signal quality of the early abdominal fetal ECG, clinicians experimented with multiple devices to record the FHR directly from the fetus. Hon developed a disposable fetal scalp electrode in 1972 that successfully obtained a direct fetal ECG; this remains the basis for the devices used today. In 1964, Callagan adapted Doppler ultrasound technology to indirectly assess fetal heart motion through the maternal abdomen. This external measurement technique became widespread in both antepartum and intrapartum settings, with progressive engineering improvement in the signal quality and accuracy.

Uterine Activity

Clinical assessment of UA with technological devices actually began a little earlier than FHR technology. In 1872, Schatz reported measuring UA by placing balloons within the uterus to record intrauterine pressures on a graph called a "pain tracing." Two decades later, Schaeffer measured UA externally by placing a hood with a tube connected to a spirometer over the pregnant woman's abdomen. These early investigators examined normal UA and uterine response to drugs such as epinephrine, ether, and morphine. By 1947, an external device, the tocodynamometer, was designed to detect and eventually to continuously record tension changes in the abdomen resulting from uterine contractions. This device provided a visual wave displaying the frequency, duration, and relative strength of uterine contractions.

The first internal assessment of UA was reported by Williams and Stallworthy in 1952; they inserted a polyethylene catheter through the cervix of a woman in labor but concluded, "No instrument was as discerning as the experienced hand in assessing the quality of uterine contractions." Also in 1952, Caldeyro-Barcia reported inserting catheters into the uterus directly through an amniocentesis needle in the abdominal wall. Caldeyro-Barcia coined the term "Montevideo units" (see Glossary) as a quantifiable measure of intrauterine pressure. Eventually, a commercial intrauterine pressure catheter was developed to be inserted into the uterus through the cervix and attached to an external strain gauge transducer to record pressure changes. With advances in microchip computers, a small, solid-state transducer to detect pressure changes was placed at the tip of the intrauterine pressure catheter, replacing the strain gauge transducer.

Electronic Fetal Monitoring (EFM)

The simultaneous measurement of FHR and uterine contractions came to be called either cardiotocography (CTG) or electronic fetal monitoring (EFM). Hammacher and Hewlett-Packard developed the first commercially available electronic FHR monitor in 1968, initially using external microphone phonocardiography and later adding external ultrasound and internal fetal ECG devices (Freeman, Garite, & Nageotte, 2003). Today, the term "phonocardiography" refers to the reflected sound wave from ultrasound technology. The computerized sampling of the raw ultrasound signal, the mathematical calculation of rate, and the visual representation all progressively improved. As ultrasound FHR signal sampling and calculation were improved through engineering (autocorrelation techniques), the devices came to be called "second-generation monitors" (see Chapter 4). Wireless transmission of the ultrasound signal later enabled ambulatory telemetry. Today, it is assumed that all ultrasound FHR signal processing uses autocorrelation, and FHR interpretation is based on this assumption (Macones, Hankins, Spong, Hauth, & Moore, 2008).

An important result of electronic technology was the conversion of an auditory signal into a visual waveform and the creation of a continuous visual pattern of the FHR, permanently recorded on paper. Thus, FHR assessment changed from unassisted auscultation using auditory skills to visual assessment of data generated by an electronic fetal monitor. The development of EFM dramatically altered obstetric practice. In many settings, EFM became the primary technique for FHR monitoring and intermittent auscultation became a screening or secondary technique. In some settings, auscultation remained the primary technique for FHM.

Technology and Intrapartal Nursing Practice

With the introduction of technological advances, nurses had to make EFM fit into their clinical practice. Nurses who experienced the introduction of EFM in their clinical settings were challenged to reconcile the conflict between using technology for greater biomedical objectivity and personalized, non-technologically assessed childbirth (Sandelowski, 2000). The profession of perinatal nursing has had to focus to ensure that constant attention to the glamour of new technology does not overshadow the fundamental practices of labor support. With research showing no benefit of EFM when compared with IA for low-risk mothers, nurses should consider the mother's informed consent and choice regarding monitoring method (Wood, 2003).

Adjunct Surveillance Methods

EFM was originally intended as screening methodology to identify or predict fetal compromise early enough to accomplish intervention that would prevent adverse neurologic outcome or death related to oxygen deprivation. The accuracy of any screening test is measured by sensitivity and specificity (Table 1-2). A normal EFM tracing (See Box 1-1) correctly identifies an oxygenated fetus with a high level of sensitivity and is unlikely to have false-negative interpretations (i.e., incorrectly identify a compromised fetus as adequately oxygenated). When a tracing is normal, clinicians usually agree with the interpretation that the fetus is adequately oxygenated. However, a category II EFM tracing is in-

determinate, has a low level of specificity, and may have false-positive interpretations (i.e., incorrectly identify an oxygenated fetus as compromised). Category II tracings are not predictive of abnormal acid-base status, but also cannot be classified as category I or category III (Macones et al., 2008). Therefore, clinicians may differ in opinion about interpretation and need more information to assess oxygenation and avoid unnecessary intervention. Adjunct surveillance methods were developed to provide additional information, and may be especially helpful with the interpretation and management of category II tracings. Category III EFM patterns are defined as abnormal (Macones et al., 2008). The positive predictive value of an abnormal FHR tracing is also quite low. However, in the case of abnormal tracings there is general consensus among experts that the risk of fetal

Table 1-2 Research Term Definitions Related to Fetal Heart Monitoring

TERM	DEFINITION	FHR EXAMPLE
Sensitivity	Correct identification of the compromised fetus as compromised and not as oxygenated. Reported as a percent. False-negative results are incorrect identification of a compromised fetus as an oxygenated fetus.	A normal FHR tracing has high sensitivity and is unlikely to incorrectly identify a compromised fetus as one who is oxygenated. When a tracing is normal, this indicates the fetus is adequately oxygenated.
Specificity	Correct identification of the oxygenated fetus as oxygenated and not as compromised. Reported as a percent. False-positive results are incorrect identification of an oxygenated fetus as a compromised fetus.	A category II tracing is indeterminate, has poor specificity and may incorrectly identify an oxygenated fetus as compromised. When an indeterminate tracing indicates a compromised fetus, the fetus may actually be adequately oxygenated.
Reliability	The measurement technique is accurate or consistent. There is agreement when two observers measure (inter-rater reliability) or when one observer makes two separate measurements (intra-rater reliability). Reported as a kappa coefficient.	Two clinicians agree on the interpretation of an FHR tracing; or one clinician agrees with his or her own previous interpretation.
Validity (predictive or concurrent)	The measurement of a particular characteristic is statistically associated with the outcome of interest.	An FHR tracing interpretation is related to a newborn outcome (e.g., metabolic acidosis, healthy newborn, poor Apgar score, adverse neurologic outcome, or death).
Efficacy	The intervention to prevent or treat a particular outcome has true effects on the outcome.	The FHR tracing interpretation and management have an effect on newborn outcome.

FHR, Fetal heart rate.

BOX 1-1   2008 Three-Tier Fetal Heart Rate Interpretation System

CATEGORY I

*Category I fetal heart rate (FHR) tracings include **all** of the following:*

- Baseline rate: 110–160 beats per minute (bpm)
- Baseline FHR variability: moderate
- Late or variable decelerations: absent
- Early decelerations: present or absent
- Accelerations: present or absent

CATEGORY II

Category II FHR tracings include all FHR tracings not categorized as Category I or Category III. Category II tracings may represent an appreciable fraction of those encountered in clinical care. Examples of Category II FHR tracings include any of the following:

Baseline rate:
- Bradycardia not accompanied by absent baseline variability
- Tachycardia

Baseline FHR variability
- Minimal baseline variability
- Absent baseline variability not accompanied by recurrent decelerations
- Marked baseline variability

Accelerations:
- Absence of induced accelerations after fetal stimulation

Periodic or episodic decelerations
- Recurrent variable decelerations accompanied by minimal or moderate baseline variability
- Prolonged deceleration ≥2 minutes but <10 minutes
- Recurrent late decelerations with moderate baseline variability
- Variable decelerations with other characteristics, such as slow return to baseline, "overshoots," or "shoulders"

CATEGORY III

Category III FHR tracings include either

- Absent baseline FHR variability and any of the following:
  - Recurrent late decelerations
  - Recurrent variable decelerations
  - Bradycardia
- Sinusoidal Pattern

Note From: "The 2008 National Institute of Child Health Human Development Workshop Report on Electronic Fetal Monitoring: Update on Definitions, Interpretations, and Research Guidelines," by G. A. Macones, G. D. Hankins, C. Y. Spong, J. D. Hauth, & T. Moore, 2008, *Journal of Obstetric, Gynecologic and Neonatal Nursing, 37,* 510-515; *Obstetrics & Gynecology, 112,* p. 665. Copyright 2008 by the American College of Obstetricians and Gynecologists. Reprinted with permission.

acidemia is high enough to warrant intervention despite the low positive predictive value of the tracing.

Adjunct methods were developed to complement the assessment of the FHR, not only during labor but also in the late antepartum period. These innovations enhanced FHM techniques, provided additional information about fetal oxygenation status, or improved FHM information management. Fetal assessment in late pregnancy introduced a new field of care: antepartum fetal surveillance. This expansion of fetal evaluation led to the development of specialized antepartum testing centers and a new obstetric subspecialty practice, Perinatal Medicine, also known as Maternal-Fetal Medicine.

In the 1960s, clinicians observed that late decelerations during labor were associated with an increased risk of metabolic acidosis. In the 1970s, physicians began using low-dose oxytocin in antepartum testing, and the term "oxytocin challenge test" (OCT) was introduced (Freeman, 1975). Clinicians observed that the FHR response to mild induced contractions could predict the FHR response to the stress of labor. The technique was broadened to become the "contraction stress test" using either oxytocin or stimulation of the breast or nipple (breast stimulation test). Use of the CST has been criticized because of its high false-positive rates.

Schifrin and colleagues adopted the observations by Hammacher and Kubli to create the nonstress test (NST) as a noninvasive predictor of fetal well-being (Rochard et al., 1976). The NST was based on spontaneous FHR accelerations occurring without inducing contractions. The NST required electronic monitors available only in hospitals or at fetal testing centers; however, manufacturers developed more portable monitors specifically suited for antepartum testing in clinicians' offices and in homes. In 1986, Paine and colleagues reported an auscultated acceleration test (AAT) using a fetoscope to graph FHR and accelerations for a 6-minute period (Paine, Zanardi, Johnson, Rorie, & Barger, 2001). A reactive AAT was at least one increase in FHR of at least two beats per 5-second sampling period above baseline during the six minute procedure. The test was shown to be a valid and better predictor than the NST for both favorable and poor outcomes. This "low-tech" AAT has been tested internationally and is recommended for settings without EFM technology (Paine et al., 2001).

Ultrasound was first used in the late 1950s to measure the fetal biparietal diameter. By the 1970s, ultrasound became widely used to identify fetal and placental structure and position. Real-time scanning technology was added, and evaluation of the fetal heart became possible. The biophysical profile was pioneered in the 1970s (Manning, Platt, & Silos, 1980) and became a standard fetal assessment test by the 1980s. Ultrasonography, or Doppler velocimetry (Doppler flow), is now used to measure blood flow in the uterine artery, umbilical arteries, and fetal middle cerebral artery as indicators of vascular status and fetal compensatory responses.

Saling reported a technique to assess the presence or absence of fetal acidosis through scalp blood pH sampling in 1961, long before continuous EFM was widely used in labor. The analysis of fetal capillary blood correlated with subsequent umbilical cord blood samples taken at birth, and together these biochemical assessments of pH were viewed as primary physiologic measures of fetal status. Scalp sampling later fell into disfavor because the technique was invasive and technically challenging, often requiring a prolonged maternal supine position, and resulting pH measures had poor specificity (Clark & Paul, 1985).

Several investigators identified methods to stimulate an FHR acceleration now known to be associated with a nonacidotic fetus. Clark and colleagues reported that an FHR acceleration following the stimulation of the scalp during a fetal blood sampling procedure (puncture) was associated with a nonacidotic fetus (Clark, Gimovsky, & Miller, 1982, 1984). These researchers found that an FHR acceleration following fetal scalp stimulation with pinching and pressure was also associated with a nonacidotic fetus. Prior to Clark's work, Read and Miller (1977) reported that an FHR acceleration in response to abdominal acoustic stimulation correlated with OCT outcomes and fetal wellbeing. This association was later tested using an artificial larynx for intrapartum acoustic stimulation (or vibroacoustic stimulation) and fetal scalp pH levels for measures of fetal well-being (Smith, Ngyguen, Phelan, & Paul, 1986). FHR accelerations were consistently shown to be associated with the absence of acidosis. Both scalp stimulation and acoustic stimulation are now recognized as effective assessments of fetal well-being.

Fetal pulse oximetry, developed and commercially available in Europe in the 1990s, was conditionally approved for use in the United States in 2000 (Bloom et al., 2006). Adult pulse oxygen saturation technology (pulse oximetry) was adapted for fetal use with a single, thin, fetal sensor that both emits and receives light. In an effort to reduce unnecessary cesarean births and improve newborn outcomes, fetal oxygen saturation has been used as an adjunct to EFM to assess oxygen status when the EFM tracing is category II (indeterminate) or uninterpretable. The American College of Obstetricians and Gynecologists (ACOG; 2001) and the Society of Obstetricians and Gynaecologists of Canada (SOGC; 2002) did not endorse fetal pulse oximetry as a standard of care because the preliminary research was not convincing. A federally funded multisite postapproval trial found no benefit; neither the rate of cesarean births nor newborn outcomes were improved with the use of fetal pulse oximetry (Bloom et al., 2006). The manufacturer ceased sales of the fetal pulse oximeter just before the study was published because of a lack of demand.

Because human visual analysis is subjective and limited by human sensory capacities, even the earliest electronic monitors used computer technology to aid human pattern recognition. One early device had flashing yellow and red lights for detection of "ominous FHR patterns" (Yeh, Jilek, & Hon, 1974). Computer analysis of the FHR uses artificial intelligence (AI) to objectively analyze the auditory signal according to predetermined criteria to alert care providers, interpret patterns, and even suggest management options. Automated analysis has provided objective, standardized, and reproducible data for research on FHR responses in the antepartum and intrapartum setting. There are a number of published studies about automated methods of fetal assessment in North America (McCartney, 2000). Several investigators have compared computer analysis to visual analysis and generally found similar or better performance with computer analysis in assessing FHR characteristics. In 1978 in England, Dawes and colleagues began to develop software and rules (Dawes-Redman criteria), now available in some commercial monitors, which have been used for CTG analysis in numerous studies around the world.

A recently developed adjunct for analysis of nonreassuring intrapartum EFM tracing characteristics is fetal electrocardiogram ST-segment analysis (STAN). Fetal hypoxemia causes an elevation in the ST-segment and T-wave amplitude, suspected to be an early indicator of myocardial ischemia. Implementation of standardized guidelines for STAN interpretation and structured training in this surveillance method has been shown to reduce unnecessary interventions and improve newborn outcomes (Devoe et al., 2006); however, because this technique is in development, its future clinical application is unclear at the time of this publication.

Obstetric clinical information systems, also known as perinatal information systems, became commercially available in the 1990s. Although originally perceived as being useful for "central fetal monitoring," these powerful computer systems are capable of more than simultaneous displays of EFM tracings. Information systems interface with EFM devices and can be used to enter, display, transmit, query, analyze, archive, and retrieve FHR data in hospital and ambulatory settings. Perinatal systems have great potential for clinical data collection and research about FHR assessment and management.

EVIDENCE FOR FHR ASSESSMENT

When clinicians first experimented with FHM techniques, they recorded their observations as evidence for practice. This kind of anecdotal reporting gradually evolved into the current expectations for (1) rigorous research methods in both observational and interventional clinical trials and (2) complete descriptions of the methods and results in publications.

The initial purpose of EFM was to identify unfavorable FHR characteristics that indicated a fetus at risk for asphyxia, thus enabling intervention to prevent poor outcomes. Years of research and practice with FHM have produced considerable information about favorable and unfavorable FHR characteristics and implications; as well as elucidating the limitations of EFM technology to predict fetal outcomes. Currently, FHM is used to identify FHR characteristics indicating fetal well-being as well as those suggesting risk. Information about normal FHR characteristics is equally helpful in clinical care.

As the practice of FHM (both auscultation and electronic) developed, researchers began to study the accuracy of interpretation by clinicians (reliability) and the relationship between FHR interpretations and neonatal outcomes (validity) (see Table 1-2). Research about the reliability, validity and efficacy of both auscultated and electronic FHR assessment has stimulated discussion and debate in the literature. Both methods were originally incorporated into clinical practice without sufficient research evidence confirming the benefits and risks of the respective methodologies.

Early proponents of EFM promoted its benefits compared with auscultation. Two early studies on auscultation skill and outcomes have been widely cited in the literature, despite concerns raised about their methodologies. The first study is only briefly described in a paragraph within the beginning of a paper by Hon (1958). This paragraph is all that was ever presented, and this original source is not a complete report. Hon proposed that periodic auscultatory sampling between contractions was inaccurate, therefore, he engaged 15 obstetricians to "count" eight rates recorded on a magnetic audiotape (ranging from 75–204 bpm). The counted values varied within a range of 6 to 68 bpm of the true, recorded FHR. Hon subsequently concluded that human auditory interpretation of the FHR had poor reliability and that electronic techniques could prevent human error. The report did not describe the counting method, the nature of the recording, or the obstetricians' experience with auscultation.

The second report was a federally funded, multicenter, prospective observational study on auscultated FHR related to "fetal distress," titled the "Collaborative Study of Cerebral Palsy, Mental Retardation, and Other Neurological Diseases and Blindness" (Benson, Shubeck, Deutschberger, Weiss, & Berendes, 1968). In this study, the FHR was auscultated by observers who were specially trained (but whose qualifications were not identified) every 15 minutes during the first stage of labor. The FHR was not obtained during a contraction or for 30 seconds following a contraction, and FHRs obtained during the second stage of labor were not used in the final study analysis. The short report states that four auscultated FHR measures (based on Von Winckel's 1893 criteria) were related to "fetal distress" (p. 259) based on the computer analysis of the data. However, the author could not identify one auscultatory FHR measure that was a reliable indicator of "fetal distress" except for bradycardia, which the authors call "save in extreme degree" (p. 262). The authors acknowledged that the study was limited because "even a generally acceptable definition of fetal distress based upon the fetal heart rate is yet to be achieved" (p. 262) but concluded that auscultated FHR findings had poor validity. These two studies have been commonly cited as support for the rejection of auscultation and increased use of electronic monitoring. A number of subsequent publications have examined individuals' skill in assessing FHR, rhythm, and accelerations; compared auscultatory devices such as Doppler and Pinard devices (Mahomed, Nyoni, Mulambo, Kasule, & Jacobus, 1994); and compared the cost-effectiveness of auscultation to EFM in labor (Feinstein, Sprague, & Trepanier, 2008; Miller, Pearse, & Paul, 1984) (see Chapter 4).

As the use of EFM increased in the late 1970s, clinicians and consumers considered the invasive nature and high equipment costs associated with EFM and questioned the widespread application of an untested technology (Banta & Thacker, 2001). Skepticism grew when the first EFM clinical trials failed to show any benefit over auscultation in low-risk births. The first reports on randomized clinical trials comparing EFM and auscultation, from Haverkamp, Thompson, McFee, and Cetrulo (1976) and the Dublin Trial (1985), showed that although the use of EFM reduced neonatal seizures, there was no difference in a number of neonatal outcome measures (including cerebral palsy) and there was an increase in the rate of cesarean and operative births. Supporters of EFM debated the methodology of these studies and their implications. Collectively, the findings from 12 randomized controlled trials (RCTs) published between 1976 and 1994 and subsequent meta-analyses of these RCTs demonstrated no benefit with EFM when compared with auscultation (Thacker & Stroup, 1999; Thacker, Stroup, & Chang, 2006).

Clinicians continue to research relationships between EFM patterns and outcomes. Parer, King, Flanders, Fox, and Kilpatrick (2006) used the standardized 1997 National Institute of Child Health and Human Development (NICHD) EFM definitions to review previously reported research to identify relationships between FHR patterns and fetal acidemia and/or newborn vigor. The authors concluded that despite the limitations of a retrospective study, there were relationships between FHR patterns and neonatal outcomes. Graham, Petersen, Christo, and Fox (2006) also used the 1997 NICHD definitions in a retrospective review and found no relationships between EFM tracings and perinatal brain injury or death.

Studies on reliability (accuracy of clinicians' measurements) with EFM patterns show that clinicians differ in their interpretations of an EFM pattern (inter-rater or interobserver reliability) and that the same clinician may give different interpretations of the same EFM pattern when it is reviewed at different times (intra-rater or intraobserver reliability). One study compared the analysis of clinicians using NICHD definitions with the analysis of a computerized fetal monitor alerting system and found that the standardized definitions did not reduce human interobserver differences in pattern interpretation (Devoe et al., 2000).

Perinatal health care professionals generally agree that additional research is needed to validate the efficacy of FHM practice. Areas for further research include examining clinician education and FHM assessment, interpretation, and intervention. The research needed about assessment includes investigation of clinicians' skills with each monitoring method, clinician reliability, optimal assessment frequency, and computer analysis. Research needed about interpretation includes describing the relationships between FHR characteristics and neonatal outcomes. The research needed about intervention includes testing relationships among interpretations, interventions, and neonatal outcomes. Researchers may capitalize on the opportunity to collect data using perinatal information systems. More evidence is needed to design clinician education and competence validation that is based on knowledge and skill development, differences between a novice and an expert, and effective instruction and evaluation methods.

Despite research and guidelines recommending auscultation for low-risk women, clinicians began to question why evidence was not being translated into practice (Haggerty, 1999). A Canadian study investigated the barriers and supports that influenced successful or unsuccessful implementation of an evidence-based guideline on intermittent auscultation in low-risk births (Graham, Logan, Davies, & Nimrod, 2004). Using focus groups and interviews, these authors found that implementation was influenced by nursing and medical leadership, unit philosophy, unit policies, medicolegal concerns, equipment availability, and auscultation skill. More evidence on research translation is needed to identify the most successful approaches to accomplish changes in practice.

STANDARDIZATION AND PROFESSIONAL GUIDELINES

The Institute of Medicine (IOM) published a comprehensive report that detailed the nature and scope of circumstances within health care systems and facilities, and among health care providers that contribute to morbidity and mortality among hospitalized patients. The IOM recommended measures to reduce the incidence of health care errors and promote patient safety (Kohn, Corrigan, & Donaldson, 2000). The report cited many measures that can significantly improve safety, including the use of standardized medical terminology, standardization of education for clinicians, and use of simulation in multidisciplinary training. The IOM report specifically encourages professional organizations to facilitate patient safety by developing and promoting practice guidelines that address patient safety issues and by standardizing technology and education. The Association of Women's Health, Obstetric and Neonatal Nurses (AWHONN) publicly responded to the IOM by emphasizing its commitment to solutions that ensure maternal-fetal safety, including the Fetal Heart Monitoring Principles and Practices (FHMPP) workshop (AWHONN, 2000). The efforts taken to move toward consensus and standardization in FHM are summarized in the next section.

Standardized Language, Controversy, and Consensus

Uniform FHR terminology and interpretation are necessary to facilitate meaningful communication, appropriate documentation, establishment of functional information databases, and sound research. A standardized approach to both auscultation and electronic monitoring requires criteria that are quantifiable, objectively measurable, unambiguous, reproducible, and generally accepted.

Historically, clinicians and researchers have sometimes disagreed about elements of FHR assessment, interpretation, and intervention. For example, physicians began to describe slight variations in baseline FHRs using different terminology, as early as the 1950s. The FHR pattern definitions used in current practice evolved from the pioneering work of Hon, Hammacher, and Caldeyro-Barcia and colleagues during the 1950s

and 1960s. These physicians agreed on descriptions of characteristics but disagreed on terms (baseline rates, changes from the baseline rate [called "accelerations" and "decelerations"], and fluctuations of the baseline rate [called "variability"] as classified by the amplitude of the FHR changes and the number of cycles of change per minute) (Freeman et al., 2003). Some international agreement on deceleration patterns was first achieved at the Fifth World Congress of Gynecology and Obstetrics in 1967. An international panel on fetal monitoring convened in 1971 in the United States and again in 1972 in Amsterdam to develop consensus on terminology and measurement (Freeman et al., 2003). The panel agreed on the terminology of baseline "variability," and "early, late, and variable" decelerations. No agreement was reached on a monitor paper scale or speed or on the categorization of variability. Consequently, discrepant terminology and categorizations of variability evolved, for example, oscillations, variability, beat-to-beat variability, and variation.

In 1995, the NICHD convened an international panel of researchers and clinicians that developed standardized, quantitative definitions for EFM to be used for both visual and computer interpretation. These definitions published simultaneously in nursing and medical specialty journals, were recommended to improve the reliability of pattern interpretation in studies and to better compare findings among studies. In 2005, both AWHONN and ACOG incorporated the NICHD definitions into practice resources (ACOG, 2005a; AWHONN, 2005). In 2008 the NICHD, ACOG, and the Society for Maternal-Fetal Medicine (SMFM) jointly sponsored an interdisciplinary workshop to review and update the 1997 NICHD definitions and to assess the need for a standardized system for interpretation of intrapartum EFM findings in the United States (Macones et al., 2008) (described in Box 1-1 and Chapter 5). Key changes resulting from this meeting include revised terminology for excessive uterine activity (Box 1-2) and the adoption of a three-tiered system for classifying EFM find-

---

BOX 1-2 Uterine Activity

Uterine contractions are quantified as the number of contractions present in a 10-minute window, averaged over 30 minutes. Contraction frequency alone is a partial assessment of uterine activity. Other factors such as duration, intensity, and relaxation time between contractions are equally important in clinical practice. The following represents terminology to describe uterine activity:

A. Normal: ≤ 5 contractions in 10 minutes, averaged over a 30-minute window.
B. Tachysystole: > 5 contractions in 10 minutes, averaged over a 30-minute window.
C. Characteristics of uterine contractions:
- Tachysystole should always be qualified as to the presence or absence of associated FHR decelerations.
- The term tachysystole applies to both spontaneous or stimulated labor. The clinical response to tachysystole may differ depending on whether contractions are spontaneous or stimulated.
- The terms hyperstimulation and hypercontractility are not defined and should be abandoned.

Note From: "The 2008 National Institute of Child Health Human Development Workshop Report on Electronic Fetal Monitoring: Update on Definitions, Interpretations, and Research Guidelines," by G. A. Macones, G. D. Hankins, C. Y. Spong, J. D. Hauth, & T. Moore, 2008, *Journal of Obstetric, Gynecologic and Neonatal Nursing, 37,* 510-515; *Obstetrics & Gynecology, 112,* p. 662. Copyright 2008 by the American College of Obstetricians and Gynecologists. Reprinted with permission.

---

ings (Box 1-1 and Chapter 5). The definitions resulting from the 2008 meeting are incorporated throughout this text.

Some automated analysis systems, such as the Sonicaid system and the SisPorto project (SisPorto; Oporto University, Portugal) apply standard criteria for computer analysis. The SisPorto project was an Internet-accessible database for an international multicenter study using automated analysis of antepartum and intrapartum CTG with standardized terms from the International Federation of Gynecology and Obstetrics (FIGO) (Ayres-de Campos, Ber-

nardes, Garrido, Marques-de-Sa, & Pereira-Leite, 2000). Commercial perinatal information systems may incorporate standardized pattern criteria for recognition and alerting functions or allow the individual users to define their own criteria.

In the 1970s, nurses began to work on a standardized language or classification system for nursing practice that could be used in a computerized database and to help nurses document their contributions to patient care, including intrapartum care (Eganhouse, McCloskey, & Bulechek, 1996). One example of standardized nursing language is the Nursing Intervention Classification (NIC) system, which includes the relevant intervention "6772: Electronic Fetal Monitoring: Intrapartum Intervention." This intervention is defined and detailed with actions that are supported with this FHMPP textbook as a reference (Dochterman & Bulechek, 2004). This standard intervention could be used for FHM nursing practice (uniform documentation) and nursing research (relating nursing interventions to newborn outcomes).

Standardized nomenclature is necessary for many aspects of clinical practice, including the following examples used in documentation, reimbursement, and bibliographic databases. Experts have expressed concern about the continued use of imprecise terms such as "fetal distress" and "birth asphyxia." In 1998, ACOG recommended that the term "fetal distress" be replaced with "nonreassuring fetal status," followed by a description of the assessment findings (ACOG, 1998, 2005b). This recommendation is likely to change based on the publication of the 2008 NICHD definitions, and clinicians should apply the updated language to most accurately reflect the EFM findings present in specific tracings. The term "fetal distress" and all-inclusive terms for "fetal distress" except "metabolic acidemia" were removed from the perinatal International Classification of Disease code (ACOG, 1998). In 2008 the NICHD Workshop participants also recommended use of the term "tachystystole" to describe excessive uterine activity and recommended the terms "hyperstimu-lation" and "hypercontractility" be abandoned due to lack of consistent definitions (Box 1-2) (Ma-cones et al., 2008).

The standard language used to organize and effectively search bibliographic databases (Medical Subject Headings [MeSH]) assigns the standard terms "fetal heart rate," "fetal monitoring," "cardiotocography," and "phono-cardiography" for articles on FHR assessment (National Library of Medicine, 2007).

Professional Guidelines

As FHM developed, professional organizations issued a number of guidelines to promote stan-dardization and competence in fetal heart assess-ment. These resources are periodically revised on the basis of new research findings, techno-logical developments, and practice changes. Some resources focus on a specific assessment technique, whereas others are comprehensive. Some resources are interdisciplinary or interna-tional in scope.

Professional guidelines have been useful for establishing consistency in FHR assessment in labor. Several guidelines address the choice of FHM method. No professional association of providers involved in childbirth has ever au-thored a guideline recommending EFM over intermittent auscultation for low-risk births. Be-cause clinical trials have demonstrated that aus-cultation is as effective as EFM, guidelines in-clude the option of intermittent auscultation for low-risk births (ACOG, 1995, 2005a). AWHONN supports the use of fetal auscultation as well as the "judicious application of intrapar-tum EFM" and does not support the use of EFM as a substitute for appropriate professional nurs-ing care (AWHONN, 2009, p. 1). Furthermore, AWHONN recommends that each facility de-velop a policy regarding appropriate use of each FHR monitoring method. SCOG states that in-termittent auscultation is the recommended method of FHR surveillance for women at low risk during labor (SOGC, 1995, 2002, 2007).

FETAL MONITORING EDUCATION

Implementation of EFM requires skilled per-sonnel at the bedside to interpret patterns throughout labor, and this responsibility be-came part of nurses' work. Nurses quickly found themselves in need of new knowledge and skills to use this technology. Collectively and diligently, nurses initially addressed their immediate needs for education and later emerged as the leaders in fetal monitoring edu-cation. Comprehensive professional education should include the knowledge and skills for FHR assessment by both auscultation and elec-tronic fetal heart monitoring.

Development of FHM Education

When EFM was introduced in the 1960s, most nurses learned basic skills through on-the-job and vendor-sponsored training. Textbooks and journals did not include basic instruction on EFM until the late 1970s. Nurses began to develop and teach EFM education programs throughout the United States. These indepen-dent educators were instrumental in early EFM instruction and continue to be primary providers of basic and advanced instruction today. Some educators went on to develop train-the-trainer programs that prepared other nurses with the knowledge and skills neces-sary to teach basic EFM (Adelsperger, 1990). However, the content, style, and emphasis in these education programs had become quite diverse. Nurses identified the need for re-sources to (1) identify a standard core of FHM knowledge and skills and (2) establish a mech-anism for validating knowledge and skills. Nurses turned to professional organizations such as AWHONN (formally know as NAACOG) to meet these needs.

NAACOG responded with a technical bulletin on EFM, followed by a joint position statement with ACOG, and educational guidelines. These resources were followed in the years to come with numerous other position statements, standards, guidelines, and educational resources on EFM and FHM for nurses. AWHONN remains the recognized source for FHM guidelines and education, including the AWHONN Fetal Heart Monitoring Program (www.awhonn.org).

Competence Validation and Certification

Competence validation is the process of evaluating an individual's knowledge and clinical skills. A variety of instruction and performance evaluation tools can be used for competence validation. Certification is recognition awarded by an accredited credentialing body to an individual who meets predetermined criteria, usually limited to testing of knowledge, demonstrated by means of a psychometrically sound exam. The advantages and disadvantages of subspecialty certification in didactic EFM knowledge have been debated (Afriat, Simpson, Chez, & Miller, 1994; McCartney, 1999; Murray, 1999). Currently there are no national requirements for certification, and facilities may vary in their requirements for credentialing and competence validation of staff responsible for fetal heart monitoring and assessment.

Instruction and Evaluation Methods

Competence in fetal monitoring requires both didactic knowledge and psychomotor skills. A core (basic) instructional program includes knowledge and skills needed to achieve minimal competence. An educational program for ongoing competence validation includes additional or more complex knowledge and skills. Programs for novices include the content and structure for basic assessment and intervention. Programs for experienced clinicians should provide opportunities for more advanced problem solving through case studies, discussion, and reflection. Both basic education and experience are necessary to achieve competence in clinical judgment and decision making.

Today, many continuing education resources exist for FHM didactic knowledge and some measure of skill proficiency at the basic and experienced levels. A number of providers (professional organizations, nurse entrepreneurs, commercial companies, and health care institutions) offer activities with a variety of formats (conferences; hands-on skills workshops; case studies; independent or home self-study assessment modules; journals; computerized simulation programs; online, audio, video, and satellite conferencing). Instruction and evaluation methods include examination, case-study analysis, tracing interpretation, computer-based evaluation, role-playing, policy debate, documentation audit, and skill demonstration.

Research about FHM instruction and evaluation methods is limited. Reports include studies about educational content and methods (Kinnick, 1989, 1990; Murray & Higgins, 1996; Sauer, 1993; Trepanier et al., 1996) and studies on assessment of skill (Chez et al., 1990; Haggerty, 1996; Haggerty & Nuttall, 2000; Morrison et al., 1993). Haggerty found that expert intrapartal nurses identified four clinical parameters to assess the severity of fetal stress: duration of stress, fetal reserve status, reversibility, and specific signs of stress. Later, Haggerty and Nuttall reported that the most important clinical factors that experienced nurses considered in determining fetal risk were scalp pH, maternal parity, amniotic fluid color, and long-term FHR variability. Further studies are needed to identify the best instruction and evaluation methods.

DEVELOPMENT OF THE AWHONN FETAL HEART MONITORING PROGRAM

FHM is a common obstetric procedure in North America, and clinicians need resources to practice in a safe, standardized, and competent manner. The AWHONN Fetal Heart Monitoring Program is designed to be part of an overall plan for competence validation in specialty practice for the individual or institution.

In 1990, NAACOG initiated the development of a standardized fetal monitoring course to validate the cognitive knowledge and psycho-motor skills of the experienced nurse in comprehensive FHM (both auscultation and EFM). The course would emphasize the physiologic basis of assessment and intervention and apply concepts to practice through the use of case studies and hands-on skill practice. Fetal monitoring would be taught within the nursing model as a component of overall childbirth knowledge and skills, not as an isolated technical skill.

The NAACOG Committee on Education appointed a National Steering Committee of member experts in fetal monitoring education from geographically diverse areas. This volunteer committee met regularly for 2 years and created the

2-day workshop (now the Intermediate Course) along with a printed manual, audiovisual materials, and skill models (Schmidt, 2000). A train-the-trainer plan included preparing qualified NAACOG members to be workshop instructors and instructor-trainers to prepare additional instructors. The FHMPP workshop was piloted in 1992, an Instructor Enhancement Course was added in 1994, and an Advanced FHMPP course was added in 1998. A newsletter, *The Beat Goes On,* was launched in 1997 to provide periodic program updates for instructors and instructor-trainers. Progressive course revisions led to the current comprehensive Fetal Heart Monitoring Program. The AWHONN FHM program includes

FIGURE 1-1   The Nursing Process and Fetal Heart Monitoring

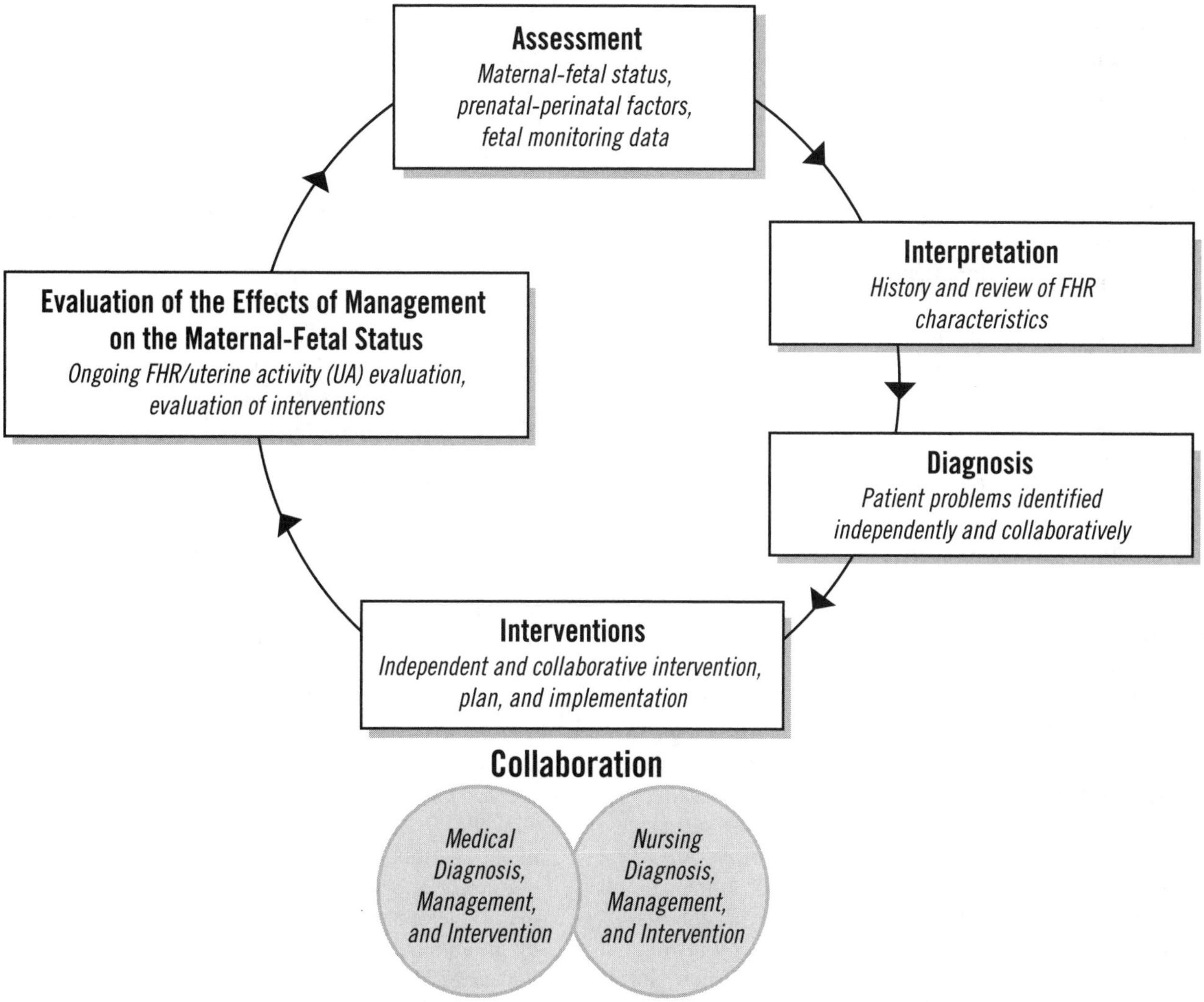

several levels: introduction, intermediate, competence assessment, and advanced. In 2007, almost 15 years after the first pilot, AWHONN had educated more than 100,000 health care professionals in FHM (AWHONN, 2008).

THE NURSING PROCESS AND THE FETAL HEART MONITORING PROGRAM

A systematic framework for providing patient care is useful for clinicians. The nursing process (assessment, interpretation, diagnosis, intervention, and evaluation) is the framework for the Fetal Heart Monitoring Program and this textbook. The nursing process is a scientific problem-solving model for decision making about FHM, and is based on the critical-thinking skills of analysis, synthesis, and evaluation. Scientific problem-solving frameworks and critical-thinking skills are similarly used across professional disciplines (Figure 1-1).

REFERENCES

Adelsperger, D. (1990). *Train the trainer program.* (Continuing Education Program). Santa Clara, CA: Hewlett Packard.

Afriat, C. I., Simpson, K. R., Chez, B. F., & Miller, L. A. (1994). Electronic fetal monitoring competency—to validate or not to validate: The opinions of experts. *Journal of Perinatal and Neonatal Nursing, 8*(3), 1–16.

American College of Obstetricians and Gynecologists. (1995). *Fetal heart rate patterns: Monitoring, interpretation, and management* (ACOG Technical Bulletin No. 207). Washington, DC: Author.

American College of Obstetricians and Gynecologists. (1998). *Inappropriate use of the terms fetal distress and birth asphyxia* (ACOG Committee Opinion No. 197). Washington, DC: Author.

American College of Obstetricians and Gynecologists. (2001). *Fetal pulse oximetry* (Committee Opinion No. 258). Washington, DC: Author.

American College of Obstetricians and Gynecologists. (2005a). *Intrapartum fetal heart rate monitoring* (ACOG Practice Bulletin No. 70). Washington, DC: Author.

American College of Obstetricians and Gynecologists. (2005b). *Inappropriate use of the terms fetal distress and birth asphyxia* (ACOG Committee Opinion No. 326). Washington, DC: Author.

Association of Women's Health, Obstetric and Neonatal Nurses. (2000). *Written statement of AWHONN to Subcommittee on Health, Committee on Ways and Means on the Institute of Medicine Report on Medical Errors.* Washington, DC: Author.

Association of Women's Health, Obstetric and Neonatal Nurses. (2005, August). NICHD terminology transition. *AWHONN's FHMPP Program Newsletter, 4.*

Association of Women's Health, Obstetric and Neonatal Nurses. (2008). *Fetal heart monitoring program.* Retrieved February 8, 2008, from www.awhonn.org

Association of Women's Health, Obstetric and Neonatal Nurses. (2009). Fetal heart monitoring (Position Statement). Washington, DC: Author.

Ayres-de Campos, D., Bernardes, J., Garrido, A., Marques-de-Sa, J., & Pereira-Leite, L. (2000). SisPorto 2.0: A program for automated analysis of cardiotocograms. *Journal of Maternal-Fetal Medicine, 9,* 311–318.

Banta, D. H., & Thacker, S. B. (2001). Historical controversy in health technology assessment: The case of electronic fetal monitoring. *Obstetrical and Gynecological Survey, 56*(11), 707–719.

Benson, R. C., Shubeck, F., Deutschberger, J., Weiss, W., & Berendes, H. (1968). Fetal heart rate as a predictor of fetal distress. A report from the collaborative project. *Obstetrics and Gynecology, 32,* 259–266.

Bloom, S. L., Spong, C. Y., Thom, E., Varner, M. W., Rouse, D. J., Weininger, S., et al. (2006). Fetal pulse oximetry and cesarean delivery. *New England Journal of Medicine, 355,* 2195–2202.

Chez, B. F., Skurnick, J. H., Chez, R. A., Verklan, M. T., Biggs, S., & Hage, M. L. (1990). Interpretations of nonstress tests by obstetric nurses. *Journal of Obstetric, Gynecologic and Neonatal Nursing, 19,* 227–232.

Clark, S. L., Gimovsky, M. L., & Miller, F. C. (1982). Fetal heart rate response to scalp blood sampling. *American Journal of Obstetrics and Gynecology, 144,* 706–708.

Clark, S. L., Gimovsky, M. L., & Miller, F. C. (1984). The scalp stimulation test: A clinical alternative to fetal scalp blood sampling. *American Journal of Obstetrics and Gynecology, 148,* 274–277.

Clark, S. L., & Paul, R. H. (1985). Intrapartum fetal surveillance: The role of fetal scalp blood sampling. *American Journal of Obstetrics and Gynecology, 153,* 717–720.

Devoe, L., Golde, S., Kilman, Y., Morton, D., Shea, K., & Waller, J. (2000). A comparison of visual analyses of intrapartum fetal heart rate tracings according to the new National Institute of Child Health and Human Development guidelines with computer analyses by an automated fetal heart rate monitoring system. *American Journal of Obstetrics and Gynecology, 183,* 361–366.

Devoe, L. D., Ross, M., Wilde, C., Beal, M., Lysikewicz, A., Maier, J., et al. (2006). United States multicenter clinical usage study of the STAN 21 electronic fetal monitoring system. *American Journal of Obstetrics and Gynecology, 195*, 729–734.

Dochterman, J. M., & Bulechek, G. M. (Eds.). (2004). *Nursing interventions classification (NIC)* (4th ed.). St. Louis: Mosby.

Eganhouse, D. J., McCloskey, J. C., & Bulechek, G. M. (1996). How NIC describes MCH nursing. *MCN: American Journal of Maternal Child Nursing, 21*, 247–252.

Feinstein, N. F., Sprague, A., & Trepanier, M. J. (2008). *Fetal heart rate auscultation*. Washington, DC: Association of Women's Health, Obstetric and Neonatal Nurses.

Freeman, R. K. (1975). The use of the oxytocin challenge test for antepartum clinical evaluation of uteroplacental respiratory function. *American Journal of Obstetrics and Gynecology, 121*, 481–489.

Freeman, R. K., Garite, T. J., & Nageotte, M. P. (2003). *Fetal heart rate monitoring* (3rd ed.). Philadelphia: Lippincott Williams & Wilkins.

Goodlin, R. C. (1979). History of fetal monitoring. *American Journal of Obstetrics and Gynecology, 133*, 323–352.

Graham, I. D., Logan, J., Davies, B., & Nimrod, C. (2004). Changing the use of electronic fetal monitoring and labor support: A case study of barriers and facilitators. *Birth, 31*, 293–301.

Graham, E. M., Petersen, S. M., Christo, D. K., & Fox, H. E. (2006). Intrapartum electronic fetal heart rate monitoring and the prevention of perinatal brain injury. *Obstetrics and Gynecology, 108*(3 Pt. 1), 656–666.

Haggerty, L. A. (1996). Assessment parameters and indicators in expert intrapartal nursing decisions. *Journal of Obstetric, Gynecologic and Neonatal Nursing, 25*, 491–499.

Haggerty, L. A. (1999). Continuous electronic fetal monitoring: Contradictions between practice and research. *Journal of Obstetric, Gynecologic and Neonatal Nursing, 28*, 409–416.

Haggerty, L. A., & Nuttall, R. L. (2000). Experienced obstetric nurses' decision-making in fetal risk situations. *Journal of Obstetric, Gynecologic and Neonatal Nursing, 29*, 480–490.

Haverkamp, A. D., Thompson, H. E., McFee, J. G., & Cetrulo, C. (1976). The evaluation of continuous fetal heart rate monitoring in high-risk pregnancy. *American Journal of Obstetrics and Gynecology, 125*, 310–320.

Hillis, D.S. (1917). Attachment for the stethoscope. *Journal of the American Medical Association, 68*, 910.

Hon, E. (1958). The electronic evaluation of the fetal heart rate. *American Journal of Obstetrics and Gynecology, 75*, 1215–1230.

Kinnick, V. G. (1989). A national survey about fetal monitoring skills acquired by nursing students in baccalaureate programs. *Journal of Obstetric, Gynecologic and Neonatal Nursing, 18*, 57–58.

Kinnick, V. (1990). The effect of concept teaching in preparing nursing students for clinical practice. *Journal of Nursing Education, 29*, 362–366.

Kohn, L. T., Corrigan, J. M., & Donaldson, M. S. (2000). *To err is human: Building a safer health system.* Washington, DC: National Academy Press.

Macones, G. A., Hankins, G. D., Spong, C. Y., Hauth, J. D., & Moore, T. (2008). The 2008 National Institute of Child Health Human Development workshop report on electronic fetal monitoring: Update on definitions, interpretations, and research guidelines. *Obstetrics & Gynecology, 112*, 661–666; and *Journal of Obstetric, Gynecologic and Neonatal Nursing, 37*, 510–515.

Mahomed, K., Nyoni, R., Mulambo, T., Kasule, J., & Jacobus, E. (1994). Randomised controlled trial of intrapartum fetal heart rate monitoring. *British Medical Journal, 308*(6927), 497–500.

Manning, F. A., Platt, L. D., & Sipos, L. (1980). Antepartum fetal evaluation: Development of a fetal biophysical profile. *American Journal of Obstetrics and Gynecology, 136*, 787–795.

McCartney, P. R. (1999). Certification in fetal heart monitoring: Is it really worth the additional effort and expense for perinatal nurses? Con position. *MCN: American Journal of Maternal Child Nursing, 24*, 10–11.

McCartney, P. R. (2000). Computer analysis of the fetal heart rate. *Journal of Obstetric, Gynecologic, and Neonatal Nursing, 29*, 527–536.

Miller, F. C., Pearse, K. E., & Paul, R. H. (1984). Fetal heart rate pattern recognition by the method of auscultation. *Obstetrics and Gynecology, 64*, 332–336.

Morrison, J. C., Chez, B. F., Davis, I. D., Martin, R. W., Roberts, W. E., Martin, J. N., Jr., et al. (1993). Intrapartum fetal heart rate assessment: Monitoring by auscultation or electronic means. *American Journal of Obstetrics and Gynecology, 168*(1 Pt. 1), 63–66.

Murray, M. L. (1999). Certification in fetal heart monitoring: Is it really worth the additional effort and expense for perinatal nurses? Pro position. *MCN: The American Journal of Maternal/Child Nursing, 24*, 10.

Murray, M. L., & Higgins, P. (1996). Computer versus lecture: Strategies for teaching fetal monitoring. *Journal of Perinatology, 16*, 15–19.

National Institute of Child Health and Human Development Research Planning Workshop (1997). Electronic fetal heart rate monitoring: Research guidelines for interpretation. *Journal of Obstetric, Gynecologic and Neonatal Nursing, 26*, 635–640.

National Library of Medicine. (2007). *Medical subject headings*. Retrieved January 15, 2007, from http://www.nlm.nih.gov/mesh/

Paine, L. L., Zanardi, L. R., Johnson, T. R., Rorie, J. A., & Barger, M. K. (2001). A comparison of two time intervals for the auscultated acceleration test. *Journal of Midwifery and Women's Health, 46*, 98–102.

Parer, J. T., King, T., Flanders, S., Fox, M., & Kilpatrick, S. J. (2006). Fetal acidemia and electronic fetal heart rate patterns: Is there evidence of an association? *Journal of Maternal-Fetal and Neonatal Medicine, 19*, 289–294.

Read, J. A., & Miller, F. C. (1977). Fetal heart rate acceleration in response to acoustic stimulation as a measure of fetal well-being. *American Journal of Obstetrics and Gynecology, 129*, 512–517.

Rochard, F., Schifrin, B. S., Goupil, F., Legrand, H., Blottiere, J., & Sureau, C. (1976). Nonstressed fetal heart rate monitoring in the antepartum period. *American Journal of Obstetrics and Gynecology, 126*, 699–706.

Sandelowski, M. (2000). Retrofitting technology to nursing: The case of electronic fetal monitoring. *Journal of Obstetric, Gynecologic and Neonatal Nursing, 29*, 316–324.

Sauer, P. (1993, June). *Interpretations of fetal heart rate tracings by obstetric nurses: Comparison of test scores with experience and education in electronic fetal rate monitoring.* Poster session presented at the annual meeting of the Association of Women's Health, Obstetric and Neonatal Nurses, Reno, NV.

Schmidt, J. V. (2000). The development of AWHONN's fetal heart monitoring principles and practices workshop. Association of Women's Health, Obstetric and Neonatal Nurses. *Journal of Obstetric, Gynecologic and Neonatal Nursing, 29*, 509–515.

Schmidt, J. V., & McCartney, P. R. (2000). History and development of fetal heart assessment: A composite. *Journal of Obstetric, Gynecologic, and Neonatal Nursing, 29*, 295–305.

Smith, C. V., Nguyen, H. N., Phelan, J. P., & Paul, R. H. (1986). Intrapartum assessment of fetal well-being: A comparison of fetal acoustic stimulation with acid-base determinations. *American Journal of Obstetrics and Gynecology, 155*, 726–728.

Society of Obstetricians and Gynaecologists of Canada. (1995). SOGC Policy Statement: Fetal health surveillance in labour. *Journal of the Society of Obstetricians and Gynaecologists of Canada, 17*, 865–901.

Society of Obstetricians, and Gynaecologists of Canada. (2002). *Fetal health surveillance in labour* (SOGC Clinical Practice Guidelines No. 112). Ottawa, Ontario, Canada: Author.

Society of Obstetricians and Gynaecologists of Canada. (2007). Fetal health surveillance: Antepartum and intrapartum consensus guideline. *Journal of Obstetrics and Gynaecology Canada, 29*, S1-S56.

Thacker, S. B., & Stroup, D. F. (1999). Continuous electronic fetal monitoring versus intermittent auscultation for assessment during labor (Cochrane Review). In *Cochrane Library,* Vol. 2, Oxford: Update Software.

Thacker, S. B., Stroup, D. F., & Chang, M. (2006). Continuous electronic heart rate monitoring for fetal assessment during labor. *Cochrane Database of Systematic Reviews*, Vol. 4.

Trepanier, M. J., Niday, P., Davies, B., Sprague, A., Nimrod, C., Dulberg, C., et al. (1996). Evaluation of a fetal monitoring education program. *Journal of Obstetric, Gynecologic and Neonatal Nursing, 25*, 137–144.

Wood, S. H. (2003). Should women be given a choice about fetal assessment in labor? *MCN: American Journal of Maternal Child Nursing, 28*, 292–298; quiz 299–300.

Wulf, K. H. (1985). History of fetal heart rate monitoring. In W. Kunzel (Ed.), *Fetal heart rate monitoring: Clinical practice and pathophysiology* (pp. 3–15). New York: Springer-Verlag.

Yeh, S. Y., Jilek, J., & Hon, E. H. (1974). On-line diagnosis of ominous fetal heart rate patterns: A warning device. *American Journal of Obstetrics and Gynecology, 118*, 559–563.

CHAPTER 2

Physiologic Basis for Fetal Monitoring

Nancy O'Brien-Abel

When the fetal heart rate (FHR) and uterine activity are assessed using intermittent auscultation or electronic fetal monitoring, the potential underlying physiology for the FHR characteristics obtained should be considered. Accurate fetal heart monitoring assessment is based on understanding the physiology of fetal heart responses to the intrauterine environment. These responses are considered indirect indicators of fetal oxygenation. Although the study of maternal and fetal physiology is an evolving science, research using animal models and ongoing clinical evaluation of associations observed between FHR tracings and fetal outcomes has led to progressive improvement in understanding the process of fetal homeostasis. Consideration of the potential underlying physiology is important for clinical decision making when the FHR characteristics or patterns are category II or III (indeterminate or abnormal). The presumed underlying physiology helps to guide the interventions and the need for further evaluation of fetal oxygenation.

Physiologic control of the FHR can be divided loosely into three types of influences: those that are extrinsic to (outside of) the fetus, those that are intrinsic to (inside of) the fetus, and those that represent the homeostatic interaction between the fetus and its environment. This chapter begins with the extrinsic influences on the fetus, including placental structure and function, uteroplacental and fetal-placental circulations, placental transfer, maternal oxygen transport, uterine blood flow, and umbilical cord and amniotic fluid structure and function. Intrinsic influences including fetal circulation, oxygenation of fetal tissues, and factors controlling FHR regulation are then discussed. Finally, fetal homeostatic responses to normal and abnormal stresses of labor and birth are illustrated in a dynamic physiologic model of FHR adaptations.

PHYSIOLOGY UNDERLYING EXTRINSIC INFLUENCES ON THE FHR

Maternal-Fetal Exchange

Placenta

Although the mature placenta contains both maternal and fetal tissue, it is primarily a fetal structure responsible for the physiologic exchange of gases, nutrients, and substances between the mother and developing fetus. Other major functions of the placenta throughout gestation include metabolism (e.g., synthesis of glycogen), endocrine secretion (e.g., human chorionic gonadotropin, human placental lactogen, estrogen, progesterone), and immunologic protection from pathogens and from physiologic maternal rejection of the "foreign" fetal tissue (Blackburn, 2007).

Moore and Persaud's (2003) schematic drawing of a transverse section through a full-term placenta is displayed in Figure 2-1. The fetal surface of the placenta is covered by a thin, transparent amniochorionic membrane, beneath which the fetal chorionic villi lie. Chorionic villi are protrusions of fetal tissue exposed to circulating maternal blood within the intervillous space. On the maternal side of the placenta, the decidua basalis forms the outer layer, which attaches to the myometrium. Significant variations exist in placental size and shape, partially because of racial and ethnic differences, altitude, maternal habits such as smoking, and diseases. The normal term placenta from which membranes and umbilical cord have been removed weighs approxi-mately 400 to 500 grams, about one-seventh the weight of the average fetus (Benirschke, 2004a).

Maternal Uteroplacental Circulation

Maternal blood reaches the intervillous space of the placenta via uteroplacental spiral arteries, which traverse the endometrium. Here, oxygen-ated blood, propelled by maternal arterial blood pressure, spurts fountain-like toward the chori-onic plate, which forms the roof of the placenta. As the pressure dissipates, maternal blood bathes

FIGURE 2-1   Schematic Drawing of a Transverse Section through a Full-Term Placenta Showing Maternal Uteroplacental Circulation and Fetal-Placental Circulation

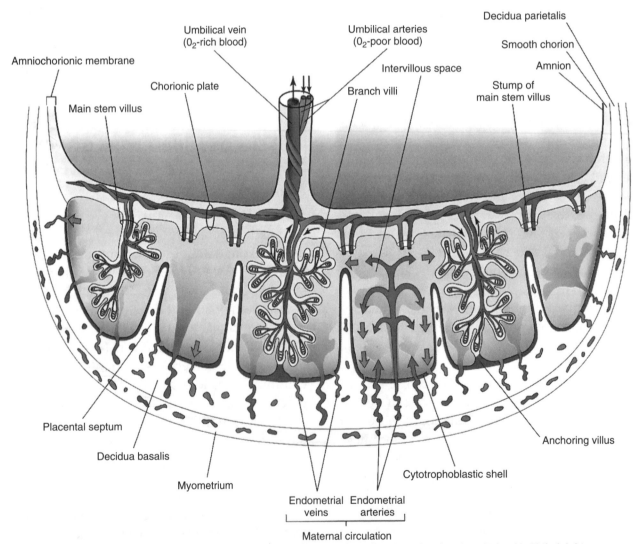

From Moore, K. L., & Persaud, T. V. N. (2003). *The developing human: Clinically oriented embryology* (7th ed.). Philadelphia: Saunders. With permission from Elsevier.

the fetal chorionic villi, allowing for exchange of substances between the maternal and fetal circulations. Eventually, deoxygenated maternal blood returns through the endometrial veins to the maternal circulation.

Fetal oxygenation depends on well-oxygenated maternal blood flow to the placenta. Both adequate maternal oxygen saturation (percent of oxygen carried on the hemoglobin, SaO_2) and adequate oxygen tension in maternal arterial blood (PaO_2) are needed to promote fetal oxygenation. Maternal arterial oxygen tension depends on adequate maternal ventilation and pulmonary integrity (Parer, Rosen, & Levinson, 2002). Although most pregnant women have adequate pulmonary function, maternal conditions that may impair oxygen delivery to the fetus include asthma, congestive heart failure, congenital cardiac defects, and severe anemia.

Fetal-Placental Circulation

Deoxygenated blood from the fetus is carried by two umbilical arteries that spiral around the umbilical vein to the placenta. As the umbilical cord enters the placenta, the umbilical arteries successively divide into smaller vessels, eventually creating an extensive arteriovenous system within each chorionic villus (Blackburn, 2007). Within this arteriovenous system, fetal blood is extremely close to the maternal blood, facilitating exchange between the fetal and maternal circulations. This newly well-oxygenated fetal blood flows into veins that follow the chorionic arteries back to the site of umbilical cord attachment. Here the veins converge, forming the large, single umbilical vein that carries the well-oxygenated blood to the fetus.

Placental Transfer

The exchange of gases, nutrients, medications, waste products, and other substances is facilitated by the large surface area of the placental membrane separating the maternal and fetal blood (Figure 2-2). As pregnancy advances, transfer of substances across the placental membrane increases because of the decreased distance between maternal and fetal blood, increased maternal and fetal blood flow, and greater fetal physiologic and metabolic demands. Placental exchange may be altered by decreased uterine blood flow, maternal diseases (e.g., hypertension, diabetes mellitus, infection), or decreased placental surface area or diffusing capacity.

Mechanisms by which substances transfer across the placental membrane include simple (passive) diffusion, facilitated diffusion, active transport, pinocytosis and endocytosis, bulk flow, breaks or leaks, independent movement, and infection. Table 2-1 summarizes these mechanisms and provides examples of substances transported by each mechanism (Blackburn, 2007; Campbell & Reece, 2005; Cunningham et al., 2005; Moore & Persaud, 2003; Ross, Ervin, & Novak, 2002).

The ability of the fetus to cope with compromises in oxygen and nutrient exchange appears as percentages of reduced blood flow in Parer's (1983) representation of placental transfer capacity (Figure 2-3). When the placental transfer capacity is near 100%, the fetus is provided with approximately twice the resources it needs to grow and be well oxygenated. This is also known as "fetal reserve". However, at less than approximately 75% of maximal transfer capacity, fetal nutrition is limited and intrauterine growth restriction may evolve. If placental function is reduced beyond approximately 50% of maximal exchange, oxygen and carbon dioxide transfer decrease and fetal compromise can result.

Maternal Oxygen Transport Physiology

The fetus depends on a constant supply of well-oxygenated maternal blood to maintain aerobic metabolism. Oxygen transport physiology involves four basic components: oxygen content, oxygen affinity, oxygen delivery, and oxygen consumption. Specifics relating to oxygen transport to fetal tissue are addressed later in this chapter.

FIGURE 2-2   Transfer of Substances between the Mother and Fetus across the Placental Membrane

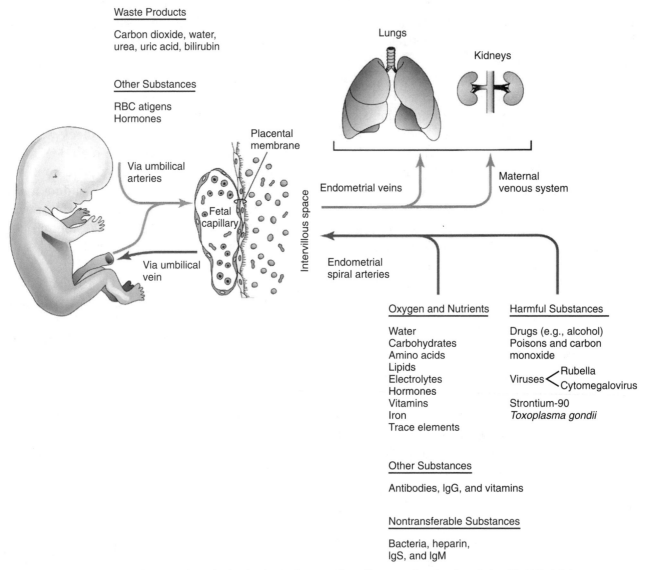

From Moore, K. L., & Persaud, T. V. N. (2003). *The developing human: Clinically oriented embryology* (7th ed.). Philadelphia: Saunders. With permission from Elsevier.

Oxygen Content

Maternal oxygen content is defined as the total amount of oxygen in the maternal arterial blood and includes two components:

1. *The amount of oxygen dissolved in plasma (PaO$_2$), also known as the "partial pressure of oxygen" or "oxygen tension."* Because oxygen is relatively insoluble in water, only 1% to 2%

of oxygen dissolves in the blood plasma. The PaO$_2$ helps bind oxygen molecules to hemoglobin. The amount of oxygen bound to the hemoglobin at any time is related, in large part, to the PaO$_2$ to which the hemoglobin is exposed. In the lungs, at the alveolar-capillary interface where the PaO$_2$ is typically high, oxygen binds readily to hemoglobin. As the

Table 2-1	Transport Mechanisms and Examples of Substances Transferred across the Placenta
TRANSPORT MECHANISMS	**EXAMPLE SUBSTANCES**
Simple (passive) diffusion Transfer down concentration gradient (higher to lower concentration)	Oxygen, carbon dioxide, water, some electrolytes, urea, uric acid, fatty acids, fat-soluble vitamins, narcotics, barbiturates, anesthetic gases, antibiotics
Facilitated diffusion Transfer facilitated by carrier molecules across concentration gradient	Glucose
Active transport Transfer against concentration gradient; carrier molecules and energy required	Amino acids, water-soluble vitamins, calcium, phosphorus, iron, iodine
Pinocytosis and endocytosis Engulfing of microdroplets of fluid (pinocytosis) or solids (endocytosis) in vesicles for transport	Immunoglobulin G (IgG), phospholipids, lipoproteins, some viruses and antibodies
Bulk flow Hydrostatic or osmotic gradient	Water, electrolytes
Breaks or leaks Transfer of substances through microscopic breaks in placental membrane	Intact blood cells
Independent movement Transfer of cells under own power	Maternal leukocytes, organisms such as *Treponema pallidum*
Infection Creates lesions or defects in membrane	Some bacteria and protozoa such as *Toxoplasma gondii*

Adapted from: Blackburn, 2007; Campbell & Reece, 2005; Cunningham et al., 2005; Moore & Persaud, 2003; Ross, Ervin, & Novak, 2002.

FIGURE 2-3   Ability of the Placenta to Transport Substances (Placental Transfer Capacity) and Effects on the Fetus

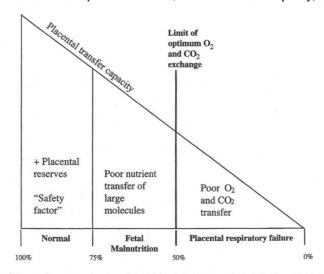

Adapted from Handbook of Fetal Heart Rate Monitoring (p. 15) by J. T. Parer, Philadelphia: W. B. Saunders. Copyright 1983 by W. B. Saunders. Adapted with permission.

blood circulates to other body tissues in which the PaO_2 is lower, the hemoglobin releases oxygen (Campbell & Reece, 2005).

2. *Oxygen saturation or the percent of oxygen carried on the hemoglobin (SaO_2).* Approximately 98% to 99% of oxygen is transported by molecules of hemoglobin in red blood cells. One molecule of hemoglobin consists of four subunits, each with a heme group that has an iron atom at its center (Campbell & Reece, 2005). The iron binds to the oxygen; thus, each hemoglobin molecule can carry four molecules of oxygen. When a hemoglobin molecule is combined with oxygen, it is called "oxyhemoglobin". The oxygen-carrying capacity is determined by the amount of hemoglobin present in the blood. Oxygen saturation is the ratio of oxyhemoglobin to the total amount of hemoglobin available, as illustrated in Figure 2-4.

Oxygen Affinity

The affinity of hemoglobin for oxygen is the means by which hemoglobin readily acquires and releases oxygen molecules. The dynamics of the uptake and release of oxygen by hemoglobin molecules is demonstrated in the sigmoid-shaped oxyhemoglobin dissociation curve, which relates oxygen saturation (SaO_2) and partial pressure of oxygen in the blood (PaO_2) (Figure 2-5).

At low PaO_2 levels (<50 mm Hg), the oxyhemoglobin curve is steep and small changes in PaO_2 result in large changes in SaO_2 (Blackburn, 2007). As blood circulates to other body tissue in which the PaO_2 is lower, hemoglobin readily releases oxygen into tissue as the affinity of hemoglobin for oxygen diminishes (Campbell & Reece, 2005).

At the upper end of the curve where it appears relatively flat (>50 mm Hg), increases in PaO_2

FIGURE 2-4   Percent Saturation of Hemoglobin

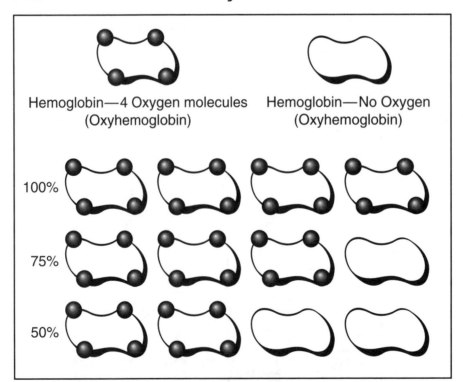

From Mandeville, L. K., & Troiano, N. H. (1999). *AWHONN's high-risk and critical care intrapartum nursing* (2nd ed., p. 68). Philadelphia: Lippincott.

FIGURE 2-5 Maternal and Fetal Oxyhemoglobin Dissociation Curves

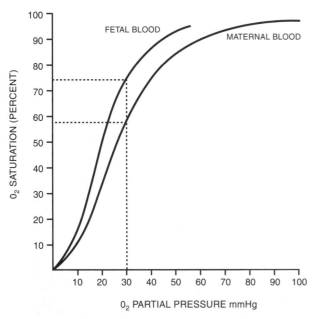

The vertical broken line illustrates the higher oxygen affinity of fetal blood. Fetal blood is more highly saturated with oxygen than maternal blood at the same oxygen partial pressure.
From Parer, J. T. (1997). *Handbook of fetal heart rate monitoring* (2nd ed.). Philadelphia: Saunders. Reprinted with permission.

produce minimal increases in SaO_2 (Blackburn, 2007). In this upper range, where the PaO_2 is typically high, oxygen binds readily to hemoglobin in the lungs.

The PaO_2 at which the hemoglobin is 50% saturated, known as the P_{50}, is typically about 26 mm Hg for a healthy adult (Blackburn, 2007). In the presence of disease or other conditions that change the affinity of hemoglobin for oxygen and, consequently, shift the curve to the right or left, the P_{50} changes accordingly. An increased P_{50} indicates a rightward shift of the standard curve, implying a decreased oxygen affinity and lower saturation at any given PaO_2. This makes it more difficult for the hemoglobin to bind to oxygen (requiring a higher PaO_2 to achieve the same oxygen saturation), but it makes it easier for the hemoglobin to release bound oxygen (e.g., acidosis, fever, elevated 2,3-diphosphoglycerate

[2,3-DPG], pregnancy) (Troiano, 1999). Conversely, conditions that lower P_{50} and shift the curve to the left (e.g., alkalosis, hypothermia, carbon monoxide, decreased 2,3-DPG, fetal hemoglobin) result in increased oxygen affinity, making it easier for the hemoglobin to pick up oxygen but harder to release it (Bobrowski, 2004; Troiano).

In pregnancy, the mother's oxyhemoglobin dissociation curve typically shifts to the right, enhancing the transfer of oxygen from the mother to the fetus (see Figure 2-5). At term, the P_{50} increases from approximately 26 to 30 mm Hg (Blackburn, 2007). Because the fetal hemoglobin has a higher affinity for oxygen compared with maternal hemoglobin, the fetal oxyhemoglobin curve shifts to the left of the mother's curve, thereby further enhancing oxygen uptake by the fetus.

Oxygen Delivery

The quantity of oxygen delivered to the tissues per unit of time is known as oxygen delivery (DO_2). Both cardiac output and arterial oxygen content (i.e., PaO_2 and SaO_2) affect the delivery of oxygen from the lungs to the tissues. Factors that increase maternal cardiac output (e.g., exercise, uterine contractions, increased metabolism) or increase total arterial oxygen content (e.g., increased carrying capacity from transfusion of packed red blood cells) increase oxygen delivery to the tissues (Troiano, 1999). Factors that decrease either maternal cardiac output or oxygen content (e.g., hypovolemia, hypotension, hypoxemia, anemia) may decrease oxygen delivery (Troiano).

Maternal hemoglobin and arterial oxygen content typically decrease as a result of the physiologic anemia of pregnancy. However, oxygen delivery is maintained at or above normal because maternal cardiac output increases 30% to 50% by the third trimester of pregnancy (Blackburn, 2007; Bobrowski, 2004). Thus, the pregnant woman, as compared with the nonpregnant patient, is more dependent on cardiac output for oxygen delivery (Bobrowski). Because the pregnant woman's oxygen delivery normally exceeds her oxygen consumption, she is usually able to maintain oxygen delivery to both herself and fetus, even during labor (Bobrowski). However, if her oxygen delivery decreases, both she and her fetus can rapidly become seriously compromised (Bobrowski).

Oxygen Consumption

Oxygen consumption refers to the quantity of oxygen consumed by the tissues each minute. Under normal conditions, the human body consumes approximately 25% of oxygen delivered (Bobrowski, 2004). When the supply of oxygen is reduced, or if oxygen consumption is high (e.g., as a result of pregnancy, hyperthermia, stress), more oxygen is extracted from the blood so that oxygen consumption is maintained. If oxygen delivery is severely reduced and the tissues are unable to sustain aerobic metabolism, oxygen consumption decreases and the tissues begin to use anaerobic glycolysis, resulting in metabolic acidosis, and eventually, irreversible tissue damage and death (Bobrowski).

Uterine Blood Flow

Adequate uterine blood flow is critical for the passage of respiratory gases and substances across the placenta (Blackburn, 2007; Cunningham et al., 2005; Parer, 1997). Uteroplacental blood flow increases progressively throughout pregnancy and in a singleton pregnancy at term is approximately 700 mL/min, or 10% to 15% of maternal cardiac output (Parer et al.; Ross et al.). Although uterine blood flow during pregnancy also supplies the myometrium, endometrium, and placenta, the intervillous space receives 70% to 90% of the total uterine blood flow near term (Parer et al., Ross et al.).

Any factor that decreases maternal cardiac output will thereby decrease uterine blood flow

and intervillous space perfusion. Factors that can potentially decrease uteroplacental perfusion include excessive uterine contractions, maternal hypotension or maternal hypertension, placental changes, and endogenous or exogenous vasoconstriction. Box 2-1 lists specific clinical factors that may decrease uteroplacental perfusion. In clinical practice, there exist few useful means of increasing uterine blood flow after it becomes suboptimal (Parer et al., 2002). Therefore, a primary goal of prenatal and intrapartum care is to minimize risk for or prevent clinical conditions that decrease uterine blood flow (e.g., maternal hypotension) or that inter-

---

BOX 2-1 Factors That May Potentially Decrease Uteroplacental Perfusion

Excessive uterine contractions or hypertonus
Abruptio placenta
Drug stimulation (e.g., oxytocin, misoprostol, prostaglandin E2)

Maternal hypotension
Supine hypotension
Sympathetic blockade (e.g., regional anesthetic)
Hypovolemic shock

Maternal Conditions
Chronic hypertension
Hypertensive disorders of pregnancy
Physical or emotional stress

Placental changes
Decreased surface area (e.g., abruptio placenta)
Degenerative (e.g., hypertension, prolonged pregnancy, diabetes)
Calcifications (e.g., smoking)
Infarcts (e.g., abruptio placenta, prolonged pregnancy)
Infection (e.g., chorioamnionitis)
Edema (e.g., erythroblastosis fetalis)

Vasoconstriction
Endogenous (sympathetic, adrenal medullary activity)
Exogenous (most sympathomimetics)

Adapted from: Blackburn, 2007; Freeman, Garite, & Nageotte, 2003; Parer, 1997

fere with uteroplacental perfusion (e.g., tachy-systole) during labor and birth.

Umbilical Cord

The umbilical cord is the vascular connection between the placenta and fetus. Normally, the umbilical cord contains three vessels: two arteries and one vein arranged in a spiral within the cord. The single umbilical vein carries the oxygen-rich blood from the placenta to the fetus; the two arteries return from the fetus carrying deoxygenated blood. Wharton's jelly, a mucoid connective tissue, helps protect the umbilical cord from compression.

The umbilical vessels twist and spiral within the umbilical cord. Coiling may protect the cord from compression, entanglement, and tension (Marino, 2004). These twists often form false knots, creating redundancies or varicosities of umbilical vessels that may protrude on the cord surface and that usually have no clinical significance (Benirschke, 2004a). True knots in the umbilical cord are uncommon, but can cause reduced blood flow to the fetus.

At term, the umbilical cord measures approximately 55 cm in length (range, 30–90 cm) (Benirschke, 2004a; Moore & Persaud, 2003). Cord length is influenced by amniotic fluid volume, fetal movement, and genetics (Marino, 2004; Cunningham et al., 2005). Frequently, the umbilical cord becomes wrapped around fetal parts, particularly the neck; this is called "nuchal cord."

Attachment of the umbilical cord is usually near the center of the fetal surface. Cord insertion at the placental margin is sometimes referred to as "Battledore placenta." With a velamentous insertion, the umbilical vessels run between the amnion and chorion without the protection of Wharton's jelly. Vasa previa occurs when the vessels from a velamentous cord insertion have a transcervical position, passing over the cervical os, or when they pass along the dividing membrane of a second twin (Benirschke, 2004b).

The umbilical cord is susceptible to entanglement, compression, and occlusion. Partial umbilical cord compression may cause occlusion of the low-pressure vein, leading to decreased return of blood to the fetal heart, decreased cardiac output, hypotension, and a compensatory FHR acceleration (Freeman et al., 2003; James et al., 1976; Lee, Di Loreto, & O'Lane, 1975). With complete cord occlusion, the two umbilical arteries become occluded, resulting in sudden fetal hypertension, stimulation of the baroreceptors, and a sudden drop in FHR (Freeman et al., 2003; Lee & Hon, 1963) (Figure 2-6).

FIGURE 2-6   FHR and Fetal Systemic Blood Pressure (FSBP) Occurring during a Uterine Contraction (UC) with Compression of Umbilical Vein (UV) and Umbilical Artery (UA)

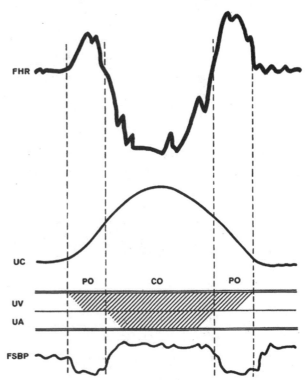

From "A study of fetal heart rate acceleration patterns," by C. V. Lee, P. C. Di Loreto, and J. M. O'Lane, Obstetrics and Gynecology, 50, p. 142. Copyright 1975 by the American College of Obstetricians and Gynecologists. Reprinted with permission.

Amniotic Fluid

Amniotic fluid provides several significant functions in the normal growth and development of the fetus (Box 2-2) (Moore & Persaud, 2003). At term, approximately 99% of amniotic fluid is water, with the remainder consisting of proteins, carbohydrates, fats, electrolytes, enzymes, hormones, urea, creatinine, bile pigments, fetal cells, lanugo, and vernix. Amniotic fluid volume is maintained by a balance of fetal fluid production (fetal urine and lung secretions) and fluid reabsorption (fetal swallowing and flow across fetal membranes and placenta). Throughout gestation, volumes increase steadily from a mean of 30 mL at 10 weeks, to 190 mL at 16 weeks, to a peak of 780 mL at 32 to 35 weeks' gestation (Brace, 2004). Thereafter, volume begins to decrease progressively, especially in postterm pregnancies.

Because amniotic fluid is readily assessed by ultrasound, two methods are available to evaluate adequacy of amniotic fluid volume. One method measures the vertical depth of the single largest pocket of amniotic fluid. The second method is the amniotic fluid index (AFI). In this method, the uterus is divided into four equal quadrants. In each quadrant, the vertical depth of the largest amniotic fluid pocket is identified and measured. The AFI is the summation of each of these four measurements reported in centimeters (Chervenak & Gabbe, 2007; Cunningham et al., 2005).

Hydramnios, or excessive amniotic fluid, is diagnosed when the vertical depth of the largest pocket exceeds 8 cm or when the AFI is 20 cm or greater at term (>95th percentile for gestational age) (Chervenak & Gabbe, 2007; Cunningham et al., 2005; Manning, 2004). In approximately 60% of women, hydramnios is idiopathic, and when diagnosed in the second trimester, approximately 50% of cases spontaneously resolve with good outcome (Blackburn, 2007; Brace, 2004). Conditions associated with hydramnios include multiple gestation; immune and nonimmune hydrops fetalis; chromosomal abnormalities; and fetal gastrointestinal, cardiac, and neural tube anomalies (Blackburn).

Oligohydramnios, or reduction in amniotic fluid, is diagnosed when the largest vertical pocket measures less than 2 cm or the AFI is less than 5 cm at term (<5th percentile for gestational age) (Chervenak & Gabbe, 2007; Cunningham et al., 2005; Manning, 2004). Conditions associated with oligohydramnios include amnion abnormalities, fetal urinary abnormalities, fetal pulmonary hypoplasia, intrauterine growth restriction, prolonged pregnancy, ruptured membranes, and umbilical cord compression (Blackburn, 2007; Cunningham et al.).

PHYSIOLOGY UNDERLYING INTRINSIC INFLUENCES ON THE FHR

Fetal Circulation

Fetal circulation differs significantly from that of the adult. In the adult, respiratory gases exchange in the pulmonary vasculature and oxygenated blood returns via the pulmonary veins to the left ventricle to be ejected into the adult circulation. In the fetus, blood does not need to enter the lungs to become oxygenated; rather, oxygenation occurs in the placenta. Another difference is that the ventricles of the fetal heart work in parallel, not in a series as in the adult configuration. Well-oxygenated fetal blood enters the left ventricle, which supplies the heart and brain, and less-oxygenated blood enters the

---

BOX 2-2 Significance of Amniotic Fluid
Permits symmetric fetal growth
Enables fetus to move freely, aiding muscular development
Permits normal fetal lung development
Prevents adherence of amnion to fetus
Maintains constant temperature
Protects and cushions fetus against impacts
Acts as barrier to infection
Maintains homeostasis of fluids and electrolytes

(Moore & Persaud, 2003)

right ventricle, which supplies the rest of the body. This presence of oxygenated blood in the right and left atria and great vessels is unique to the fetus and made possible by several anatomic shunts (e. g., foramen ovale and ductus arteriosus). A third shunt, the ductus venosus, allows relatively well-oxygenated blood to enter the fetal heart directly, bypassing the liver. At birth, when circulation of fetal blood through the placenta ceases and the neonate's lungs expand, these anatomic shunts normally close rapidly and cease to function.

Fetal circulation is illustrated in Figure 2-7. Highly oxygenated, nutrient-rich blood returns from the placenta via the umbilical vein. As the umbilical vein approaches the liver, approximately 70% to 80% of the oxygen-rich blood enters the sinusoids of the liver, reflecting the

Figure 2-7   Fetal Circulation

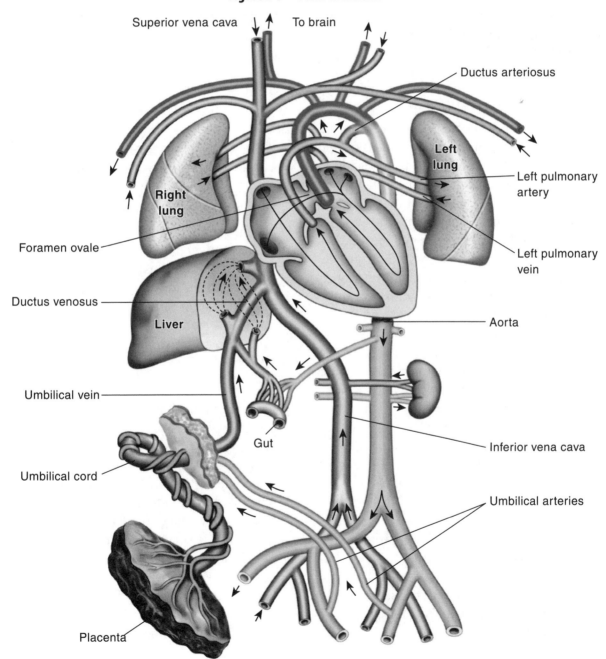

increased demand of the fetal liver near term (Blackburn, 2007; Kiserud, 2001). The blood then drains via the hepatic vein into the inferior vena cava, where it mixes with desaturated blood returning from the lower body. The remaining 20% to 30% of oxygen-rich blood in the umbilical vein is shunted via the ductus venosus directly into the inferior vena cava. This richly oxygenated blood from the umbilical vein has a greater oxygen content and kinetic energy, resulting in a distinct "stream" of blood as it enters the right atrium (Blackburn; Fineman, Clyman, & Heymann, 2004; Kiserud; Edelstone & Rudolph, 1979).

As the well-oxygenated umbilical venous blood streams preferentially across the foramen ovale into the left atrium, it mixes with a small amount of pulmonary venous return, passes through the mitral valve, and is then ejected by the left ventricle into the ascending aorta. This preferential streaming allows the most highly oxygenated umbilical venous blood to supply the coronary circulation and vessels that supply the head, neck, and upper extremities (Fineman et al., 2004; Edelstone & Rudolph, 1979). The second stream of blood, which consists of desaturated blood returning from the lower body, the liver, and some umbilical venous return, mixes in the right atrium with blood returning in the superior vena cava and coronary sinus. From here, a small amount enters the pulmonary artery and lung tissue. Most of the remaining second stream (that which does not go through the foramen ovale or to the lungs) is directed downward across the tricuspid valve, into the right ventricle, and then is shunted across the ductus arteriosus to enter the descending aorta. The descending aorta supplies the gut, kidneys, lower body, and umbilical circulation. This preferential streaming of blood returning from the superior vena cava and coronary sinus is advantageous to the fetus because it directs the desaturated blood toward the placenta for reoxygenation (Fineman et al.).

At birth, major physiologic and anatomic transitional events occur in the neonatal circulation. Oxygenation moves from the placenta to the neonate's lungs, resulting in a dramatic fall in pulmonary vascular resistance, increased pulmonary blood flow, and a rise in PO_2 levels (Blackburn, 2007). Under normal circumstances, the neonate's ventricles begin working in sequence, as in the adult configuration, rather than in parallel. Finally, fetal shunts close and cease to function. The ductus venosus functionally closes within minutes of birth because of the cessation of blood flow. Pressure changes within the cardiac chambers close the flap of the foramen ovale that separates the two atria. The ductus arteriosus begins to constrict at birth yet may remain patent for several days.

Oxygen Transport to Fetal Tissue

The fetal umbilical vein, which carries the well-oxygenated blood from the placenta to the fetus, has approximately the same amount of dissolved oxygen (partial pressure oxygen or PO_2) as in the maternal uterine vein (Meschia, 2004). Despite a low PO_2, the fetal blood transports large amounts of oxygen from the placenta to the body tissues. Several physiologic adaptations make this possible (Meschia; King & Parer, 2000; Parer 1997; Martin & Gingerich, 1976):

- Fetal blood has a higher hemoglobin concentration than adult blood, allowing for greater oxygen-carrying capacity.
- Fetal hemoblobin has a higher affinity for oxygen compared with the mother's blood, an important adaptation to the low PO_2 at which the placenta oxygenates the fetus. The fetal oxyhemoglobin dissociation curve favors a higher saturation of the hemoglobin with oxygen at any given PO_2. (Figure 2-5 compares the oxygen dissociation curves for the maternal and fetal blood.) At a PO_2 of 30 mm Hg and blood pH of 7.4, fetal blood is approximately 74%

saturated with oxygen, whereas maternal blood is only 58% saturated (Figure 2-7).

- The fetus has a higher cardiac output and heart rate than the adult, resulting in rapid circulation.

These adaptations support efficient exchange of respiratory gases and normal fetal aerobic metabolism. In addition, the normal placenta has a "safety factor" allowing the fetus to maintain normal aerobic metabolism (fetal reserve) until the available oxygen in the intervillous space of the placenta decreases to 50% of normal levels (Parer et al., 2002). When the PO_2 drops significantly, as in acute hypoxia, the normoxic fetus compensates with the following mechanisms enabling temporary survival without decompensation of vital organs (Meschia, 2004; Parer & Nageotte, 2004; Parer et al., 2002; Cohen, Sacks, Heymann, & Rudolph, 1974):

- *Redistribution of fetal blood flow favoring vital organs.* Blood flow to the heart, brain, and adrenal glands is increased; blood flow to the gut, spleen, kidneys and limbs is decreased (Figure 2-8).
- *Decrease in total O_2 consumption.* As the FHR decreases, the myocardium consumes less oxygen.

If these temporary compensatory measures do not supply sufficient oxygen for metabolic needs, anaerobic metabolism follows with accumulation of lactic acid, resulting in metabolic acidosis in the tissues. With sustained hypoxemia or severe asphyxia, decompensation may occur, during which fetal cardiac output, arterial blood pressure, and blood flow to the brain decrease, followed by tissue damage and, ultimately, fetal death (Parer, 1997; Parer & Nageotte, 2004).

FIGURE 2-8   **Schematic Illustration of the Redistribution of Blood Flow that Occurs during Fetal Hypoxia**

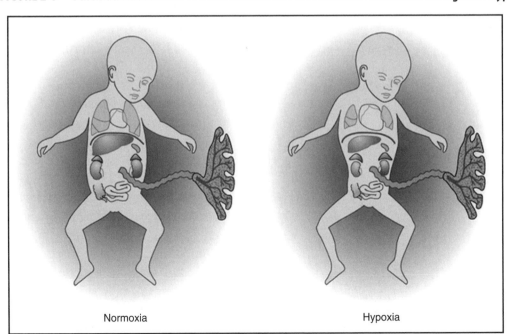

Normoxia   Hypoxia

Fetal Heart Rate Control

The source of integration for FHR control is the cardioregulatory center (CRC), a loosely defined collection of neurons in the ventral and lateral surface of the medulla oblongata (Blackburn, 2007; Manning, 1995) (Figure 2-9). The CRC receives input from a variety of sources, and these signals interact with neurons to alter output. Output from the CRC radiates throughout most organ systems and to adjacent higher centers within the fetal brain. The integration of these influences from the CRC exerts control over FHR. Baseline rate, variability, and various FHR patterns provide indirect insights into the functioning of the central nervous system.

Parasympathetic and the sympathetic branches of the autonomic nervous system, baroreceptors, chemoreceptors, fetal hormones, sleep-wake cycles, breathing movements, painful stimuli, sound and vibrations, and temperature interact with the CRC to influence FHR. Research using animal models, coupled with the ongoing clinical evaluation of associations observed between FHR tracings and fetal outcomes, has led to progressive improvement in our understanding of how these factors regulate heart rate in humans. Major factors believed to

FIGURE 2-9   Cerebral Influences on Fetal Heart Rate

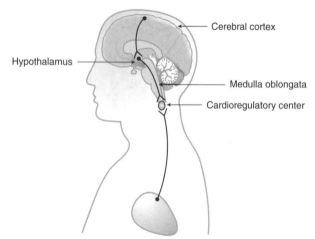

Cerebral cortex

Hypothalamus

Medulla oblongata

Cardioregulatory center

Adapted from: Parer, J. T. (1976). Physiologic regulation of fetal heart rate. *Journal of Obstetric, Gynecologic, and Neonatal Nursing, 5,* 265–295.

influence the integration of FHR control are outlined in Table 2-2.

Parasympathetic Nervous System

The parasympathetic branch of the autonomic nervous system is perhaps the most important controlling mechanism of the FHR. Parasympathetic supply to the heart travels from the CRC in the ventral surface of the fetal medulla via the vagus or 10th cranial nerve. The right and left branches of the vagus nerve innervate the sinoatrial (SA) and atrioventricular nodes within the fetal heart. Stimulation of the vagus nerve causes marked slowing of the FHR, an effect mediated by the release of acetylcholine from the nerve endings; this causes a decrease in the firing of the SA node and slows the rate of transmission to the ventricles (Parer & Nageotte, 2004).

The slow, gradual decrease in FHR observed with advancing gestational age is due to the increased dominance of parasympathetic influence on the fetal heart (Renou, Newman, & Wood, 1969; Dalton, Dawes, & Patrick, 1983). The fetal heart is similar to the adult heart, with the SA node functioning as the intrinsic pacemaker, setting the rate in the normal heart. The average baseline FHR in the normal fetus at 20 weeks' gestation is 155 beats per minute (bpm); at 30 weeks, 144 bpm; and at term before labor, 140 bpm (normal range, 110–160 bpm) (Parer & Nageotte, 2004). Although resting FHR decreases with advancing gestational age because of increased parasympathetic tone, the difference in baseline FHR between 28 and 30 weeks' gestation and term is approximately 10 bpm. Therefore, any preterm fetus with a baseline FHR greater than 160 bpm should be evaluated further to rule out fetal compromise, rather than just assuming the tachycardia is secondary to prematurity (Freeman et al., 2003).

The second primary function of the vagus nerve is the transmission of beat-to-beat irregularity or variability resulting from the irregular fluctuations in time between consecutive fetal cardiac cycles. Blocking the vagus nerve with

Table 2-2	Factors Influencing FHR Control	
INFLUENCE	**ACTION**	**FHR EFFECT**
Cardioregulatory Center: • Collection of neurons in ventral and lateral surface of medulla oblongata	• Integrating source for control of FHR • Interacts with parasympathetic and sympathetic nervous systems, baroreceptors, chemoreceptors, fetal hormones, sleep-wake cycles, breathing movements, painful stimuli, sound, vibrations, and temperature to influence FHR	• Baseline rate, variability, and various FHR patterns provide indirect insights into functioning of central nervous system • Presence of FHR variability represents an intact nervous pathway through cerebral cortex, midbrain, vagus nerve, and normal cardiac conduction system
Parasympathetic Branch of the Autonomic Nervous System: • Originates in medulla oblongata • Vagus nerve (10th cranial) innervates SA and AV nodes	• Stimulation releases acetylcholine • Pathway for transmission of variability	• ↓ FHR • Slow, gradual ↓ FHR with ↑ gestational age (approximately 10 bpm difference in baseline FHR between 28 weeks and term) • Maintains transmission of beat-to-beat variability • Moderate variability indicates absence of severe hypoxia or metabolic acidosis • Modulates baseline FHR with sympathetic
Sympathetic Branch of the Autonomic Nervous System: • At term, nerve fibers widely distributed throughout myocardium	• Stimulation releases catecholamines (e.g., norepinephrine, epinephrine) • Reserve mechanism to improve the heart's pumping ability during intermittent stress • Catecholamines can also cause fetal vasoconstriction and hypertension	• ↑ FHR • Blocking with propranolol results in ↓ FHR of approximately 10 bpm • Modulates baseline FHR with parasympathetic nervous system
Baroreceptors: • Protective, stretch receptors • Located in aortic arch and carotid sinuses at bifurcation of external and internal carotid arteries	• When ↑ arterial BP, the baroreceptors quickly detect amount of stretch, sending impulses via vagus nerve to midbrain • Impulses return via vagus nerve, causing sudden ↓ FHR, ↓ CO, and ↓ blood pressure, thereby protecting fetus	• Abrupt ↓ FHR • Abrupt ↓ CO • Abrupt ↓ blood pressure • Variable decelerations with moderate variability are baroreceptor influenced

Chemoreceptors:
• Central—located in medulla oblongata
• Peripheral—in aortic arch and carotid sinuses
	In the adult:
	• When arterial blood perfusing chemoreceptors contains ↑ PCO_2 or ↓ PO_2:
	  – Central—chemoreceptors respond with reflex tachycardia and hypertension, most likely in an attempt to circulate blood and ↓ the PCO_2
	  – Peripheral—chemoreceptors, respond with bradycardia
		In the fetus:
		• Interaction of central and peripheral chemoreceptors poorly understood
		• Combined effect is slowing of FHR
		• Described in mechanism of late decelerations and in variable decelerations resulting from umbilical arterial occlusion coupled with hypoxemia
		• When blood flow is below threshold for normal respiratory gas exchange, ↑ PCO_2 stimulates chemoreceptors to slow FHR

Continued

Table 2-2	Factors Influencing FHR Control—cont'd	
INFLUENCE	**ACTION**	**FHR EFFECT**
Hormonal Regulation: • Epinephrine and norepinephrine secreted from the adrenal medulla	• In response to stressful situations, compensatory response shunts blood away from less vital organs and toward brain, heart, and adrenal glands	• ↑ FHR, ↑ strength of cardiac contractions, ↑ CO, ↑ arterial BP
• Arginine vasopressin secreted from posterior pituitary	• In adult, responds to ↓ plasma volume, ↑ plasma osmolarity • In fetal sheep, hypoxemia most potent stimulus; distributes blood flow	• ↑ FHR, ↑ cardiac output, ↑ arterial BP • Sinusoidal heart rate pattern in experimental studies
• Renin-angiotensin-aldosterone secreted from kidneys	• Responds to ↓ plasma volume or ↓ BP; protects fetus from hemorrhagic stress by stimulating vasoconstriction	• ↑ FHR, ↑ cardiac output, ↑ arterial BP
Frank-Starling Mechanism: • In the adult, CO = HR × SV • Stroke volume is influenced by Frank-Starling mechanism which states ↑ inflow of blood into heart stretches cardiac muscle, thereby resulting in ↑ force of contraction and ↑ SV	• In the fetus, this mechanism has not been found to apply on the basis of studies involving fetal and adult lambs • Compared with adult, fetal SV does not fluctuate significantly	• Fetal CO ≈ HR • Modest variations in baseline FHR probably have little effect on fetal CO • However, during FHR > 240 bpm or FHR < 60 bpm, fetal CO is substantially decreased

AV, Atrioventricular; BP, blood pressure; bpm, beats per minute; CO, cardiac output; FHR, fetal heart rate; HR, heart rate; PCO_2, partial pressure of carbon dioxide; PO_2, partial pressure of oxygen; SA, sinoatrial; SV, stroke volume.

atropine (a substance that blocks the effects of acetylcholine) results in the disappearance of beat-to-beat variability (Dalton et al., 1983; Parer & Nageotte, 2004).

FHR variability is a reflection of neuromodulation of an active central nervous system (CNS) and normal cardiac responsiveness. The presence of FHR variability represents an intact nervous pathway through the cerebral cortex, the midbrain, the vagus nerve, and the normal cardiac conduction system (Parer, 1983, 1997). When the fetus is alert and active, the CNS responds with moderate FHR variability. If fetal brain function is reduced, FHR variability decreases. Potential causes of decreased variability include fetal sleep cycles, medications (e.g., narcotics, barbiturates, tranquilizers, general anesthetics), extreme prematurity, previous neurologic insult, or anatomic brain damage. Because severe hypoxia and metabolic acidosis will decrease CNS function, the presence of moderate FHR variability reliably indicates a well-oxygenated fetus without metabolic acidosis (Garite, 2007).

Sympathetic Nervous System

The sympathetic nervous system provides a reserve mechanism to improve the heart's pumping ability during intermittent stress (Blackburn, 2007). Nerve fibers from the sympathetic branch of the autonomic nervous system are widely distributed throughout fetal myocardium at term. Stimulation of these nerve fibers releases catecholamines (e.g., norepinephrine, epinephrine), causing an increase in FHR. Blocking the action of these sympathetic nerve fibers with propranolol results in a decrease in FHR of approximately 10 bpm (Parer & Nageotte, 2004). The effect of sympathetic stimulation in the fetus is not easily understood. Most observed FHR changes represent an integration of a variety of stimulant and inhibitory inputs. Although catecholamines have an accelerative effect on the FHR, these sympathetic agents also cause fetal vasoconstriction and fetal hypertension, which excite baroreceptor discharge and may cause reflex slowing of the FHR (Manning, 1995).

Although the parasympathetic and sympathetic nervous systems appear to work together to modulate baseline FHR, it is unclear whether they have a distinctly separate or combined role in the transmission of FHR variability (Parer & Nageotte, 2004). Animal research has demonstrated important species differences in the influence of the sympathetic nervous system on FHR variability. Parasympathetic stimulation appears to have a greater influence than sympathetic regulation on the transmission of FHR variability (Parer & Nageotte).

Baroreceptors

Baroreceptors are protective stretch receptors located in the aortic arch and the carotid sinuses at the bifurcation of the external and internal carotid arteries (Figure 2-10). When fetal arterial blood pressure increases, the baroreceptors quickly detect the amount of stretch and send impulses via the vagus nerve to the midbrain. Returning impulses via the vagus nerve cause a sudden decrease in FHR, cardiac output, and blood pressure, thereby protecting the fetus from the deleterious effects of excessive arterial pressures.

Lee et al.'s (1975) classic illustration of a variable deceleration (see Figure 2-6) depicts the relationship between the variable deceleration, a uterine contraction, umbilical cord compression, and fetal blood pressure. As a contraction begins, partial umbilical cord compression causes occlusion of the low-pressure vein and decreased return of blood to the fetal heart, resulting in decreased cardiac output, hypotension, and a compensatory FHR acceleration (Freeman et al., 2003; James et al., 1976; Lee et al.). With complete umbilical cord occlusion, the two umbilical arteries also become occluded, resulting in sudden fetal hypertension, stimulation of the baroreceptors, and a sudden drop in FHR (Freeman et al.; Lee & Hon, 1963). As the contraction begins to dissipate, the umbilical arteries open first, and a transient increase in FHR (a "secondary acceleration") may be seen. Finally, the contraction subsides and all three umbilical vessels are open, returning the FHR to predeceleration values.

Chemoreceptors

Chemoreceptors primarily function to regulate respiratory activity and control circulation by responding to changes in arterial PO_2, partial pressure of carbon dioxide (PCO_2), and acid-base balance. Central chemoreceptors are located in the medulla oblongata, and peripheral chemoreceptors are found in the carotid sinuses and aortic arch (see Figure 2-10). The interaction of the central and peripheral chemoreceptors is better understood in the adult than in the human fetus.

FIGURE 2-10   The Peripheral Chemoreceptors and Baroreceptors and Their Input to the Cardiac Regulating Center in the Medulla Oblongata

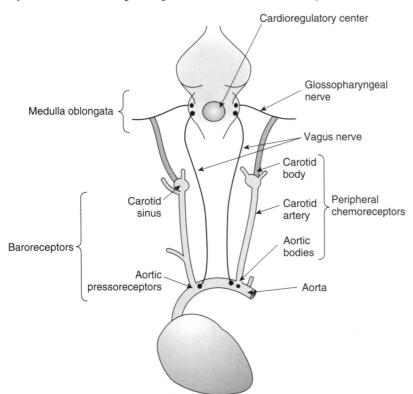

Adapted from Parer, J. T. (1976). Physiologic regulation of fetal heart rate. *Journal of Obstetric, Gynecologic, and Neonatal Nursing, 5,* 265–295.

In the adult, when arterial blood perfusing the central chemoreceptors contains increased PCO_2 or decreased PO_2, reflex tachycardia and hypertension occur, most likely in an attempt to circulate blood and decrease the PCO_2. In contrast, when increased PCO_2 or decreased PO_2 are detected by the peripheral chemoreceptors, bradycardia ensues (Parer & Nageotte, 2004).

In the fetus, the function of central and peripheral chemoreceptors are not well understood. Fetal chemoreceptor stimulation has been described in the mechanism of late decelerations and in the mechanism of variable decelerations resulting from umbilical arterial occlusion coupled with hypoxemia (Freeman et al., 2003). In both situations, when blood flow falls below the threshold for normal respiratory gas exchange, increased PCO_2 stimulates the chemoreceptors, resulting in activation of the CRC, slowing the FHR.

Hormonal Influences

The release of hormones by the adrenal glands, sympathetic nerves, hypothalamus, pituitary gland, and other fetal organs is believed to play an important role in fetal hemodynamic compensatory responses to stressors. The fetus responds to stress by releasing hormones that play a role in fetal circulatory regulation, allowing maximal perfusion to vital organs, primarily the fetal brain, heart, and adrenal glands. Key hormones that influence fetal circulation and FHR control include epinephrine, norepinephrine, arginine vasopressin, and hormones in the renin-angiotensin-aldosterone system.

When the fetus is stressed, catecholamines (e.g., epinephrine, norepinephrine) are secreted from the adrenal medulla. Epinephrine and norepinephrine increase FHR, increase force of myocardial contractions, and increase arterial blood pressure, similar to sympathetic stimulation (Parer & Nageotte, 2004). This compensatory response shunts blood away from the less vital organs and toward the brain, heart, and adrenal glands.

In the adult, arginine vasopressin (antidiuretic hormone) is released from the posterior pituitary gland in response to decreases in plasma volume and increases in plasma osmolarity. In fetal sheep, hypoxemia is the most potent stimulus known for arginine vasopressin secretion (Ross et al., 2002). Arginine vasopressin has been shown to affect the distribution of blood flow, thereby increasing FHR, cardiac output, and arterial blood pressure (Ross et al.). Murata et al. (1985) implicated arginine vasopressin in the sinusoidal heart rate pattern after finding increased levels of vasopressin and the sinusoidal pattern in fetal sheep during hemorrhage.

The renin-angiotensin-aldosterone system is a complex hormone system that responds to decreases in plasma volume or blood pressure. In the fetus, angiotensin II and aldosterone levels do not increase in proportion to changes in the plasma renin, in contrast to what occurs in the newborn or adult. This uncoupling of the fetal renin-angiotensin-aldosterone system is most likely due to increased placental clearance of angiotensin II, limited angiotensin-converting enzyme available as a result of reduced pulmonary blood flow in the fetus, and the direct inhibition of aldosterone (Ross et al., 2002). The net effect of this hormone system is to protect the fetus from hemorrhagic stress by stimulating vasoconstriction (Parer & Nageotte, 2004).

FHR and Cardiac Output

In the adult, heart rate (HR) is related to cardiac output (CO) and stroke volume (SV) in the following equation: $CO = HR \times SV$. Stroke volume is influenced by the Frank-Starling mechanism, which states that an increased inflow of blood into the heart stretches the cardiac muscle, thereby resulting in a greater force of contraction and increased stroke volume. In the fetus, this mechanism has not been found to apply on the basis of studies involving fetal and adult lambs (Rudolph, 1985). Because stroke volume in the fetus does not fluctuate significantly, fetal cardiac output is essentially rate dependent (Fetal

CO ≈ HR). In clinical practice, modest variations in baseline FHR probably have little effect on fetal cardiac output; however, cardiac output is substantially decreased with fetal tachycardia above 240 bpm or bradycardia below 60 bpm (Fineman et al., 2004; Parer & Nageotte, 2004).

Fetal State Patterns

The FHR may also be influenced by fetal sleep-wake patterns or fetal behavioral states. Behavioral state organization is thought to mirror neurologic development of the fetus, and analysis of fetal behavior may provide information about fetal CNS development, function, and maturity. Fetal state can be determined by regularity of FHR, presence of eye movements, and fetal movement (Blackburn, 2007). In early pregnancy, fetal movement is largely continuous; however, with increasing maturation, quiet periods emerge. By 28 to 32 weeks' gestation, the fetus switches between distinct periods of quiescence and activity that become more regular and rhythmic (Blackburn). The FHR cycles with alternate periods of activity and nonactivity (Peirano, Algarin, & Uauy, 2003), and fetal eye movement and gross body movements begin to show coordination (Visser, Poelmann-Weesjes, Cohen, & Bekedam, 1987). This cycling between activity and rest periods is the fetal version of alternations in rapid eye movement (REM) sleep (fetal state F2) and quiet sleep (fetal state F1).

REM or active sleep may be characterized by rapid darting eye movements, periodic body movements, normal baseline FHR, moderate variability, FHR accelerations, and a reactive non-stress test (NST). In quiet or non-REM sleep, the fetus may be observed to have absent eye movements, infrequent or absent body movements, normal FHR baseline, minimal FHR variability, and a nonreactive NST and can respond to external stimuli (e.g., vibroacoustic stimulation) (Blackburn, 2007; Manning, 1995). Box 2-2 lists characteristics of fetal REM sleep

---

BOX 2-2 Characteristics of Fetal Quiet and REM Sleep States

Quiet sleep (state F1) :
- Eye movements absent
- Movements infrequent or absent
- Fetal tone present, but reduced
- Normal baseline FHR, minimal variability, no accelerations
- Nonreactive NST
- Response to external stimuli (e.g., vibroacoustic stimulation)

REM sleep (state F2):
- Rapid darting eye movements
- Periodic active body movements
- Fetal tone increased
- Normal baseline FHR, moderate variability, accelerations
- Reactive NST
- Unresponsive to external stimuli

FHR, Fetal heart rate; NST, non-stress test; REM, rapid eye movement.

---

and quiet sleep. The mean time period of cycling between active and quiet sleep is 20 minutes; however, the duration of a given behavioral state may last longer than 1 hour (Parer, 1997).

During quiet sleep, a fetus will most likely demonstrate minimal FHR variability and no accelerations. Whereas moderate variability indicates adequate fetal oxygenation, minimal or absent variability alone does not necessarily indicate insufficient oxygenation. In this situation, the clinician should review the preceding hour or two of FHR tracing for the presence of accelerations and FHR variability and absence of decelerations and bradycardia. However, if on admission the initial FHR tracing has minimal FHR variability and no accelerations, rapid further assessment is required. Interviewing the mother about perceived fetal movement over the past several hours and days or performing vibroacoustic stimulation or NST per unit protocol may provide additional information to differentiate between normal quiet and active sleep cycles versus insufficient fetal oxygenation. Vibroacoustic stimulation is discussed in Chapter 11.

FETAL HOMEOSTATIC RESPONSES

Fetal monitoring is an ongoing indirect assessment of physiologic factors, both extrinsic and intrinsic to the fetus, that affect fetal oxygenation. The fetus depends on well-oxygenated uteroplacental blood flow, adequate placental exchange, adequate umbilical blood flow, oxygen transport to tissue, and finally, innate compensatory factors to control FHR when challenged by labor and other stressors. With a decrease in PO_2 and an increase in PCO_2, the normoxic fetus initiates compensatory mechanisms that usually maintain physiologic integrity without damage to vital organs. Redistribution of fetal blood flow favoring the heart, brain, and adrenal glands is increased, whereas blood flow to the gut, spleen, kidneys, and limbs is decreased (see Figure 2-7). As the FHR decreases, the myocardium consumes less oxygen. If these temporary compensatory measures do not supply sufficient oxygen to meet metabolic needs, anaerobic metabolism follows

with accumulation of lactic acid, resulting in metabolic acidosis in the tissues. With sustained hypoxemia or severe acidemia, decompensation may occur, during which fetal cardiac output, arterial blood pressure, and blood flow to the brain decrease, followed by tissue damage and, ultimately, fetal death (Parer, 1997; Parer & Nageotte, 2004). The fetal homeostatic responses to normal and abnormal stresses of labor and birth are illustrated in a dynamic physiologic model of FHR adaptations (Figure 2-11).

Interpretation of these physiologic responses to fetal oxygenation is reflected in an ongoing assessment of the continuum of FHR characteristics presented by the fetus; the relationship of these characteristics to maternal history, physical findings, and laboratory findings; and their evolution over time. A well-oxygenated fetus will demonstrate moderate FHR variability, a normal baseline rate, and no late or variable decelerations. Accelerations, and early decelerations may or may not be present in the tracing of a well-oxygenated fetus. The fetus unable to sustain compensatory responses to decreased oxygenation may demonstrate ab-

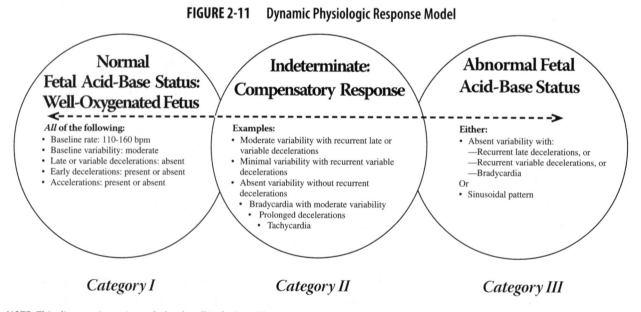

FIGURE 2-11   Dynamic Physiologic Response Model

Normal Fetal Acid-Base Status: Well-Oxygenated Fetus

All of the following:
- Baseline rate: 110-160 bpm
- Baseline variability: moderate
- Late or variable decelerations: absent
- Early decelerations: present or absent
- Accelerations: present or absent

Category I

Indeterminate: Compensatory Response

Examples:
- Moderate variability with recurrent late or variable decelerations
- Minimal variability with recurrent variable decelerations
- Absent variability without recurrent decelerations
- Bradycardia with moderate variability
- Prolonged decelerations
- Tachycardia

Category II

Abnormal Fetal Acid-Base Status

Either:
- Absent variability with:
  —Recurrent late decelerations, or
  —Recurrent variable decelerations, or
  —Bradycardia
Or
- Sinusoidal pattern

Category III

NOTE: This diagram is not intended to be all inclusive. All patterns must be treated with interventions that are based on the suspected underlying physiologic causes and ongoing evaluation of individual patient presentation.

sent FHR variability combined with either recurrent variable, or late decelerations, or bradycardia. However, many fetuses exhibit characteristics falling between these two extremes, as illustrated in Figure 2-11. In summary, FHR interpretation requires an understanding of the evolution of FHR patterns in relation to fetal oxygenation, knowledge of maternal factor that may influence fetal oxygenation, and ongoing assessment of FHR characteristics throughout labor and birth. FHR pattern interpretation is discussed in further detail in Chapter 5.

REFERENCES

Benirschke, K. (2004a). Normal early development. In R. K. Creasy, R. Resnik, & J. Iams (Eds.), *Maternal-fetal medicine: Principles and practice* (5th ed., pp. 37–44). Philadelphia: Saunders.

Benirschke, K. (2004b). Multiple gestation: The biology of twinning. In R. K. Creasy, R. Resnik, & J. Iams (Eds.), *Maternal-fetal medicine: Principles and practice* (5th ed., pp. 55–67). Philadelphia: Saunders.

Blackburn, S. T. (2007). *Maternal, fetal, and neonatal physiology: A clinical perspective* (3rd ed.). St. Louis: Saunders.

Bobrowski, R. A. (2004). Maternal-fetal blood gas physiology. In G. A. Dildy, M. A. Belfort, G. R. Saade, J. P. Phelan, G. V. Hankins, & S. L. Clark (Eds.), *Critical care obstetrics* (4th ed., pp. 43–59). Malden, MA: Blackwell Science.

Brace, R. A. (2004). Amniotic fluid dynamics. In R. K. Creasy, R. Resnik, & J. Iams (Eds.), *Maternal-fetal medicine: Principles and practice* (5th ed., pp. 45–53). Philadelphia: Saunders.

Campbell, N. A., & Reece, J. B. (2005). *Biology* (7th ed.). Upper Saddle River, NJ: Pearson Prentice Hall.

Chervenak, F. A., & Gabbe, S. G. (2007). Obstetric ultrasound: Assessment of fetal growth and anatomy. In S. G. Gabbe, J. R. Niebyl, & J. L. Simpson (Eds.), *Obstetrics: Normal and problem pregnancies* (5th ed.). Philadelphia: Churchill Livingstone.

Cohn, H. E., Sacks, E. J., Heymann, M. A., & Rudolph, A. M. (1974). Cardiovascular responses to hypoxemia and academia in fetal lambs. *American Journal of Obstetrics and Gynecology, 120,* 817–824.

Cunningham, F. G., Leveno, K. J., Bloom, S. L., Hauth, J. C., Gilstrap, L. C., & Wenstrom, K. D. (2005). *Williams obstetrics* (22nd ed.). New York: McGraw-Hill.

Dalton, K. J., Dawes, G. S., & Patrick, J. E. (1983). The autonomic nervous system and fetal heart rate variability. *American Journal of Obstetrics and Gynecology, 146,* 456–462.

Edelstone, D. I., & Rudolph, A. M. (1979). Preferential streaming of ductus venosus blood to the brain and heart in fetal lambs. *American Journal of Physiology, 237*(6), H724–H729.

Fineman, J. R., Clyman, R., & Heymann, M. A. (2004). Fetal cardiovascular physiology. In R. K. Creasy, R. Resnik, & J. Iams (Eds.), *Maternal-fetal medicine: Principles and practice* (5th ed., pp. 169–180). Philadelphia: Saunders.

Freeman, R. K., Garite, T. J., & Nageotte, M. P. (2003). *Fetal heart rate monitoring* (3rd ed.). Philadelphia: Lippincott Williams & Wilkins.

Garite, T. J. (2007). Intrapartum evaluation. In S. G. Gabbe, J. R. Niebyl, & J. L. Simpson (Eds.), *Obstetrics: Normal and problem pregnancies* (5th ed., pp. 364–395). Philadelphia: Churchill Livingstone.

James, L. S., Yeh, M. N., Morishima, H. O., Daniel, S. S., Caritis, S. N., Niemann, W. H., & Indyk, L. (1976). Umbilical vein occlusion and transient acceleration of the fetal heart rate. Experimental observations in subhuman primates. *American Journal of Obstetrics and Gynecology, 126,* 276–283.

King, T., & Parer, J. (2000). The physiology of fetal heart rate patterns and perinatal asphyxia. *Journal of Perinatal and Neonatal Nursing, 14*(3), 19–39.

Kiserud, T. (2001). The ductus venosus. *Seminars in Perinatology, 25,* 11–20.

Lee, C. Y., Di Loreto, P. C., & O'Lane, J. M. (1975). A study of fetal heart rate acceleration patterns. *Obstetrics and Gynecology, 45,* 142–146.

Lee, S. T., & Hon, E. H. (1963). Fetal hemodynamic response to umbilical cord compression. *Obstetrics and Gynecology, 22,* 553–562.

Manning, F. A. (1995). *Fetal medicine: Principles and practice.* Norwalk, CT: Appleton & Lange.

Manning, F. A. (2004). General principles and applications of ultrasonography. In R. K. Creasy, R. Resnik, & J. Iams (Eds.), *Maternal-fetal medicine: Principles and practice* (5th ed., pp. 315–355). Philadelphia: Saunders.

Marino, T. (2004). Ultrasound abnormalities of the amniotic fluid, membranes, umbilical cord, and placenta. *Obstetrics and Gynecology Clinics of North America, 31,* 177-200.

Martin, C. B., Jr., & Gingerich, B. (1976). Uteroplacental physiology. *Journal of Obstetric, Gynecologic, and Neonatal Nursing, 5*(Suppl. 5), 16s–25s.

Meschia, G. (2004). Placental respiratory gas exchange and fetal oxygenation. In R. K. Creasy, R. Resnik, &

J. Iams (Eds.), *Maternal-fetal medicine: Principles and practice* (5th ed., pp. 199–207). Philadelphia: Saunders.

Moore, K. L., & Persaud, T. V. N. (2003). *The developing human: Clinically oriented embryology* (7th ed.). Philadelphia: Saunders.

Murata, Y., Miyake, Y., Yamamoto, T., Higuchi, M., Hesser, J., Ibara, S. et al. (1985). Experimentally produced sinusoidal fetal heart rate patterns in the chronically instrumented fetal lamb. *American Journal of Obstetrics and Gynecology, 153,* 693–702.

Parer, J. T. (1997). *Handbook of fetal heart rate monitoring* (2nd ed.). Philadelphia: Saunders.

Parer, J. T. (1983). *Handbook of fetal heart rate monitoring.* Philadelphia: Saunders.

Parer, J. T., & Nageotte, M. P. (2004). Intrapartum fetal surveillance. In R. K. Creasy, R. Resnik, & J. Iams (Eds.) *Maternal-fetal medicine: Principles and practice* (5th ed., pp. 403–427). Philadelphia: Saunders.

Parer, J. T., Rosen, M. A., & Levinson, G. (2002). Uteroplacental circulation and respiratory gas exchange. In S. C. Hughes, G. Levinson & M. A. Rosen (Eds.), *Shnider and Levinson's anesthesia for obstetrics* (4th ed., pp. 19–40). Philadelphia: Lippincott Williams & Wilkins.

Peirano, P., Algarin, C., & Uauy, R. (2003). Sleep-wake states and their regulatory mechanisms throughout early human development. *The Journal of Pediatrics, 143,* S70–S79.

Renou, P., Newman, W., & Wood, C. (1969). Autonomic control of fetal heart rate. *American Journal of Obstetrics and Gynecology, 105,* 949–953.

Ross, M. G., Ervin, M. G., & Novak, D. (2002). Placental and fetal physiology. In S. G. Gabbe, J. R. Niebyl, & J. L. Simpson (Eds.), *Obstetrics: Normal and problem pregnancies* (4th ed., pp. 37–62). New York: Churchill Livingstone.

Rudolph, A.M. (1985). Distribution and regulation of blood flow in the fetal and neonatal lamb. *Circulation Research, 57,* 811–821.

Troiano, N. (1999). Invasive hemodynamic monitoring in obstetrics. In L. K. Mandeville & N. H. Troiano (Eds.), *AWHONN's high-risk and critical care intrapartum nursing* (2nd ed., pp. 66–83). Philadelphia: Lippincott.

Visser, G. H., Poelmann-Weesjes, G., Cohen, T. M., & Bekedam, D. J. (1987). Fetal behavior at 30 to 32 weeks of gestation. *Pediatric Research, 22,* 655–658.

SECTION TWO

Maternal-Fetal Assessment

1. Read This Book
2. Take the On-Line Test
3. Earn Continuing Nursing Education Credit

www.awhonn.org/fhm

AWHONN is accredited as a provider of continuing nursing education by the American Nurses Credentialing Center's Commission on Accreditation.

CHAPTER 3

Maternal-Fetal Assessment

Dodi Gauthier

INTRODUCTION TO MATERNAL-FETAL ASSESSMENT

Accurate assessment of the pregnant woman depends on a thorough understanding of the normal physiologic adaptations to pregnancy (see Chapter 2). Virtually all maternal systems are affected by the physiologic changes associated with the developing fetus. Because the well-being of the fetus depends on the well-being of the mother, a key focus of maternal assessment is to determine how maternal physiologic changes or her physical condition may affect the fetus. Ongoing maternal-fetal assessment begins during the prenatal period and continues throughout the intrapartum period (Figure 3-1). This chapter focuses on assessment of the woman presenting for antepartum or intrapartum care in inpatient settings or in labor and delivery or birth center triage. The maternal-fetal database should be current and reflect the status of the maternal and fetal dyad on a continuum. The goals of maternal assessment are to:

- Identify the woman and fetus at risk for developing complications.
- Promote appropriate, safe care and interventions.

Data collection methods include review of the prenatal record, interviews during admission, and initial and ongoing assessments of the maternal-fetal dyad. A review of the maternal medical, surgical, obstetric, gynecologic, and family histories should be included in the data collection and reviewed with each outpatient assessment or admission. Assessment data provide information about the mother's current health status and identification of risk factors for maternal or neonatal morbidity or mortality.

Box 3-1 provides a summary of maternal-fetal assessment components. A more detailed discussion of key assessments components follows.

PRENATAL RECORDS

The prenatal record provides an important source of information that directs the assessment of the maternal-fetal dyad. These include basic initial laboratory results, trended vital signs, weight records, and documentation of significant events. Availability of the prenatal chart varies per institution. Access to current information can streamline a comprehensive patient assessment and help ensure appropriate care. Web-based prenatal records are used in some institutions, making information available wherever the woman seeks care within the system.

INTERVIEWS

Pregnancy is a dynamic state; both psychosocial and physical changes may occur from day to day. Building on the information already available in the prenatal record often contributes to a smooth transition through the continuum of

FIGURE 3-1   The Nursing Process and Fetal Heart Monitoring: Assessment

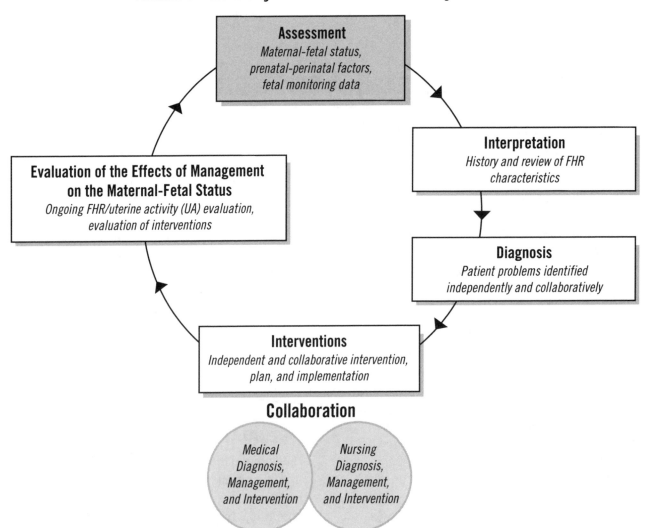

care. Interviewing women and using interactive bedside computers to access records can provide additional, up-to-date information that may not be available in the prenatal record. Interviews should be conducted at prenatal visits and at each admission to any health care facility.

Privacy should be maintained during the interview process. Ideally, women should be interviewed without significant others present to increase the ease of answering sensitive questions on topics such as domestic violence or undisclosed sexual history or pregnancies. However, if a woman is unable to provide information because of an altered level of consciousness, significant others may be able to provide critical

and reliable information. Whenever possible, conduct the interview in a language the woman is most comfortable speaking and understanding. Health care facilities should have protocols that accommodate language interpretation and prevent language barriers to care.

Attention to basic patients' rights can ultimately improve the quality of data collection, decrease maternal and family anxiety, and allow the woman to concentrate on the work of childbearing. For example, women with physical challenges should be provided with the resources needed to participate as fully as possible in the births of their infants. If the mother is hearing impaired, she may require a sign language interpreter. If the woman is blind, she may require instructions in Braille as well as tactile orientation to the environment. The cultural and spiritual needs of both the patient and her family should be identified and respected to facilitate the family's full participation in the birth.

HISTORICAL DATA

Maternal-fetal historical data are gathered from demographic and socioeconomic information; psychosocial assessments; medical, surgical, obstetric, and gynecologic histories; and physical assessment of both the mother and the fetus.

Demographic Factors

Data that may directly affect the outcome of the pregnancy include race, age, number of pregnancies, place of residence, and workplace. For example, pregnancy occurring before age 19 or after age 35 places mother and fetus at increased risk for age-related complications, including preeclampsia, intrauterine growth restriction (IUGR), low birth weight, hemorrhagic disorders, and preterm birth (Johnson & Niebyl, 2003).

Socioeconomic Factors

Socioeconomic data are important and may be useful when beginning the process of discharge planning for the mother and her infant. Clinicians should identify the presence of risk factors and assess the extent to which they may influence the outcome of the pregnancy or infant and family well-being. Socioeconomic data include but may not be limited to the following (Smith, 2004):

- Exposure to domestic violence
- Number of sexual partners
- Adequacy of housing arrangements
- Financial resources to provide food, clothing, and other infant needs

- Access to appropriate health care and social services
- Fears or anxieties regarding pregnancy, delivery, and neonatal care

The individual's residence and employment directly affects quality of life and consequent availability and accessibility of needed services. For example, undocumented immigrant families may not seek prenatal care for fear of deportation. Environmental conditions may increase the risk of environmental toxin exposure and may increase the potential for fetal problems, including altered fertility, genetic defects, stillbirth, miscarriage, growth restriction, congenital malformations, and developmental disabilities (Wotring, 2004).

After assessment of potential risk factors in the current pregnancy, the clinician is better prepared to identify services needed and to help address or solve ongoing problems. Collection of such data will help the care provider develop a comprehensive plan with the family to address their needs appropriately, thereby promoting positive family coping and adaptation.

Medical and Surgical History

Although the prenatal record should contain the woman's medical and surgical history, admission to labor and delivery provides another opportunity for clinicians to complete or update data. The onset of labor often results in the communication of information that may not have been obtained during the prenatal period. Chronic medical conditions should be assessed and recorded because they may have an effect not only on the pregnancy, labor, and birth outcomes, but also on the postpartum recovery. Using a systems approach provides an organized and efficient method of collecting data. Health care facilities often have documentation systems that provide cues for assessment and documentation of patient information. Individual circumstances may influence conditions un-

BOX 3-1   Outline of Maternal-Fetal Assessment

I. Prenatal record review

II. Patient and family interviews

III. Maternal-fetal historical data
  A. Demographic factors
  B. Socioeconomic factors
  C. Medical and surgical history
  D. Obstetric history
    1. Past
    2. Current
    3. Gestational age assessment
    4. Fetal activity
    5. Leopold's maneuvers
      a. Fetal lie
      b. Fetal attitude
      c. Fetal presentation
      d. Fetal presenting part
  E. Psychosocial assessment
    1. Cultural diversity
    2. Resources and support systems
    3. Domestic violence screening
    4. Substance abuse screening
    5. Health coping mechanisms

IV. Physical examination
  A. Clinical assessment of maternal vital signs
    1. Temperature
    2. Pulse
    3. Blood pressure
    4. Respirations
    5. Pain
  B. Maternal height, weight, weight gain
  C. Nutritional status
  D. Uterine activity
    1. Contraction assessment
    2. Fetal response to contractions
  E. Membrane status
    1. Intact
    2. Ruptured
      a. Time of rupture
      b. Color of fluid
      c. Amount of fluid
      d. Odor of fluid
  F. Vaginal examination
    1. Vaginal bleeding or discharge
      a. Color
      b. Amount
      c. Precipitating factors
      d. Timing
      e. Odor
    2. Cervical examination
      a. Dilation
      b. Effacement
      c. Station
      d. Presenting part
  G. Biochemical assessment (may vary depending on institutional policy and patient condition)
    1. Labs
      a. Complete blood count
      b. Blood group, Rh, and antibody screening
      c. Glucose screening
      d. Toxicology screen, if indicated
      e. Urinalysis
      f. Dipstick urine for protein and glucose
      g. Fetal fibronectin (24–35 weeks)
      h. Analysis of membrane status
      i. Sickle cell status
    2. Infectious disease evaluation
      a. Chlamydia
      b. Cytomegalovirus
      c. Group B streptococcus (GBS)
      d. Hepatitis A, B, and C
      e. Herpes simplex virus
      f. Human immunodeficiency virus
      g. Rubella
      h. Syphilis
      i. Toxoplasmosis
      j. Trichomonas
      k. Tuberculosis
      l. Chicken pox (varicella)

V. Fetal assessment
  A. Gestational age determination
    1. Last menstrual period
    2. Fundal height and McDonald's measurement
    3. Fetal movement assessment
    4. Dating sonogram
  B. Fetal activity
    1. Fetal movement by maternal report
    2. Fetal movement felt through palpation
  C. Antenatal assessment
    1. Nonstress test
    2. Contraction stress test
    3. Biophysical profile (BPP) or modified BPP
    4. Ultrasound
      a. Limited: Fetal number, presentation(s), cardiac activity, placental location, and amniotic fluid index (along with the BPP)
      b. Basic: same as limited and additionally

BOX 3-1   Outline of Maternal-Fetal Assessment—cont'd

includes gestational age, fetal anatomy for gross malformations, nuchal translucency, and maternal pelvic masses
   c. Comprehensive: examination of specific anatomic structures; may include an echocardiogram performed by a specialist
   d. Cervical length
   e. Serial ultrasounds for fetal growth and follow up for known abnormalities
   f. Amniocentesis results for genetic testing or fetal lung maturity
   D. Method of monitoring
      1. Auscultation
         a. Rate
         b. Rhythm
         c. Increases or decreases in fetal heart rate (FHR)
         d. Interventions
         e. Response to interventions
      2. External
         a. Ultrasound

(1) Baseline FHR
(2) Variability
(3) Accelerations or decelerations
(4) Interventions
(5) Response to interventions
   b. Tocodynamometer
      (1) Relative duration and relative frequency
3. Internal
   a. Fetal spiral electrode
      (1) Baseline FHR
      (2) Variability
      (3) Accelerations or decelerations
      (4) Interventions
      (5) Response to interventions
   b. Intrauterine pressure catheter
      (1) Fluid-filled
      (2) Sensor-tipped
         a. Intensity in mm Hg
         b. Duration
         c. Frequency
         d. Resting tone in mm Hg

Adapted from Association of Women's Health, Obstetric and Neonatal Nurses [AWHONN]. (2008). *Basic, high-risk and critical care intrapartum nursing: Clinical competencies and education guide* (3rd ed.). Washington, DC: Author. Reprinted with permission.

---

der which patient data is collected. Pregnant women with congenital diseases or chronic illnesses usually require additional targeted assessment. Therefore, information specific to disease state, related surgeries, hospitalizations, and medications should be obtained. For example, patients with sickle cell disease or cystic fibrosis require not only a complete history including disease state, but also information such as disease specific medications taken during pregnancy and the various specialists who have consulted with the primary obstetrician.

Data collection should include the use of prescribed medications as well as herbs, vitamins, teas, tonics, tinctures, or any other substances that were taken during the pregnancy. Use of complementary alternative medicines, including herbal therapies, has increased significantly in the past decade. Few studies have been conducted regarding herbal use and safety in pregnancy (Born & Barron, 2005). There are some

known possible side effects and drug interactions for some alternative medicines and herbs and examples can be found at http://www.asahq.org/patientEducation/herbPhysician.pdf (American Society of Anesthesiologists, 2003).

Obstetric History
Current and Past

Past pregnancy experiences and outcomes may significantly influence the plan of care and outcome of a current pregnancy. History of previous pregnancy complications such as preeclampsia, gestational diabetes, preterm labor, placental abnormalities, and difficult or operative births can provide valuable insight into potential problems for the current pregnancy. Table 3-1 provides a summary of selected medical, obstetric, and psychosocial conditions and risk factors with associated implications for fetal and neonatal well-being.

Table 3-1	Selected Maternal Conditions or Risk Factors with Associated Fetal and Neonatal Implications*		
MATERNAL CONDITIONS	**POTENTIAL FETAL/NEONATAL RISKS OR RISK FACTORS**		**POTENTIAL FHR ALTERATIONS**

Cardiac
Underlying disease
  History of insufficiency
Hypertensive disorders
  Chronic hypertension
  Preeclampsia
  Kidney disease
  HELLP syndrome
	SGA/IUGR
	Hydrops
	Hypoxemia
	Decreased amniotic fluid
	Preterm labor/birth
	Placenta abruption
			Bradycardia
			Decreased variability
			Lack of accelerations
			Late decelerations
			Sinusoidal pattern

Respiratory Smoking Asthma Infections	SGA/IUGR Hypoxemia Presence of meconium Preterm labor/birth		Tachycardia Bradycardia Decreased variability Late decelerations
Neurologic Stroke Underlying neurologic disease	Placental abruption Hypoxemia		Bradycardia Decreased variability Late decelerations
Renal Infection Calculi Fluid/electrolyte imbalance Anemia Dialysis complications	SGA/IUGR Decreased amniotic fluid Decreased/reversed umbilical blood flow Preterm labor/birth		Tachycardia Decreased variability Variable decelerations Late decelerations Prolonged decelerations
Gastrointestinal Nutritional compromise Constipation/hemorrhoids Gall bladder disease Electrolyte imbalance	SGA/IUGR Altered electrolytes may adversely affect fetus if prolonged		Bradycardia Decreased variability
Hematologic Anemia Deep vein thrombosis Antiphospholipid antibody syndrome Thrombocytopenia	SGA/IUGR Preterm labor/birth Hypoxemia		Bradycardia Late decelerations Decreased variability

Psychosocial/Mental Health
Lack of prenatal care
Effects of prescribed or nonprescribed medications
Malnutrition
Substance abuse
  Tobacco
  Alcohol
  Illicit drugs
Increased stress
Domestic violence
	SGA/IUGR
	Congenital anomalies
	Poor tolerance of labor
	Placental abnormalities
	Preterm labor/birth
	Neonatal infection
	Decreased amniotic fluid
	Hypoxemia
			Tachycardia
			Marked variability
			Decreased variability
			Variable decelerations
			Late decelerations

*This is not an all-inclusive summary, nor does it imply cause and effect. This summary is presented to illustrate some of the potential fetal or neonatal implications of selected maternal conditions as risk factors.

FHR, Fetal heart rate; FHRV, fetal heart rate variability; HELLP, hemolysis, elevated liver enzymes and low platelet count; SGA/IUGR, small for gestational age/intrauterine growth restriction.

Adapted from: Gabbe, S. G., Neibyl, J. R., & Simpson, J. L. (2003). *Obstetrics: Normal and problem pregnancies* (4th ed.). New York: Churchill-Livingston.

Mandeville, L., & Troiano, N. (1999). *High risk and critical care intrapartum nursing* (2nd ed.). Philadelphia: Lippincott.

Simpson, K. R., & Creehan, P. A. (2008). *Perinatal nursing* (3rd ed.). Philadelphia: Lippincott.

When a woman presents to the birth center, the assessment history should include:

- Estimated due date (EDD)
- Reason for seeking medical attention
- Allergies to medications or foods
- Perceptions of fetal movements
- Perceptions of rupture of membranes (ROM) or bleeding
- Medications, prescribed and over-the-counter, and complementary alternative medicines taken during pregnancy (time, dosage, frequency, and reason for taking)
- History of chronic illness or past surgeries
- Total number of times she has been pregnant (gravida) and the results (para) of previous pregnancies (live births, elective terminations, and miscarriages)
- Length of gestation of previous pregnancies
- Type of births she has experienced and the outcomes (i.e., vaginal, assisted operative vaginal birth with forceps or vacuum extractor, cesarean, vaginal birth after cesarean)
- Any known complications experienced by the mother or infant
- Current and prepregnancy weight, including any recent significant change in weight
- History of any sexually transmitted infections and treatment and any other infections
- Group B streptococcus (strep; GBS) history and results of culture if obtained
- Plans and expectations for pain management during labor and the postpartum period
- Plans and expectations for breastfeeding

Questions regarding obstetric history will assist in formatting a targeted physical examination and optimizing intake data. The specifics of the woman's birth plan should also be discussed.

Gestational Age Assessment

Assessment of the gestational age at the time of admission helps direct care and prioritization of interventions. A primary clinical estimator of gestational age is an accurate LMP (first day of the last menstrual period) (Johnson & Niebyl,

2003). The initial assessment of the EDD is performed at the first prenatal visit. Use of Naegele's rule (the date of the last normal menstrual period, minus 3 months, plus 7 days) provides an initial estimate of EDD. In addition to the LMP, there are other tools to assist the provider in estimating the gestational age. Abdominal palpation and fundal height measurement are preformed to assess uterine size and fetal position.

Fundal height is determined by measuring the uterus from the symphysis pubis to the top of the fundus (over the curve), and approximates the gestational age from 16 to 38 weeks within 3 cm (Johnson, Gregory, & Niebyl, 2007). By 20 weeks' gestation, the fundus usually reaches the lower border of the umbilicus and increases in height approximately 1 cm per week until weeks 34 to 36, when the fundus is at the height of the xiphoid process. Maternal obesity and multiple gestations are examples of conditions that may reduce the reliability of the fundal height. "Quickening," the first perception of fetal movement by the mother, commonly occurs at predictable times during the pregnancy. During a first pregnancy, quickening is usually noted at approximately 19 weeks' gestation; in subsequent pregnancies, it occurs about 2 weeks earlier. Fetal heart tones are most often detected at 19 to 20 weeks with a fetoscope and are often heard by 12 weeks with the use of an electronic Doppler device (Johnson et al.).

Ultrasound is used to estimate gestational age in the first half (20 weeks) of pregnancy. Between 7 and 13 weeks, the crown-rump length, measurement of the length of the fetus from the top of the head to the bottom of the buttocks, is used to assess gestation. After 13 weeks, measurement of the biparietal diameter and femur length more closely correlates with age (Johnson et al., 2007). As pregnancy advances, dating the pregnancy using ultrasonography is much less accurate. It can, however, be useful for other assessments, such as a follow-up for growth parameters, amniocentesis for fetal lung maturity, or a biophysical profile (BPP).

Fetal Activity

The mother's perception of fetal movement provides valuable information and should be assessed on admission. Nonperception of movement coupled with a history of conditions that may affect placental well-being should heighten the suspicion of fetal physiologic compromise or demise. Clinicians should ascertain time and quality of the last perceived fetal movements. See Chapter 11 for a more detailed discussion of fetal movement counting.

Leopold's Maneuvers

Leopold's maneuvers are an abdominal assessment technique used to determine the presentation, position, and lie of the fetus, which then may be confirmed by a vaginal examination. *Fetal lie* is the position of the long axis of the fetus and is described as being longitudinal, transverse, or oblique. *Fetal presentation* refers to the part of the fetus that is entering the pelvis and is described as cephalic, breech, or shoulder. *Fetal position* describes the relationship of the presenting part to the pelvis and is described as anterior, posterior, or transverse. Leopold's maneuvers include assessment of four components:

1. Fetal part in the fundus
2. Location of the fetal back
3. Presenting part (Pallach's maneuver)
4. Descent and attitude of the presenting part

These four maneuvers provide a systematic approach to identify the point of maximal sound intensity of the fetal heart. In general, the optimal fetal heart sounds are heard over the curved part of the fetus presenting closest to the anterior uterine wall (Tucker, 2004). In addition, the initial physical contact of obtaining Leopold's maneuvers may assist in establishing a positive clinician-patient relationship. For a complete description and discussion of Leopold's maneuvers, refer to the additional information about performing this technique in Chapters 4 and 9. Also refer to Figure 3-2.

Psychosocial Assessment

Completion of the psychosocial assessment includes data collection about cultural mores that may influence provision of care in labor and during the postpartum period. Cultural diversity should be addressed during the prenatal period to facilitate appropriate care practices. Interventions that are culturally relevant to the needs of the woman and her family decrease the possibility of conflict or misunderstanding arising between people of different backgrounds (Mattson, 2004).

History of exposure to risk-taking behaviors such as smoking or tobacco use, alcohol or chemical dependency, or history of multiple unprotected sexual encounters may be identified. Other issues, such as the planning and spacing of pregnancies, emotional acceptance of the current pregnancy, and past or present psychiatric problems (e.g., depression, postpartum psychosis, bipolar or schizophrenic disorders, or eating disorders), may be revealed though ongoing assessment.

Screening for domestic violence is an important component of both the psychosocial and physical assessment. The reported incidence of abuse during pregnancy has a wide range of 1% to 20% (American College of Obstetricians & Gynecologists [ACOG], 2006). Domestic violence often begins during pregnancy, or if there is a previous history, may escalate during both the pregnancy and the postpartum period (ACOG, 2005). ACOG recommends screening every pregnant woman for partner violence at the first prenatal visit, at least once per trimester, and again at the postpartum visit. Frequent screenings provide increased opportunities to disclose partner violence or intimidation. Each institution should have policies that address the assessment of domestic violence. Screening for domestic violence should be conducted in private, whenever possible, rather than in the presence of a woman's partner or other family members (ACOG, 2005, 2006; AWHONN, 2007).

FIGURE 3-2   The Four Steps in Performing Leopold's Maneuvers

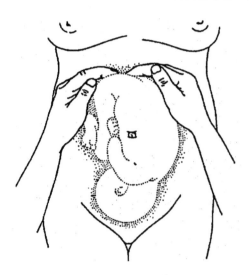

1st Maneuver
Assess part of fetus
in the upper uterus

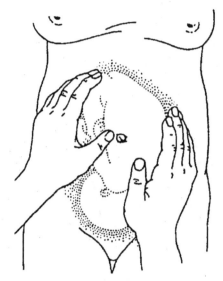

2nd Maneuver
Assess location
of the fetal back

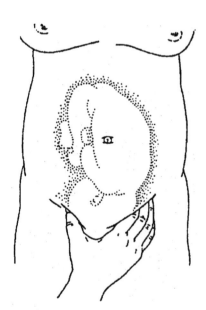

3rd Maneuver
Identify presenting part

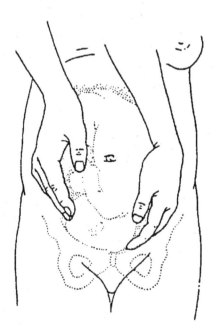

4th Maneuver
Determine the descent
of the presenting part

PHYSICAL EXAMINATION

The physical examination includes a complete physical assessment of the woman, focusing on four of the essential forces of labor:

- Power (assessment of uterine contractions)
- Passage (vaginal and pelvic examination)
- Passenger (fetal assessment)
- Psyche (assessment of maternal emotional status)

The physical examination includes assessment of maternal vital signs, uterine activity and fetal well-being, assessment of fetal presentation and station, membrane status, estimated fetal weight, and presence or absence of vaginal bleeding and laboratory evaluation. Maternal-fetal condition may influence the prioritization of elements of the physical assessment. The primary obstetric provider should be notified in a timely manner when the physical examination reveals risk factors (AAP & ACOG, 2007) such as:

- Vaginal bleeding
- Acute abdominal/flank pain
- Temperature ≥100.4° F (38° C)
- Preterm labor
- Preterm, premature rupture of membranes
- Hypertension (>140 systolic or 90 diastolic)
- Diffuse, vague symptoms, including headache, epigastric pain, visual changes, nausea and vomiting, difficulty urinating
- Category II or III fetal heart rate pattern (See Chapter 5)

Identification and assignment of women to high-risk status have significant implications to her care. Each institution should have interdisciplinary policies addressing the assessment of risk and the assignment of women to low-risk, at-risk or high-risk status.

Clinical Assessment of Maternal Vital Signs

Vital signs include temperature, blood pressure, pulse, respiration, and pain assessment; ongoing assessments are based on clinical findings and facility protocol. Vital signs outside of the normal range for pregnancy should be reported to the primary obstetric care provider. The *Guidelines for Perinatal Care* (AAP & ACOG, 2007) suggest focused maternal assessments including vital signs a minimum of every 4 hours, with increased frequency of surveillance as needed.

Vital signs outside of the normal range for pregnancy and unrelieved or unusual pain should be reported to the primary obstetric care provider. Evaluation of the effectiveness of pain management strategies should be performed at regular intervals during labor and birth. Assessing pain on a continuum yields information about unusual manifestations of pain, such as epigastric pain or unremitting uterine contractions that may indicate potential maternal-fetal compromise.

Pain assessment should include information about acute and chronic sources of pain, effectiveness of coping techniques for pain management, and an assessment of the woman's and family's expectations regarding pain relief or control during labor.

Maternal Height, Weight, and Weight Gain

Assessment of maternal height and weight, the weight of previous infants (if applicable), and current pregnancy weight gain may provide clinicians with additional information that may identify potential risks for the laboring woman (Table 3-2). Prepregnancy weight and weight gain during pregnancy are related to the infant's weight at birth. Because women who are either overweight or underweight are at risk for a variety of adverse pregnancy outcomes, height and weight should be measured at the first prenatal visit and a body mass index (BMI) calculated. Discussion of the women's target pregnancy weight gain should be based on evaluation of the BMI. BMI is calculated by using this formula:

$$\left(\frac{\textit{weight in pounds divided by height in inches}}{\textit{height in inches}} \right) \times 703$$

Table 3-2	Recommended Total Weight Gain in Pregnancy (IOM)
Pre-Pregnancy BMI	**Recommended Weight Gain**
Underweight (BMI < 18.5)	28–40 pounds
Normal weight (BMI 18.5–24.9)	25–35 pounds
Overweight (BMI 25–29.9)	15–25 pounds
Obese (BMI ≥30)	15 pounds

From Committee on Nutritional Status During Pregnancy and Lactation, IOM (1990). Copyright 1990 by the National Academies Press. Reprinted with permission.

There are many co-morbidities associated with obesity in pregnancy. In a large prospective population-based cohort study, when mothers who were "morbidly obese" (defined as those with a BMI >40) were compared with normal weight mothers, there was an increased risk for a variety of adverse pregnancy outcomes (Cedergren, 2004). These outcomes, compared with outcomes of normal weight mothers included gestational hypertension or preeclampsia, antepartum stillbirths after 28 weeks gestation, gestational diabetes, prolonged labors, induction of labor, and cesarean birth. Underweight women are at higher risk for preterm birth and low birth weight (Ehrenberg, Dierker, Milluzzi, & Mercer, 2003). Low-carbohydrate or low-calorie diets are ketogenic and may cause glucose deprivation to the fetal brain and ketonuria, which have been correlated with preterm labor (Bond, 2004).

Uterine Activity

Subjective and objective data are used to assess uterine contraction status. The mother should be asked about the onset, timing (frequency and duration), and intensity of her contractions. Clinicians should also assess contraction frequency, duration, intensity, and resting tone by directly palpating the uterus before, during, and after contractions. Con-traction *frequency* is measured from the beginning of one contraction to the beginning of the next contraction and is described in minutes. *Duration* is the length of the contraction and is described in seconds. *Intensity* refers to the strength of the contraction and is described as mild, moderate, or strong by palpation. *Resting tone* is described as soft or firm by palpation (Simpson, 2008).

Membrane Status

Membrane status is assessed by history, objective assessment, or a combination of both. The mother may report ROM as a gush of fluid or a small leak. Time of suspected ROM or onset of leaking should be determined, along with assessment of the color of fluid, presence or absence of blood, and odor. When frank amniotic fluid is not discernible, a sterile speculum examination may be performed, and fluid from the vaginal vault may be tested with Nitrazine paper or placed on a microscope slide for a ferning test (ACOG, 2007). Amniotic fluid is alkaline. Nitrazine paper indicates the pH of a fluid and will turn blue or blue-green if the membranes have ruptured. However, the reliability of a Nitrazine test can be compromised by the presence of blood, urine, semen, vaginal infection, or incorrect application. A ferning testing may also be performed to assess the status of the membranes. For this method, the vaginal fluid obtained from the speculum examination is applied to a slide, dried, and evaluated under a microscope. A distinct, fern-like crystallization pattern known as "ferning" is observed when membranes are ruptured.

Another method of determining ROM is a rapid immunoassay test for a protein, placental alpha microglobulin-1 (PAMG-1), that is abundant in amniotic fluid (Norwitz & Park, 2005). This test for PAMG-1 is useful at any gestational age (15–42 weeks) and does not require a sterile speculum examination. A summary of methods to determine ROM is found in Table 3-3.

The treatment of premature ROM depends on gestational age and the presence or absence of infection or labor. After the membranes rupture, the risk for infection and chorioamnionitis increases. Therefore, vaginal examinations should be performed only as indicated by maternal or fetal status rather than at regularly timed intervals (AAP & ACOG, 2007).

Preterm, premature ROM arises from multiple pathways (Devlieger, Millar, Bryant-Greenwood, Lewi, & Deprest, 2006). Chronic inflammation and/or infection increase the production of hormones and cytokines in the membranes and placenta, possibly causing preterm contractions, membrane weakening, and thus membrane rupture. Repeated stretching of the amnion may make the membranes less elastic and more susceptible to preterm rupture. Relaxin levels may also be elevated, causing extracellular matrix degradation leading to rupture (Devlieger et al.). Another pathway associated with premature ROM relates to the attachment of bacteria ascending from the vagina to the amniotic membranes. Attachment of bacteria to the membranes in this circumstance has been shown to produce certain proteases that cause weakening of the membrane and this ultimately may lead to ROM (Garite, 2007). When the woman is in labor following ROM, her temperature should be obtained frequently to assess for early signs of amnionitis. If the woman is not in labor but being expectantly managed, her temperature should be obtained every 4 hours. Attention to perineal hygiene is important and may help decrease the risk of infection (AAP & ACOG, 2007). Signs of chorioamnionitis at any gestational age may include (ACOG, 2007):

- Maternal fever ($\geq$100.4° F [38° C])
- Maternal or fetal tachycardia

Table 3-3	**Clinical Tests to Confirm Rupture of Membranes**	
Name of Test	**Methodology**	**Special Considerations**
Pooling	A sterile speculum examination is performed to visualize pooling of fluid in the posterior fornix of the vagina.	Urine, semen, and other fluids may be mistaken for amniotic fluid.
Nitrazine	A speculum examination is performed to obtain fluid from the posterior fornix of the vagina. Nitrazine paper is used to indicate the pH of the fluid. Amniotic fluid is alkaline. Rupture of the membranes is suspected if the nitrazine paper turns blue.	False-positive results may occur as a result of cervicitis, vaginitis, alkaline urine, blood, semen, or antiseptics.
Ferning	A speculum examination is performed to obtain fluid from the posterior fornix of the vagina. Fluid specimen is swabbed onto a slide and allowed to dry. The slide is viewed through a microscope. Crystallization of dry amniotic fluid in a "fern like" pattern is observed when membranes are ruptured.	False-positive results may occur as a result of fingerprints on slide, blood, semen, or cervical mucus.
Blue dye	An amniocentesis is performed, and dilute indigo carmine is instilled into amniotic cavity. Membranes are ruptured if the dye leaks into vagina within 20–30 minutes.	Invasive, may result in bleeding, infection, and loss of pregnancy.
Rapid immunoassay for placental alpha microglobulin-1 (PAMG-1)	A speculum exam is not needed. A manufacturer's "kit" is needed, and the instructions in the kit should be followed.	Semen, urine, blood, or vaginal infections do not affect results.

- Elevated maternal white blood cell count (this is a nonspecific sign, however)
- Uterine tenderness
- Foul-smelling vaginal discharge

Vaginal Examination

Vaginal Bleeding or Discharge

Assessment should include evaluation of vaginal bleeding or discharge and identification of related potential risk factors in the patient's history. The underlying cause of vaginal bleeding may be bloody show (blood-tinged mucus accompanied with mucous strands), which is a normal indicator of cervical dilation. However, vaginal bleeding may result from more serious disorders, such as placenta previa, placental abruption, or ruptured uterus, that can alter uteroplacental perfusion and significantly compromise maternal and fetal well-being. Hemorrhage can occur unexpectedly during any stage of the perinatal period. If the woman states that she has vaginal bleeding, vaginal examinations should not be performed until further evaluation by the primary care provider is undertaken to ascertain the source of bleeding such as placenta previa. In addition, the clinician should question the woman regarding the onset of bleeding; amount, color, and type of blood (i.e., presence or absence of clots); pain or absence of pain with the bleeding; and precipitating events, if any. For example, questions may include: "Was the bleeding precipitated by sexual intercourse, a fall, or blunt trauma?" "Are you now having or did you have uterine contractions with the bleeding?"

The color and character of vaginal bleeding can be important diagnostic indicators. Bright red, painless vaginal bleeding may be an indication of placenta previa or low-lying placenta. The dark red bleeding with clots or board-like abdomen typical of placental abruption may indicate accumulated blood loss. However, overt placental abruption and uterine rupture may occur without evidence of vaginal bleeding. In those instances, maternal vital signs and fetal heart rate (FHR) assessments will provide

critical information (MacMullen, Dulski, & Meagher, 2005).

Hypovolemia may result from excessive bleeding. The fetus is not protected from maternal blood loss because autoregulation of uterine perfusion does not occur. The vasoconstrictive effects often seen in hypovolemic shock also contribute to this problem. Maternal vital signs may remain unchanged until approximately 20% of blood volume is lost (Francois & Foley, 2007); and at this point, the uteroplacental perfusion may be impaired. Fetal heart rate manifestations of decreased uteroplacental perfusion may include late decelerations, increasing baseline, and decreasing variability.

A narrowing of the pulse pressure occurs in Class 2 hemorrhage with a loss of 1200 to 1500 mL of blood. Tachycardia is a hallmark sign of physiologic compensation for hypovolemia as the body attempts to increase cardiac output. Although tachypnea is a nonspecific response to volume loss, it is also a compensatory sign of volume deficit that is often overlooked (Francois & Foley, 2007). Additional important signs of Class 2 hemorrhage are increasing maternal heart rate, orthostatic blood pressure changes, prolonged capillary refill (indicating decreased perfusion of extremities), and blanching or mottling of the extremities. Overt hypotension; marked tachycardia and tachypnea; and cold, clammy skin are signs of worsening hemorrhage (Class 3), with a blood loss of 1800 to 2100 mL (Francois & Foley). The use of pulse oximetry may be helpful in assessment of maternal oxygenation, along with frequent vital signs, and FHR assessment.

Ultrasound evaluation by a qualified provider may be performed to assess the placenta and its location. A Kleihauer-Betke (KB) laboratory test is used to detect transplacental hemorrhage and can be helpful in predicting preterm labor following maternal trauma (Muench et al., 2004).

As the pregnancy nears completion, vaginal discharge normally increases. However, vaginal discharge that is copious, malodorous, or discolored may indicate infection and should be evaluated further. The woman should be questioned about the onset, color, amount, and odor of vaginal discharge and about other unusual symptoms, such as vaginal pruritus, that might indicate a monilial or other infection.

Cervical Examination

A vaginal examination is performed to assess cervical status. The examination includes assessment of the cervix for dilation, effacement, cervical position, and station of the presenting part. This is accomplished through gloved digital examination or by sterile speculum examination in the case of ruptured membranes without labor, premature ROM, (PROM), or preterm PROM (PPROM). When contractions occur between 24 0/7 to 34 6/7 weeks' gestation, it may be of benefit to obtain a fetal fibronectin (fFN) sample (Tekesin, Marek, Hellmeyer, Reitz, & Schmidt, 2005).

Fetal fibronectin (fFN) is an immunodiagnostic, biochemical marker obtained from cervicovaginal secretions. It is a helpful tool used to differentiate women who are at risk for impending preterm delivery from those who are not (Tekesin et al., 2005). A sample is collected from the secretions in the posterior fornix or external cervical os during a speculum examination using a Dacron swab included in the manufacturer's kit. The woman should have no digital examinations, intercourse, or vaginal ultrasounds for 24 hours prior to obtaining the sample, nor should she have had any vaginal medications or lubricants during that same period. A fFN concentration of greater than 50 ng/mL is considered positive (Leitich & Kaider, 2003). The presence of fFN in cervicovaginal secretions between 20 and 34 weeks' gestation is a strong predictor of preterm birth in those women with signs and symptoms of preterm labor. Its presence does not necessarily indicate the onset of labor (positive predictive value of 15%–25%); its absence, a negative result, rules out labor occurring within 7 to 14 days, with a high negative predictive value (97%–99%) in symptomatic women (Tekesin et al., 2005).

The clinician should explain the vaginal examination procedure to the woman and her partner. The woman determines whether her significant other will remain during the examination. She should be draped for minimal exposure and positioned to maximize fetal oxygenation, avoiding the supine position. It may not be necessary to place the woman in the lithotomy position; the examination can also be accomplished in alternative positions, such as side lying. Increased maternal cooperation and decreased discomfort can be gained by having the woman take slow, deep breaths through a wide-opened mouth during the examination.

Cervical dilation is reported in a range between 0 and 10 cm. Cervical dilation of 10 cm is commonly referred to as "complete" dilation. Effacement is reported as a percentage between 0% and 100%. One hundred percent effacement is also referred to as "complete" effacement. Cervical position is reported as posterior, midposition, or anterior. Fetal station is reported as a number between −5 cm (floating) and +5 cm (on the perineum); this indicates the position of the fetal head above (-5 cm to -1 cm), at (0 cm), or below (+1 cm to +5 cm) the ischial spines. The presenting part is the part of the fetus that is presenting and felt through the cervix.

Ultrasound assessment of the cervix may be a very valuable tool in predicting preterm birth (Iams, 2003). Digital assessment of cervical length has commonly been used. However, evaluating cervical length in this manner is subjective, varies between examiners, and may underestimate the true anatomic length. Of all variables assessed by digital or ultrasound examination, ultrasonic transvaginal cervical length measurement is the best predictor of preterm birth, especially when used in combination with other markers for preterm birth such as the fFN test (Iams). The relative risk of preterm labor and birth increases as the cervical length decreases. The findings of cervical length greater than 30 mm *or* a negative fFN assay can minimize false positive prediction of preterm labor. fFn and cervical length measurements are primarily useful in situations in which a negative result can avoid interventions including bed rest, tocolytics, steroids, cerclage, and long-term hospitalization (Iams).

Biochemical Assessment

Laboratory Values

Each institution should establish a policy addressing required laboratory tests for pregnant patients admitted to labor and delivery or perinatal units. Typically, the following basic tests may be performed and evaluated:

- Complete blood count or hemoglobin and hematocrit with differential
- Blood group, Rh, and antibody screen (if not already done)
- Urinalysis for protein, glucose, ketones, and specific gravity
- Rapid plasma reagin (RPR)

The maternal condition and the presence of risk factors such as preeclampsia, infection, or diabetes will determine the need for additional laboratory assessments. For example, a woman presenting with preeclampsia may have additional laboratory tests drawn, such as a comprehensive metabolic screen, including liver enzymes, renal panel, and uric acid. A coagulation panel also may be indicated.

Gestational diabetes mellitus (GDM) affects 7% of pregnant women and is recognized as any degree of carbohydrate intolerance during pregnancy (Wallerstedt & Clokey, 2004). This definition applies when either diet modification or insulin administration is used as treatment. Maternal hyperglycemia is associated with an increased fetal morbidity secondary to fetal hyperinsulinemia. Maintenance of normal glucose levels is necessary to help ensure optimal pregnancy outcome. Glucose crosses the placenta, whereas insulin does not; thus, fetal blood sugars are 70% to 80% of maternal levels (Wallerstedt & Clokey, 2004). The American Diabetes Association (2008) recommends screening based on risk. Women considered at average risk should

be screened between 24 and 28 weeks' gestation for GDM. Women at low risk generally do not need screening. The low-risk group includes women who meet **all** of the following criteria (American Diabetes Association, 2008):

- Age less than 25 years
- Normal body weight prior to pregnancy (BMI ≤25 or less)
- No family history of diabetes in first-degree relative
- No history of impaired glucose tolerance or impaired fasting glucose
- No history of poor obstetric outcome
- Not a member of a high-risk ethnic or racial group (i.e., African American, Asian, Hispanic, Pacific Islander or Native American).

Women with identified high-risk factors should undergo glucose testing as soon as feasible in the prenatal period. These risk factors include marked obesity; strong family history of type 2 diabetes; personal history of GDM; or presence of glycosuria. If the initial screening is not indicative of GDM, they should be retested between 24 and 28 weeks' gestation (American Diabetes Association, 2008).

A fasting plasma glucose level greater than 126 mg/dL or a random plasma glucose level greater than 200 mg/dL meets the criteria for the diagnosis of diabetes. Initial evaluation for gestational diabetes in women with identified high-risk factors is based on a 50-g glucose challenge test (GCT). The woman ingests 50 g of glucose and a serum glucose is drawn 1 hour later. A blood glucose level of 130 mg/dL or more requires follow-up testing with a 100-g, 3-hour oral glucose tolerance test (OGTT).

To prepare for the OGTT, the woman is instructed to eat a diet containing 150 g of complex carbohydrates for 3 days prior to the test. She should remain NPO (nothing by mouth) for 8–14 hours prior to the test. A fasting serum glucose is drawn. The woman drinks a 100-g glucose solution. Serum glucose samples are then drawn at 1, 2, and 3 hours. A diagnosis of gestational diabetes is made if two or more glucose levels exceed the normal values defined by the American Diabetes Association. The normal serum values for an OGTT using 100-g glucose solution in pregnancy are (American Diabetes Association, 2008):

- Fasting   <95 mg/dL
- 1 hour   <180 mg/dL
- 2 hour   <155 mg/dL
- 3 hour   <140 mg/dL

The results of glucose screening should be available on the prenatal record (AAP & ACOG, 2007).

Group B Streptococcus Prevention and Prophylaxis

Despite significant progress in the reducing the rate of GBS since the 1990s, GBS remains the leading infectious cause of neonatal morbidity and mortality (Centers for Disease Control and Prevention, 2002). The Centers for Disease Control and Prevention 2002 guidelines were created using a culture-based screening approach, and thus, recommend universal prenatal screening for GBS colonization by vaginal-rectal culture between 35 and 37 weeks' gestation. Indications for antibiotic prophylaxis during the intrapartum period are listed in Box 3-2, including indications for those women who were not screened prenatally. Routine intrapartum antibiotic pro-

phylaxis for GBS-colonized women undergoing planned cesarean births without preceding labor or membrane rupture is not recommended (www. cdc.gov/groupbstrep). Penicillin remains the first-line agent for intrapartum antibiotic prophylaxis, with ampicillin an acceptable alternative. Because of the emergence of clindamycin- and erythromycin-resistant GBS isolates, the second-line agents for use in those women with penicillin allergies have been revised as described in Box 3-3.

Infectious Disease Evaluation

When a woman presents with symptoms or a history of sexually transmitted infection or other infection during her pregnancy, testing should be completed. Health care facilities should determine infectious disease policies appropriate for perinatal patient population consistent with federal, state, and local regulatory agency requirements.

FETAL ASSESSMENT

The assessment of fetal status is a key component of perinatal care. Fetal assessment begins at the first prenatal visit with gestational age determination and continues during subsequent visits to include fetal activity assessment, antenatal testing (as indicated by maternal or fetal needs), and, finally, assessment of the fetus during labor.

BOX 3-2 Indications for Intrapartum Antibiotic Prophylaxis for GBS

- Previous infant with invasive GBS disease
- GBS bacteriuria during current pregnancy
- Positive GBS screening during current pregnancy (unless a planned cesarean birth in the absence of labor or rupture of membranes)
- Unknown GBS status *and* any of the following:
    * Labor and birth at less than 37 weeks' gestation
    * Rupture of membranes for greater than 18 hours
    * Intrapartum temperature greater than 100.4° F (38° C)

GBS, Group B streptococcus (strep).
Adapted from: Centers for Disease Control and Prevention. (2002). Prevention of perinatal group B streptococcal disease. Retrieved November 16, 2007, from http://www.cdc.gov/groupbstrep/docs/RR5111.pdf

BOX 3-3 Intrapartum Antibiotic Prophylaxis for Group B Streptococcus (GBS)	
Recommended	Penicillin G, 5 million units IV initial dose, then 2.5 million units IV every 4 hours until delivery
Alternative	Ampicillin, 2 g IV initial dose, then 1 g IV every 4 hours until delivery
If penicillin allergic[†]	
Patients not at high risk for anaphylaxis	Cefazolin, 2 g IV initial dose, then 1 g IV every 8 hours until delivery
Patients at high risk for anaphylaxis[§]	
GBS susceptible to clindamycin and erythromycin[¶]	Clindamycin, 900 mg IV every 8 hours until delivery
	OR
	Erythromycin, 500 mg IV every 6 hours until delivery
GBS resistant to clindamycin or erythromycin or susceptibility unknown	Vancomycin,** 1 g IV every 12 hours until delivery

IV, Intravenous.

Note: From Centers for Disease Control and Prevention. (2002). Prevention of perinatal group B streptococcal disease. Retrieved November 16, 2007, from http://www.cdc.gov/groupbstrep/docs/RR5111.pdf

* Broader-spectrum agents, including an agent active against GBS, may be necessary for treatment of chorioamnionitis.

† History of penicillin allergy should be assessed to determine whether a high risk for anaphylaxis is present. Penicillin-allergic patients at high risk for anaphylaxis are those who have experienced immediate hypersensitivity to penicillin including a history of penicillin-related anaphylaxis; other high-risk patients are those with asthma or other diseases that would make anaphylaxis more dangerous or difficult to treat, such as persons being treated with beta-adrenergic–blocking agents.

§ If laboratory facilities are adequate, clindamycin and erythromycin susceptibility testing should be performed on prenatal GBS isolates from penicillin-allergic women at high risk for anaphylaxis.

¶ Resistance to erythromycin is often but not always associated with clindamycin resistance. If a strain is resistant to erythromycin but appears susceptible to clindamycin, it may still have inducible resistance to clindamycin.

** Cefazolin is preferred over vancomycin for women with a history of penicillin allergy other than immediate hypersensitivity reactions, and pharmacologic data suggest it achieves effective intraamniotic concentrations. Vancomycin should be reserved for penicillin-allergic women at high risk for anaphylaxis.

Antenatal Assessment

A variety of methods are available that enable ongoing assessment of fetal well-being during pregnancy. The methods include but are not limited to the nonstress test (NST), contraction stress (CST), biophysical profile (BPP) and modified BPP. An in-depth discussion of antepartum assessment methods is presented in Chapter 11. In addition, ultrasound performed by a skilled and credentialed sonographer can provide critical information regarding amniotic fluid index (AFI) and amniotic fluid volume (AFV). Evidence of oligohydramnios (AFI < 5 cm) may result in variable decelerations resulting from of a lack of cushioning of the umbilical cord. If oligohydramnios is present, clinicians can be prepared to intervene with amnioinfusion if indicated (Tucker, 2004). If there is evidence of polyhydramnios (AFI > 25 cm), clinicians should be aware of the increased risk for umbilical cord compromise if ROM occurs prior to engagement of the presenting part.

In addition to AFI/AFV determination, an ultrasound can provide important information about placental location. Such information should be reviewed when the patient presents with undiagnosed vaginal bleeding or documented low-lying placenta accompanied by vaginal bleeding.

Method of Fetal Monitoring

The method of fetal monitoring used to assess fetal status during labor (auscultation; or external or internal modes with EFM) should be identified and documented. Each method has benefits and limitations, as discussed in Chapter 4. When using auscultation, the clinician can assess the FHR, rhythm, and increases and decreases of the FHR. Uterine activity is assessed by palpation. On the basis of those findings, interventions are planned, and responses to interventions are assessed and documented.

When using external and internal modes of monitoring, the baseline FHR, variability, accelerations and decelerations, and evolution of the tracing over time can be assessed. When the internal mode of monitoring (i.e., fetal spiral electrode and intrauterine pressure catheter) is used, the information obtained on the uterine activity panel on the fetal monitor should be validated by the clinician through palpation. Interpretation of the data obtained with auscultation or the electronic fetal monitor, coupled with ongoing assessment of maternal physical and emotional status, can be used to plan interventions and assess maternal-fetal responses. Chapter 6 includes a detailed discussion of interventions related to fetal assessment by auscultation and palpation and electronic fetal monitoring.

SUMMARY

Maternal-fetal assessment begins at the first prenatal visit and continues through birth as a process on a continuum of care. Ongoing assessment of the physical and emotional condition of the mother and the physical condition of the fetus are keys to ensuring appropriate care during the perinatal period. Gathering essential data assists the nursing and medical staff in formulating the plan of care for the family, anticipating potential problems, and intervening on behalf of mother and fetus in a timely manner. Maternal-fetal assessment data are derived from many sources including, but not limited to, the prenatal record and information gathered through test results and interviews. Accessing a variety of information sources may be necessary to gain a clear understanding of the physical and psychosocial needs of the mother and her fetus.

REFERENCES

American Academy of Pediatrics (AAP) & American College of Obstetricians and Gynecologists (ACOG). (2007). *Guidelines for perinatal care* (6th ed.). Elk Grove, IL: Authors.

American College of Obstetricians and Gynecologists. (2005). Intimate partner violence and domestic violence. In *Special issues in women's health* (pp. 169–188). Washington, DC: ACOG.

American College of Obstetricians and Gynecologists. (2006). Psychosocial risk factors: Perinatal screening and intervention (ACOG Committee Opinion Number 343). *Obstetrics and Gynecology, 108*, 469–477.

American College of Obstetricians and Gynecologists. (2001). Gestational diabetes (ACOG Practice Guideline Number 30). *Obstetrics and Gynecology, 98*, 525–538.

American College of Obstetricians and Gynecologists. (2007). Premature rupture of membranes (ACOG Practice Bulletin Number 80). *Obstetrics and Gynecology, 109*, 1007–1019.

American Diabetes Association. (2008). Diagnosis and classification of diabetes mellitus. *Diabetes Care, 31*(Suppl. 1), S55–S58.

Association of Women's Health, Obstetric and Neonatal Nurses. (2007). *Mandatory reporting of intimate partner violence* (Position Statement). Washington, DC: Author.

Association of Women's Health, Obstetric and Neonatal Nurses. (2008). *Basic, high-risk, and critical care intrapartum nursing: Clinical competencies and education guide*. Washington, DC: Author.

American Society of Anesthesiologists. (2003). Considerations for anesthesiologists: What you should know about your patient's use of herbal medicines and other dietary supplements. Retrieved March 19, 2008 from: http://www.asahq.org/patientEducation/herbPhysician.pdf

Bond, L. (2004). Physiology of pregnancy. In S. Mattson & J. E. Smith (Eds.), *Core curriculum for maternal newborn nursing* (3rd ed., pp. 96–123). St. Louis: Saunders.

Born, D., & Barron, M. L. (2005). Herb use in pregnancy: What nurses should know. *MCN: American Journal of Maternal Child Nursing, 30*, 201–206; quiz 207–208.

Cedergren, M. I. (2004). Maternal morbid obesity and the risk of adverse pregnancy outcome. *Obstetrics and Gynecology, 103,* 219–224.

Centers for Disease Control and Prevention. (2002). *Prevention of perinatal group B Streptococcal disease*. Retrieved November 16, 2007, from: http://www.cdc.gov/groupbstrep/docs/RR5111.pdf

Cousins, L. M., Smok, D. P., Lovett, S. M., & Poeltler, D. M. (2005). AmniSure placental alpha microglobulin-1 rapid immunoassay versus standard diagnostic methods for detection of rupture of membranes. *American Journal of Perinatology, 22*, 317–320.

Devlieger, R., Millar, L. K., Bryant-Greenwood, G., Lewi, L., & Deprest, J. A. (2006). Fetal membrane healing after spontaneous and iatrogenic membrane rupture: A review of current evidence. *American Journal of Obstetrics and Gynecology, 195*, 1512–1520.

Druzin, M. L., Smith, J. F., Jr., Gabbe, S. G., & Reed, K. L. (2007). Antepartum fetal evaluation. In S. G. Gabbe,

J. L. Neibyl, & J. L. Simpson (Eds.), *Obstetrics: Normal and problem pregnancies* (5th ed., pp. 267–300). New York: Livingston.

Ehrenberg, H. M., Dierker, L., Milluzzi, C., & Mercer, B. M. (2003). Low maternal weight, failure to thrive in pregnancy, and adverse pregnancy outcomes. *American Journal of Obstetrics and Gynecology, 189*, 1726–1730.

Francois, K. R., & Foley, M. R. (2007). Antepartum and postpartum hemorrhage. In S. G. Gabbe, J. R. Niebyl, & J. L. Simpson (Eds.), *Obstetrics: Normal and problem pregnancies* (5th ed., pp. 456–485). New York: Churchill Livingstone.

Garite, T. (2007). Premature rupture of membranes. In R. K. Creasy, R. Resnick, & J. D. Iams (Eds.), *Maternal-fetal medicine: Principles and practices* (5th ed., pp. 723–739). Philadelphia: Saunders.

Iams, J. D. (2003). Prediction and early detection of preterm labor. *Obstetrics and Gynecology, 101*, 402–412.

Johnson, T. R., Gregory, K. D., & Niebyl, J. R. (2007). Preconception and prenatal care: Part of the continuum. In S. G. Gabbe, J. R. Niebyl, & J. L. Simpson (Eds.), *Obstetrics: Normal and problem pregnancies* (5th ed., pp. 111–137). New York: Churchill Livingston.

Leitich, H., & Kaider, A. (2003). Fetal fibronectin—how useful is it in the prediction of preterm birth? *British Journal of Obstetrics and Gynaecology, 110*(Suppl. 20), 66–70.

MacMullen, N. J., Dulski, L. A., & Meagher, B. (2005). Red alert: Perinatal hemorrhage. *MCN: American Journal of Maternal Child Nursing, 30*, 46–51.

Mattson, S. (2004). Ethnocultural considerations in the childbearing period. In S. Mattson & J. E. Smith (Eds.), *Core Curriculum for Maternal-Newborn Nursing* (3rd ed., pp. 75–95). St. Louis: Saunders.

Muench, M. V., Baschat, A. A., Reddy, U. M., Mighty, H. E., Weiner, C. P., Scalea, T. M., et al. (2004). Kleihauer-Betke testing is important in all cases of maternal trauma. *Journal of Trauma, 57*, 1094–1098.

Norwitz, E., & Park, J. (2005). Technical innovations in clinical obstetrics. *Contemporary OB/GYN Technology*. Retrieved November 16, 2007, from http://pharmexec. mediwire.com/main/Default.aspx?P=Content&Article ID=181112

Quinn, L. A., Thompson, S. J., & Ott, M. K. (2005). Application of the social ecological model in folic acid public health initiatives. *Journal of Obstetric, Gynecologic and Neonatal Nursing, 34*, 672–681.

Simpson, K. R. (2008). Labor and birth. In K. R. Simpson & P. A. Creehan (Eds.), *Perinatal nursing* (3rd ed., pp 300–398). Philadelphia: Lippincott.

Simpson, K. R., & Creehan, P. A. (2008). *Perinatal nursing* (3rd ed.). Philadelphia: Lippincott.

Smith, J. (2004). Age-related complications. In S. Mattson & J. E. Smith (Eds.), *Core curriculum for maternal-newborn nursing* (3rd ed., pp. 147–169). St. Louis: Saunders.

Tekesin, I., Marek, S., Hellmeyer, L., Reitz, D., & Schmidt, S. (2005). Assessment of rapid fetal fibronectin in predicting preterm delivery. *Obstetrics and Gynecology, 105*, 280–284.

Tucker, S. M. (2004). *Fetal monitoring and assessment* (5th ed.). St. Louis: Mosby.

Wallerstedt, C., & Clokey, D. (2004). Endocrine and metabolic disorders. In S. Mattson & J. E. Smith (Eds.), *Core curriculum for maternal-newborn nursing* (3rd ed., pp. 660–702). St. Louis: Saunders.

Wotring, R. (2004). Environmental hazards. In S. Mattson & J. E. Smith (Eds.), *Core curriculum for maternal-newborn nursing* (3rd ed., pp. 201–224). St. Louis: Saunders.

CHAPTER 4

Techniques for Fetal Heart Assessment

Karen M. Harmon

INTRODUCTION

The aim of intrapartum fetal surveillance is to assess fetal well-being and the fetal heart rate (FHR) response to labor in order to make appropriate, physiologically based clinical decisions. The goal of fetal heart rate assessment is to identify those fetuses at risk for hypoxia and provide timely intervention to avoid adverse outcomes. Many factors should be taken into consideration when selecting methods of fetal monitoring. These may include maternal and fetal status, maternal preferences, institutional policies, and national guidelines. Regardless of the fetal heart monitoring (FHM) method selected for a given woman, the clinician is accountable for knowing how to recognize and respond to auditory and electronically obtained FHR data. FHR data are incomplete without uterine activity assessment, and the clinician should also recognize and respond to both palpated and electronically obtained uterine activity data. The development of skills in these monitoring methods enables the clinician to select and combine the most appropriate techniques for individual patients.

This chapter focuses on a variety of techniques for assessing the FHR and uterine activity and addresses the current state of the science for auscultation, palpation, and electronic fetal monitoring (EFM). Techniques, capabilities, limitations, procedures, and troubleshooting strategies for each monitoring method are also discussed.

AUSCULTATION

Auscultation of fetal heart characteristics requires attention to the audible characteristics of the FHR. The majority of the following discussion of fetal heart rate auscultation is adapted with permission from Feinstein, Sprague, and Trépanier (2008).

Auscultation as Compared with EFM

Although IA has been used for many years, EFM has been the predominant method of intrapartum fetal surveillance since its inception in the 1960s. However, EFM was adopted into clinical practice prior to scientific validation of its presumed benefits (Banta & Thacker, 2001; Parer, 2003). In 2002, EFM was noted to be the most common obstetric procedure, and 85% of live births in the United States were assessed using EFM (Martin et al., 2003). As discussed in Chapter 1, the expected improvements in neonatal outcomes have not been demonstrated despite the pervasive use of EFM in labor. EFM has been shown to increase the incidence of cesarean and operative vaginal birth rates without generating a corresponding reduction in perinatal mortality or childhood morbidity (Schwartz & Young, 2006; Smith & Onstad, 2005). In a recent U.S. national survey of women, 93% reported having fetal monitoring during their labor (Declercq, Sakala, Corry, & Applebaum, 2006). Most of the women reported having continuous electronic monitoring, whereas only 6% stated that a handheld Doppler device or stethoscope was used exclusively to monitor their fetus. In Canada, EFM was used for 75% to 90% of laboring women (Davies et al., 1993, 2002; Levitt, Hanvey, Avard, Chance, & Kaczorowski, 1995).

The available evidence supports IA as an appropriate primary method of fetal heart rate surveillance during labor for women without risk factors (American Academy of Pediatrics [AAP] & American College of Obstetricians & Gynecologists [ACOG], 2007; ACOG, 2005; Feinstein, et al, 2008; Society of Obstetricians and Gynaecologists of Canada [SOGC], 2007). Sources are conflicting on their position regarding use of IA in women with risk factors. (AAP/ACOG; ACOG). In Canada, the SOGC has stated that IA is recommended as the preferred method of fetal surveillance in healthy pregnancies during the active phase of labor (SOGC).

Auscultation Devices

Nonelectronic devices for auscultation (e.g., fetoscope or Pinard-type stethoscope) allow the practitioner to hear the fetal heart sounds associated with the opening and closing of ventricular valves via bone conduction. In contrast, a Doppler device uses ultrasound (US) technology (similar to the external US transducer) to detect the motion of the heart walls or valves. The US device then converts the information into sounds representing cardiac events. The two methods obtain information differently; however, both are appropriate choices in most clinical auscultation situations (Feinstein et al., 2008).

To minimize the risk associated with reliance on potentially inaccurate data, it is important for the practitioner to evaluate the capabilities of each device (Table 4-1). A fetoscope or Pinard-type stethoscope allows the practitioner to hear the actual fetal heart sounds, including opening and closing of the ventricular valves (Goodwin, 2000). These devices can be used to detect the FHR baseline, rhythm, and changes from the baseline. Baseline rhythm is assessed for

regularity and is described as either regular or irregular. The fetoscope can also be used to further clarify the presence of an irregular rhythm. When an irregular heart rate is audible by Doppler US, assessment with a fetoscope-type device is warranted to rule out artifact. A Doppler cannot be used reliably to verify the presence of an irregular rhythm because of its technical limitations in information processing. For example, if a fetus has a supraventricular tachycardia, the Doppler device could halve the FHR because the rapid rate is higher than the rate that the device can accurately detect (Freeman, Garite, & Nageotte, 2003). In this situation, using the stethoscope device allows the practitioner to hear the actual heart sounds and rate. If an arrhythmia is suspected, further evaluation by other methods (e.g., formal US, cardiography) may be required to determine the type of arrhythmia present. Although most arrhythmias are benign and often revert to a normal rhythm during or after birth, all irregular FHRs should be reported to the primary care provider. Further discussion regarding arrhythmias can be found in Chapter 12.

Auscultation is also a useful method for assessing the FHR prior to initiation of EFM and for validating EFM findings (Murray 2004; Parer, 1997). Maternal and fetal heart rates can be differentiated by palpating the maternal pulse at the same time the FHR is auscultated. This is an important assessment because both the US and the fetal spiral electrode can transmit the maternal heart rate (MHR) signal in the case of a fetal demise (Murray). Auscultation along with verification of maternal pulse can clarify the source of the signal and may assist in ruling out artifact.

Some practitioners use the external US transducer of the fetal monitor as an auscultation device without generating a tracing, rather than using a handheld Doppler device. Practitioners should be aware that some EFM computerized systems automatically archive any data obtained, whether or not the paper tracing is turned on. Although theoretically the intermittent brief segments of EFM data could be retrieved, data generated would be of too short a duration to

Table 4-1	Capabilities of Auscultation Devices	
The Fetoscope can:		**The Doppler can:**
• detect FHR baseline		• detect FHR baseline
• detect FHR rhythm		• detect FHR rhythm
• verify the presence of an irregular rhythm		• detect increases (accelerations) and decreases (decelerations) from FHR baseline
• detect increases (accelerations) and decreases (decelerations) from FHR baseline		
• clarify double counting or half-counting by EFM		

EFM = Electronic fetal monitor(ing); FHR = fetal heart rate.
From: *Fetal Heart Rate Auscultation* (p. 14), by N. F. Feinstein, A. Sprague, and M. J. Trépanier, 2008, Washington DC: Association of Women's Health, Obstetric and Neonatal Nurses. Copyright 2008 by the Association of Women's Health, Obstetric and Neonatal Nurses. Used with permission.

be interpretable. Ideally, it is best to use a hand-held Doppler or fetoscope. These issues should be addressed by institutional policies and procedures.

Benefits and Limitations of Auscultation

Auscultation has a number of benefits and limitations. Depending on patients' preferences and practitioners' viewpoints, some properties may fit into either category (Table 4-2). Auscultation may be less costly and less constricting than EFM. It increases freedom of movement; and also permits assessments of the FHR with the woman immersed in water. Use of a fetoscope may limit the ability to hear the FHR, and some women may feel that the technique is more intrusive because of the frequency of assessment. The protocols in the randomized controlled trails (RCTs) comparing EFM and IA during the active and second stages of labor used a 1:1 nurse–patient ratio. Therefore, it is reasonable to recommend that, optimally, a 1:1 nurse–patient ratio be maintained during the active and second stages of labor. Staffing may need to be realigned to meet this recommendation (Feinstein, et al., 2008; SOGC, 2007). The results of one RCT comparing women's responses to IA versus EFM during labor revealed no difference between the two groups regarding their perceived labor experience (Killien & Shy, 1989). However, in the

same study, the women's evaluations of their labor experiences were significantly affected by the level of perceived nursing support received during labor.

IA does not provide a continuous record of the FHR characteristics. From a legal perspective, some perceive this as a benefit, whereas others argue that this is a limitation. A meta-analysis (Alfirevic, Devane, & Gyte, 2006) found that continuous EFM does not lead to significant differences in cerebral palsy, infant mortality, or other standard measures of neonatal well-being. Current evidence does not support the idea that the use of EFM is "safer" than IA, so practitioners should feel confident that they are practicing evidence-based care when obtaining auditory FHR data with IA, provided they are following recommended practice guidelines. Such guidelines include the appropriate indications for IA and EFM and the appropriate monitoring methods, interpretation, and documentation.

Auscultation Procedure

Both auscultation of the FHR and palpation of the uterus are necessary to evaluate the fetal heart status when IA is used as the primary method of fetal heart assessment (Table 4-3). Abdominal palpation is used to assess the resting tone of the uterus and characteristics of uterine contractions, whereas Leopold's maneu-

Table 4-2	Benefits and Limitations of Auscultation
BENEFITS	**LIMITATIONS**
• Based on current RCTs, neonatal outcomes are comparable to those monitored with EFM. • Lower cesarean birth rates have been associated with auscultation than with EFM in some RCTs. • The technique is noninvasive. • Widespread application is possible. • Freedom of movement and ambulation are increased. • The equipment is less costly than EFM equipment. • Hands-on time and one-to-one support are facilitated because the caregiver must be present at the bedside for frequent assessments.	• Use of a fetoscope may limit the ability to hear the FHR (e.g., in cases of obesity, increased amniotic fluid volume, maternal/fetal movement, and with uterine contractions). • Certain FHR characteristics associated with EFM (e.g., variability and types of decelerations) cannot be assessed. • Some women may feel that auscultation is more intrusive. • Documentation on paper is not automatic (as is the case with EFM and which may be perceived as an important component by some practitioners). • There is a potential need to increase or realign staff to meet the 1:1 nurse-to-patient ratio recommended on the basis of RCTs comparing auscultation and EFM use. • Education, practice, and skill in auditory assessment are required.

EFM = Electronic fetal monitor(ing); FHR = fetal heart rate; RCT = randomized controlled trial.
From: *Fetal Heart Rate Auscultation* (p. 15), by N. F. Feinstein, A. Sprague, and M. J. Trépanier, 2008, Washington, DC: Association of Women's Health, Obstetric and Neonatal Nurses. Copyright 2008 by the Association of Women's Health, Obstetric and Neonatal Nurses. Used with permission.

vers are performed to assess the details of fetal position. Leopold's maneuvers help identify the fetal back and optimal location for application of the auscultation device. (A detailed review of the technique for conducting Leopold's maneuvers can be found in Chapter 9).

In relation to FHM, using Leopold's maneuvers provides a systematic approach to identifying the point of maximal sound intensity of the FHR. In general, the FHR is best heard over the curved part of the fetus that is closest to the anterior uterine wall. For example, if the fetus is in a vertex or breech presentation with an anterior position, the fetal heart is generally heard by placing the monitoring device over the fetal back. When there is a face or brow presentation, the FHR is often heard by placing the device over the fetal chest or small parts. After the point of maximal sound intensity is identified, the auscultation device or the Doppler US transducer can be placed in the optimal position for fetal heart assessment. Placement of the device also depends on the degree of descent of the fetal presenting part.

Auscultation Technique

After uterine activity has been assessed and fetal position determined, the bell of the fetoscope or the Doppler transducer is placed over the fetal back. While the maternal pulse is being assessed, the FHR is auscultated between uterine contractions to establish the FHR baseline. Palpation of the uterine contractions also assists the practitioner in clarifying the relationship between the FHR and the uterine activity.

Listening and Counting

The art of auscultation involves both *listening* and *counting*. Auscultation requires the ability to differentiate the sounds generated by the specific device being used. When a fetoscope or stethoscope is used, a fetal souffle (representing blood flow though the foramen ovale), a placental souffle (representing blood flow through the placental bed and synchronous with the MHR), or a funic souffle (representing blood flow through the umbilical arteries) may be heard

Table 4-3	Auscultation Procedure	
PROCEDURE	**RATIONALE**
1. Explain the procedure to the woman and her support person(s).	1. Allays fears and anxiety; offers opportunity for emotional and informational support.
2. Assist the woman to a semi-Fowler's or wedged lateral position.	2. Decreases potential for supine hypotension and promotes comfort.
3. Palpate the maternal abdomen and perform Leopold's maneuvers.	3. Locates the fetal vertex, buttocks, and back and determines the optimal location for auscultation (fetal heart sounds are best heard over the fetal back).
4. Assess uterine contractions (frequency, duration, intensity) and uterine resting tone by palpation.	4. Determines the maternal and fetal response to uterine activity.
5. Apply conduction gel to underside of the Doppler device, if used.	5. Provides an airtight seal and aids in the transmission of US waves.
6. Position the bell of fetoscope or Doppler device on the area of maximal intensity of the fetal heart sounds (usually over the fetal back). Use firm pressure if using the fetoscope.	6. Obtains the strongest FHR signal.
7. Palpate the woman's radial pulse.	7. Differentiates maternal from fetal heart rate.
8. Count the FHR *after* uterine contractions for at least 30–60 seconds.	8. Identifies the baseline FHR (in bpm), the rhythm (regular or irregular), and the presence or absence of accelerations or decelerations of the FHR between contractions.
9. In clarifying FHR changes, recounts for multiple, consecutive brief periods of 6–10 seconds (multiplied by 10 and 6, respectively) may be particularly helpful.	9. Clarifies the presence of FHR changes. Clarifies the nature and amplitude of FHR changes.
10. Interpret FHR findings and document per unit protocol.	10. Provides record of assessments.
11. Share findings with woman and support person(s) and answer questions as needed.	11. Provides informational support.
12. Promote maternal comfort and fetal oxygenation.	12. Provides physical support and promotes fetal well-being.

bpm = Beats per minute; FHR = fetal heart rate.
From: *Fetal Heart Rate Auscultation* (p. 20), by N. F. Feinstein, A. Sprague, and M. J. Trépanier, 2008, Washington, DC: Association of Women's Health, Obstetric and Neonatal Nurses. Copyright 2008 by the Association of Women's Health, Obstetric and Neonatal Nurses. Used with permission.

(Murray, 2007). Erroneous conclusions about fetal status could be reached if the maternal sounds are incorrectly considered to be fetal heart sounds, therefore, the maternal pulse should be checked whenever auscultating the FHR (Feinstein et al., 2008).

To identify the baseline rate and FHR response to contractions, it is important to begin listening and counting the FHR immediately after a uterine contraction and to listen for at least 30 to 60 seconds (Feinstein et al., 2008). Because there is no clear evidence about the best method of counting to determine the baseline rate, the practitioner's preference often dictates the method used. For example, some practitioners count for one full minute and use that number as the baseline rate in beats per minute (bpm). Others count for 30 seconds and multiply by 2. And still others may count during a few consecutive 15-second intervals, multiplying each by four to obtain an approximate baseline rate and to determine the presence of variations within that rate. None of these methods has been determined to be superior to the others, and different counting intervals may be appropriate for different conditions. For example, longer intervals may help establish the baseline, whereas repeated short sampling of the FHR may help differentiate accelerations and decelerations of the FHR (Feinstein et al).

When changes in the FHR are heard during auscultation, a technique that may assist in clarifying the nature of the audible changes is to count for multiple, brief, consecutive periods. This method consists of counting for consecutive 6-second intervals and multiplying the number of beats for each interval by 10: number of beats/6 seconds × 10 (which provides a very rough estimate of the number of bpm for each interval). This helps in providing additional information regarding the nature (increase or decrease) and amplitude of the FHR change and may assist in the decision making regarding whether to initiate EFM for further evaluation and clarification (Feinstein, et al., 2008).

Frequency of Auscultation

Professional associations (AWHONN, ACOG, American College of Nurse Midwives [ACNM], Society of Obstetricians and Gynaecologists of Canada [SOGC], AAP, Royal College of Obstetricians and Gynaecologists [RCOG]) have suggested protocols for the frequency of assessment of the fetal heart rate by auscultation to determine fetal status during labor. The suggested frequencies are typically based on protocols reported in clinical trials that compared perinatal outcomes associated with fetal heart rate auscultation and electronic fetal monitoring (Haverkamp et al., 1979; Haverkamp, Thompson, McFee, & Certulo, 1976; Kelso et al., 1978; Luthy et al., 1987; McDonald, Grant, Sheridan-Pereira, Boylan, & Chalmers, 1985; Neldam et al., 1986; Renou, Chang, Anderson, & Wood, 1976; Vintzileos et al., 1993). The range of frequency of assessment using auscultation in these studies varied from q 15 – 30 minutes during the active

phase of the first stage of labor to q 5-15 minutes during the second stage of labor. Most studies reported a 1:1 nurse to patient ratio for auscultation protocols. These studies included low-risk and/or high-risk patient populations.

Because variation exists in the original research protocols, clinicians should make decisions about the method and frequency of fetal assessment based on evaluation of factors including patient preferences, the phase and stage of labor, maternal response to labor, assessment of maternal-fetal condition and risk factors, unit staffing resources and facility rules and procedures.

Considering these factors, the suggested frequencies for fetal heart rate auscultation are within the range of every 15 - 30 minutes during the active phase of the first stage of labor and every 5-15 minutes during the active pushing phase of the second stage of labor (Table 4-4). No clinical trials have examined fetal surveillance methods during the latent phase of labor. Therefore, healthcare providers should use their clinical judgment, taking into consideration their institution's policies and procedures, when deciding the method and frequency of fetal surveillance in the latent phase.

It is also appropriate to evaluate the fetal heart characteristics before and after labor events such as medication administration, ambulation, or the initiation of labor-enhancing procedures (e.g., artificial rupture of membranes). The process of management and documentation is similar to that of EFM and should reflect assessment of the overall clinical picture, actions taken, and the evaluation of results of the interventions.

What Cannot Be Assessed via Intermittent Auscultation?

Evidence does not support the ability of an individual to accurately and reliably assess auscultated FHR baseline variability or discriminate FHR deceleration patterns (Murray, 1997; Parer, 1997). Based on the available research, it is appropriate to assess the FHR baseline rate, rhythm, and increases or decreases from the baseline. Baseline variability and types of decelerations should not be assessed with auscul-

Table 4-4	**Recommended Frequency of Auscultation**		
	LATENT PHASE	ACTIVE FIRST STAGE	ACTIVE SECOND STAGE
ACNM[a]		q 15-30 minutes	q 5 minutes
ACOG[b]		q 15-30 minutes	q 5 minutes
AWHONN[c]		q 15-30 minutes	q 5-15 minutes
RCOG[d]		q 15 minutes	q 5 minutes
SOGC[e]	At time of assessment and approximately q 1h	q 15-30 minutes	q 5 minutes

These guidelines reflect emerging clinical and scientific advances as of the date issued and are subject to change. The information should not be construed as dictating an exclusive course of treatment or procedure to be followed. Variations in practice may be warranted based on individual circumstances.
[a] American College of Nurse Midwives, 2007
[b] American Academy of Pediatrics & American College of Obstetricians and Gynecologists, 2007
[c] Association of Women's Health, Obstetric and Neonatal Nurses; Feinstein, Sprague, & Trepanier, 2008
[d] Royal College of Obstetricians and Gynaecologists, 2001
[e] Society of Obstetricians and Gynaecologists of Canada, 2007

tation because these are based on visual interpretations of the electronic FHR data. If provider concerns warrant a visual assessment of FHR information, it is appropriate to initiate EFM. Alternatively, other methods to assess fetal well-being, such as fetal stimulation (scalp or acoustic) or fetal capillary sampling, may be appropriate as adjunct assessments to IA.

Interpreting Auscultated FHR Characteristics

The new guidelines for interpretation of EFM tracings (Macones et al, 2008; see chapter 5) have implications for the interpretation and communication of FHR data obtained by intermittent auscultation. Using a common language for discussion of fetal status is a key principle of effective clinical communication and has the potential to decrease communication errors. It would be potentially confusing to have one set of terms for interpretation of auscultation and another set of terms for interpretation of EFM, especially when clinicians may at times use both methods of fetal assessment in the course of caring for the same woman. In the past, the terms "reassuring" and "nonreassuring" were used in interpreting auscultation findings. In order to maintain a consistent language for discussion of

FHR findings, two categories for interpretation of IA are presented below; Category I and Category II (Box 4-1). The definitions of these categories are consistent with the terminology used to interpret EFM patterns, but refer only to auscultation.

BOX 4-1   Interpretation of Auscultation Findings

CATEGORY I
Category I FHR characteristics by auscultation include **all** of the following:

- Normal FHR baseline between 110 and 160 bpm
- Regular rhythm
- Presence of FHR increases or accelerations from the baseline rate
- Absence of FHR decreases or decelerations from the baseline

CATEGORY II
Category II FHR characteristics by auscultation include any of the following:

- Irregular rhythm
- Presence of FHR decreases or decelerations from the baseline
- Tachycardia (baseline >160 bpm > 10 minutes in duration)
- Bradycardia (baseline <110 bpm > 10 minutes in duration)

Category I auscultated FHR characteristics are normal (Box 4-1). Normal IA findings include all of the following characteristics: FHR baseline between 110 and 160 bpm, regular rhythm, the presence of FHR increases or accelerations, and the absence of FHR decreases or decelerations. Normal FHR characteristics are predictive of fetal well-being at the time they are observed and may be followed with routine supportive measures.

Category II auscultated FHR characteristics include all findings that are not classified as normal (Box 4-1). Irregular rhythm, presence of decreases or decelerations from baseline, tachycardia and bradycardia are all indeterminate IA findings. They cannot be classified as abnormal without information about FHR variability, as the patterns identified in Category III all include assessment of variability. Category II FHR characteristics require evaluation, ongoing surveillance, and re-evaluation, consistent with the assessment of the overall clinical circumstances. This may include, but is not limited to: continuous electronic fetal monitoring, use of intrauterine resuscitation techniques, ruling out maternal heart rate, and assessment of the continuation of indeterminate findings. As with EFM, auscultation findings and management needs are interpreted in the context of the overall clinical picture. Preparations to expedite birth in emergent situations (e.g. apparent significant fetal bradycardia) should be undertaken simultaneously with efforts to ameliorate, verify and determine the precise nature of the FHR findings.

Clinical Management

Clinical decision making is a complex process and a skill acquired over time. The process involves a total assessment of a situation, development of a realistic plan of care based on the assessment, implementation of the plan, and evaluation of the effects. Haggerty (1999) advises that decisions about use of fetal surveillance cannot be made by relying on simple algorithmic rules.

Making clinical decisions about auscultated FHR findings is similar to clinical decision making with EFM. As with any woman in labor, decision making begins with a review of the woman's medical and pregnancy history to determine her risk factors. Then all aspects of the maternal and fetal status should be assessed. The plan of care is developed based on synthesis of this information.

For example, if the FHR baseline is normal and rhythmic and increases are audible, it is appropriate to continue to assess the FHR at the designated intervals while providing routine care and support for the laboring woman. When a change in the FHR baseline is auscultated, it is appropriate to reassess and confirm whether a change has occurred or if it persists. It is important to consider the potential physiologic reasons for the auscultated change (e.g., whether there is maternal fever when fetal tachycardia is noted). When a decrease from the FHR baseline is audible, it may be appropriate to reassess with the next contraction or two to confirm the finding. In addition, interventions to promote the physiologic goals of improving uterine blood flow, umbilical cord blood flow, and oxygenation and reducing uterine activity are implemented as appropriate to the individual situation (Figure 4-1).

Staffing Issues and IA

The use of IA as a primary method of fetal surveillance raises concerns related to appropriate staffing levels required and potential costs associated with the recommended staffing ratios.

Based on the research to date, the minimal staffing levels and nurse-patient ratio necessary for implementation of IA are not clear. However, the protocols in the RCTs comparing IA and EFM typically used a 1:1 nurse-patient ratio. It is important to acknowledge that this 1:1 ratio actually reflects a 1:2 nurse-patient ratio, given that there are two patients, the mother and the fetus (SOGC, 2007). Implementing auscultation as a primary method of fetal surveillance using this evidence-based 1:1 ratio is in keeping with guidelines set forth by national organizations. In addition, resources are available to assist facilities in promoting staffing based on

FIGURE 4-1   Fetal Heart Monitoring Decision Tree

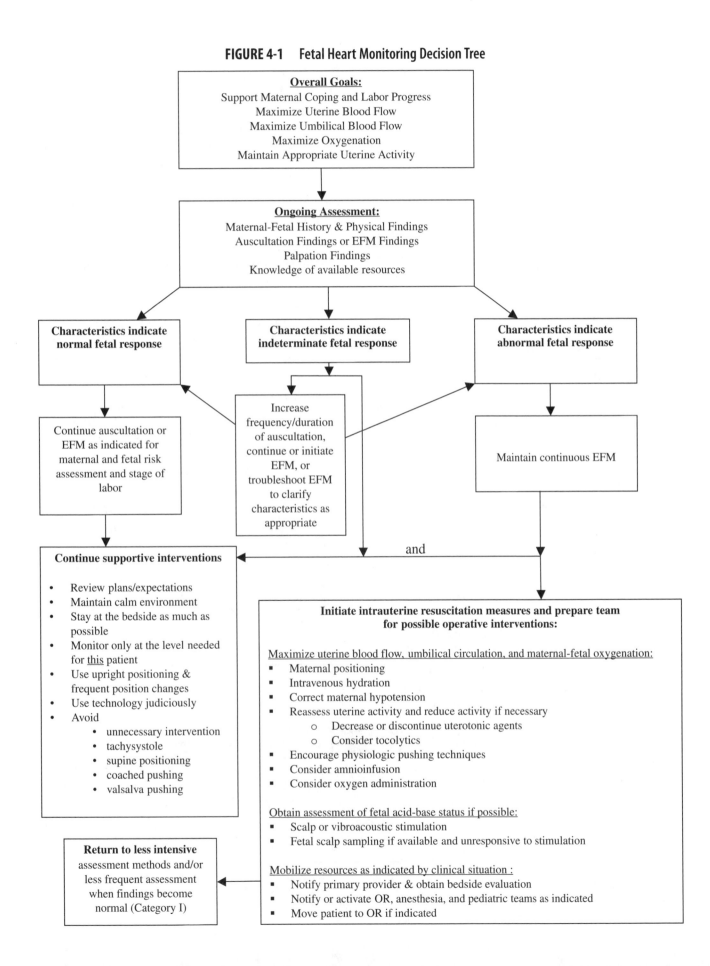

guidelines from professional organizations, including AWHONN, AAP/ACOG, American Nurses Association [ANA] (2005), and The Joint Commission (Schofield, 2003).

In Canada, the SOGC (2007) promotes the use of IA as the primary fetal surveillance method for low-risk pregnancies. In conjunction with that view, the SOGC also recognizes the need for appropriate education to prepare clinicians and support the implementation of IA. In addition to the learning materials in this text, the AWHONN FHM courses and AWHONN auscultation monograph (Feinstein et al., 2008), a Canadian self-learning manual focusing on fundamentals of IA and EFM is available (Canadian Perinatal Regionalization Coalition, SOGC, & Perinatal Educator Programs across Canada, 2002). Administrative and clinical support for the use of IA in a particular setting is helpful (Davies et al., 2002). Although further study is needed to demonstrate the cost-effectiveness of IA, there are known benefits of one-to-one labor support for women that can be used to support the need for altered staffing patterns (Hodnett, 1997). This information may be helpful to facilities investing in the use of IA during labor.

PALPATION

When the uterus contracts, its musculature becomes more firm and tense; this can be felt by the care provider when the fingertips are placed over the woman's uterine fundus. This assessment provides information regarding uterine tone and contraction frequency, intensity, and duration. In addition, direct uterine palpation can provide information about uterine tenderness, fetal size, and fetal movement. Assessment of contractions provides important contextual data when considering FHR information during labor.

Palpation Technique

Palpation should be performed throughout an entire contraction, from the beginning of the contraction to the palpation of resting tone following that contraction. Palpation is used in conjunction with auscultation of the fetal heart. It also is used to confirm and supplement findings gathered from electronic uterine activity monitoring. The actual frequency of assessment via palpation may vary depending on the status of labor, but should be at least as frequent as FHR assessments. The following steps may be used when performing palpation:

- Place fingertips on the maternal abdomen, over the area where changes in uterine firmness can be best felt (most commonly near the fundus). Fingertips are generally more sensitive than the palm of the hand.
- Firmly but gently attempt to indent the uterus with fingertips to assess uterine resting tone. Avoid sharp, jabbing movements to prevent undue discomfort to the woman.
- Assess *frequency* of contraction from the beginning of one contraction to the beginning of the next contraction.
- Assess *duration* of the contraction from the beginning of uterine tightening to its ending.
- Assess *intensity* of contractions as mild, moderate, or strong. Although there is no standard measure for determining palpated contraction intensity (strength), the following comparison approach, based on the degree to which the uterine muscle can be indented, is used by many clinicians (Table 4-5).

Benefits, limitations, and troubleshooting strategies for uterine palpation are summarized in Table 4-6.

Table 4-5	Comparison Model for Palpation of Uterine Activity	
PALPATION OF UTERUS	**FEELS LIKE**	**CONTRACTION INTENSITY**
• Easily indented	• Tip of nose	• Mild
• Can slightly indent	• Chin	• Moderate
• Cannot indent	• Forehead	• Strong

Note: Contractions should be referred to using one of the above descriptive terms; mild, moderate, strong, rather than labeled as "good" or "satisfactory."
Adapted from: Malinowski, Pedigo, & Phillips, 1989.

Table 4-6	Uterine Palpation

Capabilities
• Detect relative uterine resting tone
• Detect relative frequency, duration, and strength of uterine contractions

Benefits and Limitations	
BENEFITS	LIMITATIONS
• Noninvasive; hands-on assessment and care of patient	• Palpation cannot be used to detect actual intrauterine pressures
• Not limited by access to equipment; widely used	• Maternal size, amount of adipose tissue, uterine size, etc., may limit ability to palpate contractions
• Provides information regarding relative frequency, duration, strength, and resting tone	• Subjectivity may result in different interpretations of uterine activity characteristics
• Allows mother freedom of movement and ambulation	
• Use of touch may be reassuring to some women	

Troubleshooting/Corrective Actions	
PROBLEM	ACTION
• If uterine contractions are not readily felt over the fundal area	• Attempt palpation over a variety of areas on the uterus to find best location

ELECTRONIC FETAL HEART RATE MONITORING

Doppler Ultrasound

The Doppler US transducer is used to assess FHR characteristics and patterns. Multiple piezoelectric crystals within the US transducer generate sound waves that are transmitted toward the fetal heart and receive US waves reflected back from the fetal heart movements (Figure 4-2). The sound waves returning from moving structures are altered in frequency from those sound waves originally transmitted toward the moving structure. This frequency shift, called the "Doppler shift," is detected and amplified to produce the waveform, which is then interpreted by the computer in the fetal monitor. The monitor then produces an audible sound and tracing to reflect the detected FHR.

In the evolution of the technology of Doppler FHR assessment, advances in the electronic processing of data have led to a distinction between two generations of equipment (Boehm et al., 1986). To compensate for the complexity and variation in waveforms, the first-generation monitors employed two mechanisms: use of a refractory window and maximal peak detection. To prevent the counting of both components of the fetal cardiac waveform as separate beats, a refractory window is used (Hutson & Petrie, 1986; Klapholz, 1978). This window of time is an inhibitory period in which the system does not attempt to count the incoming signal. This time period follows the moment of detection of the fetal cardiac waveform and is presumed to be the waveform's first component. The length of time of the refractory window, measured in milliseconds, is dynamic in that the time is set to vary according to the FHR. This variance, however, has limitations. Slow FHRs below 90 bpm may cause the second component of the waveform to occur after the refractory window period. This action will produce double counting of a single waveform, leading to doubling on the FHR tracing. Rapid FHRs may cause a second waveform to occur within the refractory window period and produce halving of the FHR tracing because the second heart beat is not counted (Freeman et al., 2003).

The complexity and variability of the first-generation Doppler-generated waveforms made accurate counting of the same point in the fetal cardiac cycle difficult. The mechanism that first-generation monitors used to compensate for this problem was maximal peak detection. When the movement of the fetal heart generates a waveform, the monitor detects its maximal peak and then counts the time interval between peaks. Problems with this technique are caused by Doppler signals from other anatomy, such as the umbilical cord, as well as variations in an early or late appearance of the peak in the waveform. These problems lead to false variability in the printed fetal heart tracing. Consequently, what was viewed on the tracing with first generation monitors via the US transducer could not reliably be equated with the true FHR variability.

Second-Generation Monitors and Autocorrelation

The major alteration in Doppler signal processing associated with second-generation fetal monitors introduced in the 1980s is referred to as autocorrelation (Figure 4-2). This technique evolved from efforts to improve the quality of the processing of waveforms. Advancements in microprocessor technology facilitated the development of this technique, which entails digitizing and analyzing the reflection of US waveforms. Autocorrelation is defined by Schwartz and Young (2006) as computerized smoothing of waveforms. The internal computer averages three consecutive beat-to-beat intervals and then assigns the FHR. This averaging methodology minimizes artifact (Schwartz & Young). Autocorrelation works by matching each incoming waveform with the previous one by repetitively analyzing small segments of the waveforms. Important information will have regular form and repeat over time, whereas random noise is devoid of regularity, and artifactual waveforms are discarded (Freeman et al., 2003). This process of rejecting artifactual waveforms provides for a more accurate identification of the initiation of the fetal cardiac cycle than other techniques provide. Today, it is assumed that all ultrasound FHR signal processing uses autocorrelation techniques and interpretation of EFM data is based on this assumption (Macones, Hankins, Spong, Hauth, & Moore, 2008).

Maternal or Fetal Heart Rate?

US transducers are designed to detect waveforms from the beating fetal heart. However, the monitor may inadvertently detect and print signals from the MHR. When initiating placement of the US transducer or changing FHR modes, the clinician should palpate the mother's radial pulse and compare it with the audible signal and printed rate to rule out inadvertent recording of the MHR (Freeman et al., 2003; Murray, 2004). The recorded MHR can mimic FHR patterns (Murray, 2004), possibly resulting in the failure to diagnose fetal demise or deterioration. The MHR may be picked up by the external US transducer, especially if the fetus is active, mother's habitus is large (Schifrin, Harwell, Rubinstein, & Visser, 2001), a large maternal blood vessel is under the transducer (Sherman et al., 2002), or the MHR and FHR are similar. Elevated MHRs may be more readily confused with a FHR, particularly during maternal pushing efforts in second-stage labor. It is recommended that sudden changes in recorded heart rate be attended to and that maternal pulse be assessed at times other than just when a recorded heart rate appears to be bradycardic, especially with noncontinuous tracings, to confirm whether the mother or the fetus is the signal source (Freeman et al.; Schifrin et al.).

Today, some monitors allow for the monitoring and recording of both MHR and FHR patterns. Specific differential characteristics of the MHR

FIGURE 4-2   Linear Pictorial of Piezoelectric Effect

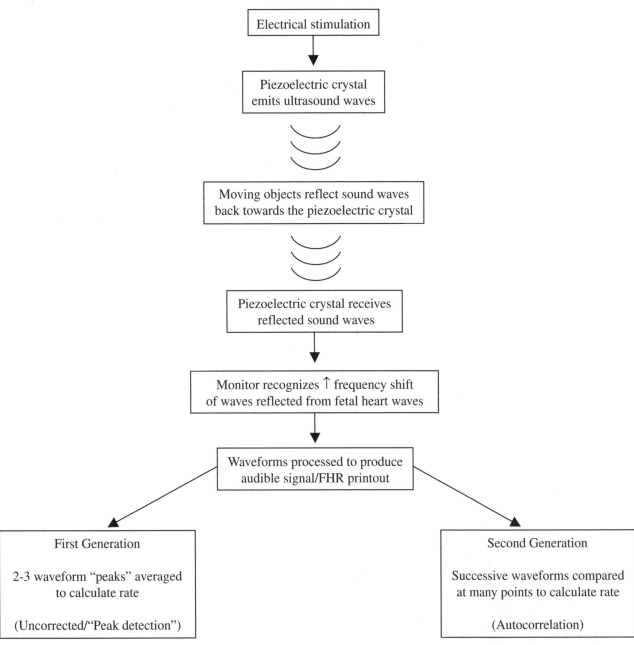

This is a linear view, but in fact, the piezoelectric crystal is emitting and receiving sound waves continually.
Adapted from: Hon (1975) and Klavan, Laver, and Boscola (1977).

and FHR have been described by Murray (2004). Major differences include the following:

• Baseline MHR was significantly lower than the FHR baseline and MHR variability significantly greater at all stages of labor. A significant drop in maternal variability was noted by Sherman et al. (2002) after the delivery of the placenta.

• MHR accelerations have higher amplitude and longer duration, especially during second stage and pushing. They tend to increase in frequency as labor progresses. Maternal accelerations have only one hump and coincide with contractions (maternal pain response). In addition, MHR accelerations have been reported to be as high as 60 bpm above the baseline in the case of a fetal demise.

- MHR baseline as it approaches 140 bpm may flatten, especially if the patient is diabetic or hemodynamically or metabolically unstable. Artifact lines that move above and below the MHR may be the result of a weak signal, interruption of signal, or loss of signal.
- In multiple reports as cited by Sherman et al. (2002), situations of fetal death and transmission of the maternal electrocardiogram (ECG) via the fetal scalp electrode found a baseline bradycardic rate to be the most consistent finding.

Artifact

Artifact is defined as "irregularities on the monitor tracing due to poor reception of the fetal heart signal which appears as scattered dots, gaps on the tracing, or lines" (Murray 2007, p. 511). "Artifact" is a term used to describe irregular variations or absence of the FHR on the fetal monitor record resulting from mechanical limitations of the monitor or electrical interference. With the use of the Doppler US, gaps and dots may be noted on the tracing when the cardiac signal is either too weak to be continually traced or is undetected. When a fetal spiral electrode (FSE) is used, artifact may be present on the tracing in the form of irregular lines with varying lengths, unlike the regular lines seen with some arrhythmias (Figure 4-3).

A number of types of artifact can occur. These include, but are not limited to, increased variability on first-generation monitors, half-counting and double counting of the FHR, and recording of the MHR. Half-counting of the FHR is most commonly seen when the FHR is rapid. Double counting may also occur with either mode of monitoring. Troubleshooting efforts to improve the FHR signal include repositioning the US transducer, ensuring that an adequate amount of coupling gel is used, and checking for adequate placement of the FSE. Signal interference can also occur causing artifact if the scalp electrode hits up against the vaginal wall (Murray, 2007).

A summary of benefits, limitations, and troubleshooting actions to address common problems with US transducer use are included in Table 4-7.

Fetal Spiral Electrode

Direct FHR monitoring, when using the spiral electrode, uses electronic logic to detect and measure R-to-R wave intervals in consecutive

FIGURE 4-3 Example of Artifact on a Fetal Heart Rate Tracing

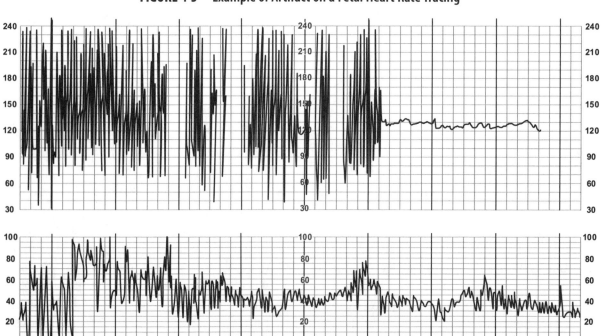

Table 4-7	Ultrasound (US) Transducer: Capabilities, Benefits and Limitations, Troubleshooting/Corrective Actions

Capabilities	
• Detect FHR variability, baseline, accelerations, and decelerations	

Benefits and Limitations	
BENEFITS	LIMITATIONS
• Is noninvasive • Does not require rupture of membranes • Provides a permanent record (depending on storage conditions; heat can deteriorate paper over time)	• Signal transmission may be influenced by maternal obesity, occiput posterior, anterior placenta, and fetal movement (e.g., weak, absent, or false signal) • May restrict maternal movement • Maternal and fetal movement may interfere with continuous recording • Monitor may half-count or double count, especially in the presence of FHR tachycardia or bradycardia

Troubleshooting/Corrective Actions	
PROBLEM	ACTIONS

• Erratic recordings or gaps on the tracing paper
 	
  ◦ Potential causes
 	
    ◦ Inadequate conduction of US signal
 	
    ◦ Transducer may be displaced
 	
    ◦ Fetal or maternal movement
 	
    ◦ Arrhythmia
 	
    ◦ Paper not loaded correctly
 	
    ◦ Equipment malfunction
	• Evaluate potential causes
	
	• Assess whether sufficient ultrasonic gel is present under the transducer
	
	• Apply ultrasonic gel to the transducer as needed until a light seal is formed
	
	• Encourage maternal position changes to improve the signal
	
	• Determine whether the belt holding the transducer is snug around the abdomen; tighten as needed to improve contact and signal detection
	
	• Reposition the transducer over the fetal back (determined by Leopold's maneuvers), as necessary
	
	• Check maternal pulse; auscultate as needed
	
	• Check the connection to the power source as well as the connections to the monitor
	
	• Check paper for proper loading
	
	• Check equipment according to manufacturer's directions
	
	• Apply FSE if clinically indicated

FHR = Fetal heart rate; FSE = fetal spiral electrode.

QRS complexes to derive the FHR. The interval is recalculated with the detection of each new R wave. In addition to the direct measurement of the FHR, other benefits and limitations are described in Table 4-8. When an FSE is being used to assess FHR, a range of problems may require troubleshooting by the clinician to correct or improve the quality of monitor data. The EFM is, like any instrument, capable of equipment malfunction or error. Use of the instrument may be subject to incorrect procedure or human error. Common situations and suggestions for troubleshooting are also included in Table 4-8.

The frequency for evaluation of the FHR with both internal and external electronic monitoring is the same as for IA (AAP/ACOG, 2007; SOGC, 2007). See Chapter 8 for discussion of documentation principles.

ST-SEGMENT ANALYSIS

Overview

Assessing the fetal ECG, specifically the ST waveform of the fetal ECG, has been shown to be a promising adjunct to EFM. The purpose of ST waveform analysis (STAN, for ST ANalysis) is to identify cases of significant hypoxia and improve the timeliness and consistency of intervention (Norén et al., 2005). Two large RCTs have supported clinical use and demonstrated positive outcomes (Rosén, 2005; Rosén, Amer-Wåhlin, Luzietti, & Norén, 2004). According to Rosén et al., other adjunctive modalities have been used to aid in the interpretation of FHR patterns; however, none has been tested as extensively by RCTs as the STAN system. The STAN method provides a more comprehensive warning in cases of fetal hypoxia than EFM alone.

Table 4-8	**Fetal Spiral Electrode: Capabilities, Benefits and Limitations, Troubleshooting/Corrective Actions**
Capabilities	
• Detect FHR variability, accelerations, decelerations, baseline	
• Provide limited information about some types of arrhythmias	
Benefits and Limitations	
BENEFITS:	LIMITATIONS:
• Provides continuous detection of FHR when clinically necessary and not achievable by US transducer • Maternal position change does not alter ability to assess FHR or quality of tracing	• Is invasive • Requires rupture of membranes, cervical dilation, and accessible/appropriate fetal presenting part • Requires moist environment for detection of FHR • Potential small risk of infection and fetal hemorrhage or injury • May record maternal heart rate in presence of fetal demise • Fetal arrhythmias may not be evident if logic or ECG button is engaged • Electronic interference and artifact may occur
Troubleshooting/Corrective Actions	
PROBLEM	ACTIONS
• Intermittent markings on the FHR tracing 　◦ Potential causes 　　◦ Artifact 　　◦ Failure to detect electrical activity 　　◦ Fetal arrhythmia 　　◦ Monitor connections improperly attached	• Evaluate potential causes • Confirm FHR with fetoscope • Check connections to the monitor, electrode cable • Check circuitry of the monitor • Turn off the logic or ECG deactivation switch • Check FSE placement on presenting part, if possible • Apply new FSE as indicated

Table 4-8	Fetal Spiral Electrode: Capabilities, Benefits and Limitations, Troubleshooting/ Corrective Actions—cont'd

Troubleshooting/Corrective Actions	
PROBLEM	**ACTIONS**

• Illegible FHR tracing
  ◦ Potential causes
    ◦ Artifact
    ◦ Faulty electronic connection or monitor placement
    ◦ Faulty loading or feeding of monitor paper
• Abnormal rate on the tracing
  ◦ Potential causes
    ◦ Doubling or halving of actual heart rate by monitor
    ◦ Actual fetal tachycardia, bradycardia, or deceleration
    ◦ Interference from maternal signal (e.g., fetal demise, FSE placement on maternal cervix)
    ◦ Artifact
	• Press the test button; check the numerical value
	• Check the connection to the power source and check all lead connections
	• Check condition of monitor paper
	• Confirm "record" button is activated
	• Confirm/establish correct rate (e.g., auscultation with fetoscope)
	• Confirm maternal pulse simultaneously with FHR
	• Refer to manufacturer's instruction manual for procedure for separating or distancing the maternal signal from the fetal ECG signal.
	• Replace the FSE if necessary

• FHR pattern compressed
  ◦ Potential causes
    ◦ Paper speed or scaling errors
	• Verify paper speed (e.g., 3 cm/min in the United States)
	  • Confirm that paper being used has the appropriate calibrations for the monitor in use

• INOP display
  ◦ Potential causes
    ◦ Signal cannot be received
    ◦ Leads not connected to leg plate
    ◦ FSE may have a poor connection to the presenting part
    ◦ Referencing electrode may not be operating
	• Check the lead connections to the monitor (gently remove the FSE wire) and check the EFM circuitry
	• Vaginal secretions may be inadequate, and an external reference electrode, if available, may need to be applied
	• Palpate the maternal pulse and compare it with the audible signal and printed rate to rule out a recording of the maternal heart rate

ECG = Electrocardiogram; EFM = electronic fetal monitor; FHR = fetal heart rate; FSE = fetal spiral electrode.

ST-Segment Pathophysiology

Theoretically, ST-segment analysis of the fetal ECG provides continuous information regarding the ability of the fetal heart to respond to stress in labor by providing information about intracardiac responses to intrapartum hypoxia (Kwee, Dekkers, van Wijk, van der Hoorn-van den Beld, & Visser, 2007; Rosén, 2005). ST-segment and T-wave changes occur with myocardial ischemia, prior to permanent cell damage (Ross, Devoe, & Rosén, 2004). Therefore, analysis of the ST segment may permit detection of myocardial ischemia and the fetus's ability to respond to stress prior to peripheral organ and central nervous system damage (Amer-Wåhlin et al., 2002; Ross et al.).

ST-segment and T-wave elevation are indicative of a fetus at risk of developing hypoxia but still capable of responding against hypoxemia.

These changes are the direct result of a catecholamine surge, beta-adrenoceptor activation, and myocardial glycogenolysis, which releases glycogen stores in the heart and acts as an extra source of energy (Norén et al., 2003; Olofsson, 2003; Rosén, 2005; Rosén et al., 2004). However, fetal ST-segment depression (biphasic ST) has been associated with the inability of the fetal heart to further respond to hypoxia, indicating that the fetus either had no time to respond or has exhausted compensatory mechanisms. ST depression is thought to reflect endocardial hypoxia (Amer-Wåhlin, Ingemarsson, Marsal, & Herbst, 2005; Kwee et al., 2007; Norén et al., Olofsson). ST depression has also been associated with infection, fetal heart malformation, and disturbances in the heart muscle function (Kwee et al.) (Fgure 4-4). Alternatively, the absence of alteration in the ST segment may aid in the determination of fetal well-being (Ross et al., 2004). Of note, fetal ST changes are thought to be clinically relevant only if they coincide with "intermediate" or "abnormal" FHR tracings because ST changes have occurred in the presence of normal FHR tracings (Kwee et al.). Another explanation for the noted ST changes with normal FHR tracings may be the catecholamine surge in response to the physical and stress forces of labor. The fetus with the ability to compensate will display an otherwise normal FHR tracing. Thus, the ST changes associated with a normal FHR tracing are more likely due to nonhypoxemic fetal stress and the surge of stress hormones (Kwee et al.).

A high-quality ECG signal is necessary to evaluate and interpret waveform analysis (Rosén et al., 2004). FSE placement and use of a STAN monitor are required to retrieve the ECG data. ST analysis requires close observation of the quality of the fetal ECG signal. If the electrode is applied improperly, signal disturbance may still allow the FHR to be recorded but not allow adequate signals for ECG ST analysis (Rosén, 2005).

Future Research and Implications for Practice

Adequate research did not occur prior to the introduction and dissemination of EFM technology in the 1960s. This has proved to be a significant disadvantage today. A Cochrane Systematic Review of the STAN methodology provides some support for the use of the ST waveform analysis when the decision has been made to perform continuous fetal monitoring during labor (Neilson, 2006). Inclusion criteria for all but one study was gestation greater than 36 weeks. Thus, further research with preterm fetuses would be valuable. In addition, information regarding long-term neurologic development of the babies included in the trials would also be valuable (Neilson). Whether the technology will be adopted widely for clinical use is unknown at this time.

ELECTRONIC UTERINE ACTIVITY MONITORING

Tocodynamometer (Toco Transducer)

The contour of the uterus and abdomen changes somewhat with contractions. The tocodynamometer is the part of the EFM that externally detects abdominal pressure or contour changes

FIGURE 4-4 Fetal Electrocardiogram: ST Segment and T Wave Changes Associated with Intrapartum Hypoxia

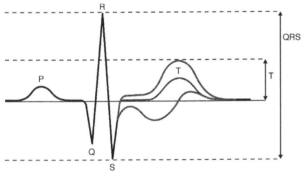

Note: From Ross, M. G., Devoe, L. D., & Rosén, K. G. (2004). ST-segment analysis of the fetal electrocardiogram improves fetal heart rate tracing interpretation and clinical decision making. *The Journal of Maternal-Fetal and Neonatal Medicine, 15,* 181–185. Copyright 2004 by Taylor & Francis Group. Reprinted with permission.

resulting from uterine contractions. The pressure sensor, usually a button-like device, should be placed on the abdomen over the uterine fundus at the point of maximal contraction intensity. The specific location is determined by abdominal palpation. The optimal location varies from woman to woman and may change during labor. Computer technology translates the degree of pressure detected by the sensor into an electrical signal that is displayed numerically on the monitor and graphically on the tracing paper. When the sensor is placed correctly, this mode of assessment is useful in determining the following:

- Approximate contraction frequency
- Approximate duration (length) of contractions
- Relative changes in abdominal pressure between uterine resting tone (tonus) and contractions

It is important to note that use of the external toco transducer does not allow for determination of the *actual* contraction strength (intensity), a fourth key element of contraction assessment. Therefore, palpation of the uterus during and between contractions, as well as input from the laboring woman, is essential for developing a complete and accurate picture of contraction quality at any given time. Palpation is used in conjunction with electronic uterine activity monitoring to validate uterine contraction intensity and confirm findings from electronic monitoring. Palpation also is used to assess uterine activity when the tocodynamometer is removed for ambulation or during procedures such as epidural placement and to validate findings from intrauterine pressure catheter (IUPC) readings.

Caldeyro-Barcia and Poseiro (1960) described contractions as being abdominally palpable at a pressure of 10 mm Hg, which is a slightly below the point at which the laboring woman feels the pain of contractions (15 mm Hg), whereas Parer (1997) states that women may often be aware of the contraction before the toco transducer detects it. In most cases, toco transducers, in concert with palpation, provide satisfactory data to adequately assess uterine contraction patterns

(LaCroix, 1968) (Figure 4-5). The uterine activity portion of the tracing paper is vertically marked in specific units of measure. Millimeters of mercury (mm Hg) are the units of measure used in North America. Kilopascals are considered the standard measure for contraction strength in some other parts of the world. These measures have utility only when an IUPC is used and will be discussed in the IUPC section.

When the external toco transducer is in use, the numbers that represent uterine contraction pressures on the uterine activity channel of the EFM are arbitrary. The uterine activity (UA) resting tone should be adjusted to 15 to 20 mm Hg between contractions in order to obtain the best tracing. A uterine activity transducer from the EFM should be used when the US transducer or FSE is in use. This simultaneous assessment of UA ensures that FHR patterns and responses can be considered in relation to the presence or absence, frequency, and duration of contractions.

FIGURE 4-5   Comparison of Uterine Contraction Assessment by Palpation, External Tocodynamometer, and Intrauterine Pressure Catheter

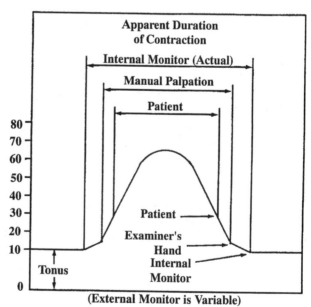

From Freeman, R. K., Garite, T. J., & Nageotte, M. P. (1991). *Fetal heart rate monitoring* (p. 81). Baltimore: Williams & Wilkins. Copyright 1991 by Williams and Wilkins. Reprinted with permission.

The current time should be documented on the tracing at regular intervals. Although most monitors currently print the time automatically, the clinician should ensure that the time is accurately and correctly shown on the EFM tracing.

Benefits, limitations, and troubleshooting strategies for using the tocodynamometer are summarized in Table 4-9. Variations in the recording of uterine contractions with a tocodynamometer are illustrated in Figure 4-6.

Table 4-9	Toco Transducer: Capabilities, Benefits and Limitations, Troubleshooting/Corrective Actions
Capabilities	
• Detect relative uterine resting tone • Detect relative frequency, duration of uterine contractions	
Benefits and Limitations	
BENEFITS	LIMITATIONS
• Is noninvasive • Is easily placed • Does not require ruptured amniotic membranes • Generates a tracing for future assessment and for a permanent medical record	• Is subjective • Is unable to detect actual uterine contraction intensity and resting tone • May be unable to accurately detect exact contraction frequency and duration, particularly if a woman is very large or is having preterm labor • Toco is location sensitive; poor placement can lead to false information • Sensitive to maternal or fetal motion that may be superimposed on the waveform • Transducer presence or position may be uncomfortable for the mother • May limit potential for maternal movement and ambulation during labor
Troubleshooting/Corrective Actions	
PROBLEM	ACTION
• Contractions not recording on the tracing	• Use manual palpation to validate presence of contractions • Confirm toco transducer is on abdomen and connected to monitor • Test calibration of the toco system by pushing firmly on the abdominal transducer button; digital monitor display should show a particular numeric display (see operating manual for the monitor type you are using to confirm what the specific number should be) • Ensure that placement of the tocodynamometer is firm, but not tight, on the maternal abdomen • Palpate the uterus for the area of strongest contraction and reposition the tocodynamometer over that point • When the uterus is relaxed, set the UA dial or button to 15–20 mm Hg

Table 4-9	Toco Transducer: Capabilities, Benefits and Limitations, Troubleshooting/ Corrective Actions—cont'd
Troubleshooting/Corrective Actions	
PROBLEM	**ACTION**

• Recording only portions of contractions
• Other problems
  ◦ Position
  ◦ Pushing
  ◦ Vomiting
	• Consider IUPC placement, if clinically indicated
	• Palpate the uterus for the area of strongest contraction intensity; reposition the tocodynamometer over that area
	• When the uterus is relaxed, set the uterine activity dial or button to 15–20 mm Hg
	• Encourage position change as needed
	• Palpate to verify uterine activity
	• If necessary, note uterine contractions on tracing using the event marker
	• Note clinical events (e.g., vomiting, pushing)

IUPC = Intrauterine pressure catheter.

Intrauterine Pressure Catheter

Internal monitoring with an IUPC is used in the management of laboring women in the United States today at a rate of 1 in every 5 women (Sciscione et al., 2005). Inserted internally into the uterine cavity via the vagina (transcervical insertion), the IUPC allows for greater quantitative measurement of uterine contraction frequency, duration, intensity or peak intrauterine pressure, and resting tone. There are currently three types of IUPCs in use: fluid-filled catheter systems, transducer-tipped catheters, and air-coupled catheters. The decision to use an IUPC should be based on the clinical need for additional uterine activity information—for example, cases in which maternal obesity or uterine overdistention inhibits the ability to assess uterine activity. Other indications for IUPC placement may include (1) need for amnioinfusion, (2) oxytocin induction or augmentation when external methods of assessing uterine activity are not producing an interpretable uterine activity tracing, and (3) lack of progress of labor when quantitative analysis of uterine activity is indicated for clinical decision making (ACOG, 2003). IUPC placement is invasive and requires the consideration of the potential risks and benefits prior to placement (Table 4-10). A physician, midwife, or registered nurse can place the catheter; however, state and provincial guidelines and hospital policies governing placement of IUPCs by registered nurses vary. The sterile, flexible catheter is inserted into the amniotic cavity of the uterus with the use of a guide. The catheter should be placed only after rupture of membranes has occurred and when adequate cervical dilatation (usually at least 2 cm) has been achieved.

The most common North American unit of IUPC measurement for contraction intensity is millimeters of mercury (mm Hg). Uterine baseline resting tone and peak intrauterine pressure intensity can be described using the mm Hg measurement from the monitor tracing.

Alternative methods of describing uterine activity strength include determining the contraction amplitude by subtracting the difference in mm Hg between the uterine contraction peak and baseline. Using this definition of amplitude, contraction strength tends to vary across a given labor, from 30 mm Hg amplitude in early spontaneous labor, to 50 mm Hg at the end of first stage, to 20 to 30 mm Hg during second stage (Caldeyro-Barcia & Poseiro, 1959).

Another approach to quantify uterine contraction strength is to use Montevideo units (MVUs), a measurement defined in 1952 by Dr. Caldeyro-Barcia and colleagues from Montevideo, Uruguay. These units are calculated by measuring

FIGURE 4-6   Tocodynamometer Variations

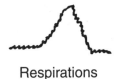

Normal

1. Uterine contraction wave form.

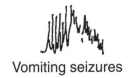

Respirations

2. Respiration may produce an undulating overlay.

Pushing

3. Valsalva maneuver with pushing effects during the second state of labor may produce blunted spikes.

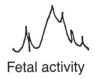

Vomiting seizures

4. Extreme maternal activity such as vomiting or a seizure may produce a series of sharp spikes.

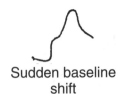

Fetal activity

5. Fetal movement may produce sharp isolated spikes.

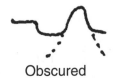

Sudden baseline shift

6. Sudden baseline shifts may be produced by maternal position change.

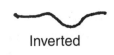

Obscured

7. Low baseline setting may obscure all but tip of contractions.

Inverted

8. Certain placements of tocodynamometer may produce reversed waveform when uterus contracts away from the tocodynamometer.

Adapted from information in Wagner and Cabaniss, unpublished

the peak intensity or amplitude (in mm Hg) for each contraction occurring in a 10-minute period of time and adding the numbers together (Caldeyro-Barcia, Pose, & Alvarez, 1957). Contraction amplitude is the difference between the resting tone and the peak of the contraction (in mm Hg). For example, if there are three contractions in 10 minutes, peaking 70, 80, and 75 mm Hg of intrauterine pressure, and a baseline uterine tone of 10 mm Hg, this would be calculated as $(70 - 10) + (80 - 10) + (75 - 10) = 60 + 70 + 65 = 195$ MVUs. It is important to note that these calculations are dependent on the accuracy of IUPC data. A contraction pattern totaling at least 200 MVUs per 10-minute period has long been considered as adequate labor (ACOG, 2003) and normal spontaneous labor activity is generally less than 280 MVUs (Caldeyro-Barcia, & Poseiro, 1959), although MVUs can vary widely across spontaneous laboring women (Caldeyro-Barcia & Poseiro, 1960). Contraction amplitude in normal labor can vary from 25 to 75 mm Hg and MVUs can vary from as low as 95 to as high as 395 per 10 minutes (ACOG). ACOG (2003) has recommended that uterine contraction patterns be at least 200 MVUs per 10 minutes for at least 2 hours without cervical change before diagnosing arrest of first-stage labor. Research findings by Rouse and colleagues (1999, 2001) suggest that at least 4 hours in active phase of labor may be more appropriate before such a diagnosis can be made. ACOG (2003) suggests that oxytocin augmentation for a minimum of 4 hours prior to cesarean birth for arrest of active labor is appropriate in the absence of other indications for surgical birth.

Friedman Curve

The Friedman Labor Curve, developed by Dr. Emanual Friedman in 1954, continues to be used today as a tool in the assessment of satisfactory labor progress and in the decision-making process regarding the implementation of labor augmentation, instrumental, and operative births. The Friedman curve depicts the relationship between cervical dilation and the duration of labor illustrated as a sigmoid curve consisting of latent, active, and second stage labor (Zhang, Troendle, & Yancey, 2002). This curve then defined the "normal" length of labor and was designed so that birth of the neonate occurred within a specified time frame associated with the best outcomes. At the time the Friedman curve was developed, extremely long labors were associated with hypoxic injuries attributable to birth trauma (Cesario, 2004).

Cesario (2004) conducted a study that suggested that the parameters used to determine whether a labor is progressing as "normal" according to Friedman may need to be expanded. This is primarily supported not only because of the change in the technology now available to assess fetal well-being but also because of the changing demographics of the population and birth environments and the frequent use of epidural analgesia.

Additional studies have also evaluated labor progression. A study conducted by Vahratian, Zhang, Troendle, Sciscione, and Hoffman (2005) found that labor progression differed substantially for women in spontaneous labor versus women with an elective induction of labor. The investigators also noted that nulliparous women with an unfavorable cervix who were being induced had a high rate of arrest of labor, significantly longer latent and early active phases of labor, and a two-fold to three-fold increase in the incidence of operative birth. Rouse, Owen, Savage, and Hauth (2001) reported that labors augmented with oxytocin proceed substantially more slowly than those of spontaneous labor and argue that the criterion of labor arrest at 2 hours is insufficient for the performance of cesarean birth if MVUs are sustained at 200. In this study, 61% of women who experienced labor arrest of 2 hours despite adequate MVUs went on to give birth vaginally when oxytocin augmentation was continued. These data suggest that parameters as defined by Friedman's curve do not apply to oxytocin-augmented patients or patients receiving epidural analgesia, which may prolong the active

Table 4-10	Intrauterine Pressure Catheters: Capabilities, Benefits and Limitations, Troubleshooting/ Corrective Actions

Capabilities

Intrauterine pressure catheters can be used to:

- Detect actual uterine resting tone
- Detect actual frequency, duration, and strength/intensity of uterine contractions
- Withdraw amniotic fluid for testing
- Perform amnioinfusion

Benefits and Limitations

BENEFITS	LIMITATIONS
General	General
• Is an objective method of assessing accurate uterine contraction frequency, duration, intensity, and resting tone	• Requires rupture of membranes and adequate cervical dilation
• May provide a more accurate assessment of timing of FHR changes with uterine activity when an accurate tracing cannot be obtained externally	• Is invasive
• Generates a tracing that is a permanent part of the medical record	• Has increased risk of uterine infection, uterine or placental perforation
	• Limits potential for maternal ambulation during labor
	• May be contraindicated with infections where rupture of membranes is discouraged to prevent maternal-fetal transmission (e.g., GBS, herpes, HIV, hepatitis)
	• May be contraindicated in presence of vaginal bleeding
	• Has increased risk of uterine perforation (rupture), placental abruption or perforation, infection, or umbilical cord prolapse (Usta, Mercer, & Sabai, 1999)
	• Produces differences in readings between fluid-filled, sensor-tipped, and transducer-tipped catheters
Solid-state IUPC (transducer & sensor-tipped)	Solid-state IUPC (transducer & sensor-tipped)
• Is easily zeroed to atmospheric pressure; most can be re-zeroed	• Maternal position may change hydrostatic pressure within the uterus and may alter readings including resting tone
• Allows for amnioinfusion and aspiration of amniotic fluid (with most models)	• Pressure readings may be higher than with fluid-filled catheters
• Is designed to avoid pressure artifacts that may be caused by a catheter that may contain air or become kinked	
Fluid-filled IUPC	Fluid-filled IUPC
• Provides means for aspiration of amniotic fluid	• Catheter tip may become wedged against the uterine wall or fetal part and prevent the production of any pressure data; may produce a distorted or dampened waveform
• Provides means for amnioinfusion	• Catheter tip in relation to external pressure transducer position may affect pressures
	• Catheter may become obstructed with particulate matter such as meconium or blood
	• Although not a true limitation, pressure readings may be lower than sensor-tipped (or solid) transducers

Table 4-10	Intrauterine Pressure Catheters: Capabilities, Benefits and Limitations, Troubleshooting/Corrective Actions—cont'd

Troubleshooting/Corrective Actions	
PROBLEM	**ACTIONS**
• No contractions recorded ◦ Potential causes ◦ Displacement of IUPC ◦ Obstructed catheter ◦ Incorrectly zeroed catheter ◦ Uterine perforation	• Evaluate potential causes • Ask patient to cough or perform Valsalva's maneuver to verify the position of the IUPC; a spike should appear if the IUPC is positioned properly • Palpate to confirm presence of contractions • Check monitor for loose connections • Flush fluid-filled catheter • Verify calibration per detailed instructions in transducer manufacturer's operating manual (run monitor's self-test) • Zero/re-zero the transducer according to manufacturer's operating manual and verify the position of the IUPC • In addition to troubleshooting for placement of IUPC, observe for signs of maternal or fetal compromise
• Abnormal uterine contraction waveform appearance on tracing ◦ Potential causes ◦ The IUPC tip may be lodged against the uterine wall, placenta, or a fetal body part ◦ Fluid-filled IUPC may be dry or incompletely filled with sterile water, thus permitting air to dampen the waveform ◦ Catheter tip is above the diaphragm transducer level, creating higher pressure readings; or, if below, the reading may be artificially low ◦ Inadvertent insertion of the IUPC between the wall of the uterus and the membranes (extraovular) ◦ Uterine perforation, placental abruption, or perforation	Evaluate potential causes • Palpate uterus for contractions • Flush the IUPC, if applicable • Try rotating the IUPC 180 degrees; this may change the relationship of the pressure-sensing device to the fetus and uterus • Withdraw and reposition catheter if blood returned through catheter • In addition to troubleshooting for placement of IUPC, observe for signs of maternal or fetal compromise
• Inverse tracing of uterine contractions ◦ Potential causes ◦ Uterine perforation	• Evaluate potential causes • In addition to troubleshooting for placement of IUPC, observe for signs of maternal or fetal compromise
• Uterine resting tone or baseline tonus is elevated or not tracing • Potential causes ◦ Fluid-filled IUPC is sensitive to hydrostatic pressure and changes in hydrostatic pressure ◦ Pressures may vary in different maternal positions	• Palpate uterine resting tone • Re-zero IUPC according to manufacturer's instructions • Record the uterine resting tone in all positions on insertion, especially when using IUPCs that cannot be rezeroed after insertion

FHR = Fetal heart rate; GBS = group B streptococcus; HIV = human immunodeficiency virus; IUPC = intrauterine pressure catheter.

phase of labor compared with Friedman's original data (Alexander, Sharma, McIntire, & Leveno, 2002). A study conducted by Zhang et al., (2002) of 1329 nulliparous women at term reiterates the need to reevaluate the use of the Friedman's curve (Figure 4-7).

Fluid-Filled Intrauterine Pressure Catheter

The fluid-filled, or water column method, IUPC was the first type of catheter available and was widely used in the measurement of uterine con-

FIGURE 4-7 **A. Comparison between Friedman Curve and Pattern of Cervical Dilatation Based on Current Data**

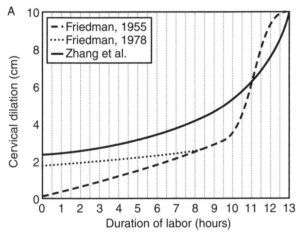

B. Patterns of Cervical Diliation (Left) and Fetal Descent (Right) in Nulliparous Women Based on Contemporary Clinical Conditions

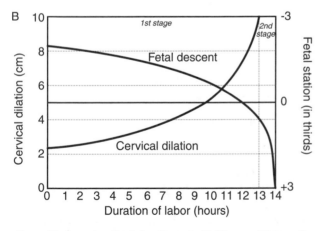

From: "Reassessing the Labor Curve in Multiparous Women," by J. Zhang, J. F. Troendle, & M. K.Yancey, 2002, *American Journal of Obstetrics and Gynecology, 187,* p. 825. Reprinted with permission.

traction intensity (Dowdle, 2003). With the use of the fluid-filled catheter, the intrauterine pressure generated by a contraction is transmitted through the water column to a transducer located away from the source of pressure, typically at the monitor site. This displaced fluid exerts pressure against a diaphragm in the transducer, generating changes in the electrical resistance of a series of wires. These electrical changes are converted to measures of pressure and displayed on the uterine activity channel of the fetal monitor tracing.

Technical problems with fluid-filled catheters include cumbersome setup and maintenance; catheter occlusion with solids (e.g., meconium or vernix) requiring intermittent flushing; kinking and entrapment of the catheter between the uterus and fetus; and artifact resulting from catheter manipulation and maternal movement. These problems produce dampened uterine waveforms and inaccurate measurement of contractions (Devoe, Smith, & Stoker, 1993; Hutson & Petrie, 1986; Klapholz, 1978). The use of fluid-filled catheters dramatically decreased after the introduction of the transducer-tipped catheter in 1987.

See Table 4-10 for an overview of capabilities, benefits, limitations, and troubleshooting issues regarding the use of the fluid-filled IUPC.

Transducer-Tipped Intrauterine Pressure Catheters

The transducer-tipped IUPC was introduced in the 1980s as an alternative to the fluid-filled catheter systems (Strong & Paul, 1989). This technology was developed to include both the pressure sensor and transducer at the catheter tip that is placed directly into the uterus (Beeson & Martens, 2005). The force exerted by a uterine contraction is then converted to an electrical signal that is transmitted through a wire system to the fetal monitor, where the uterine activity is displayed graphically on the fetal monitor strip. This catheter offers options of dual lumen versions that enable simultaneous amnioinfusion or sampling of amniotic fluid and may be re-zeroed after insertion.

The baseline reading of resting tone from a transducer-tipped IUPC can be affected by changes in maternal position and the hydrostatic pressures exerted on the catheter. The position of the IUPC tip in relation to the position of the patient may affect the amount of pressure exerted by the fluid above the catheter. Intrauterine hydrostatic pressure is altered by maternal position changes. Obtaining baseline pressure readings in the left, right, and supine with lateral tilt positions demonstrates these alterations and should be completed and documented after initial insertion (Figure 4-8). This in turn may prevent potential misinterpretations of resting tone pressures following subsequent position changes during labor. Knowing these baseline differences may prevent erroneous conclusions regarding induction or augmentation management.

Air-Coupled Intrauterine Pressure Catheters (Sensor-Tipped)

The air-coupling technology, which is a newer method of IUP monitoring, uses a distally mounted flexible balloon in the uterus connected to an external reusable transducer in the monitor cable. Similar to the technology of noninvasive blood pressure monitors, this catheter consists of a membrane sensor at the tip of the catheter that communicates pressures through a micro-column of air with an externally located transducer (Clinical Innovations, 2001).

Transducer-Tipped versus Sensor-Tipped?

The decision regarding what catheter type to use, although not all inclusive, may depend on physician or nurse preference, hospital contractual agreements, budget, or study results. Also, the ease and reliability of the various re-zeroing features of the IUPC may affect decision making regarding the type of catheter that an institution may use or chose to change to. A study conducted by Dowdle (2003) found that the two most common catheter types, transducer-tipped and sensor-tipped, yielded similar quantitative measurement of uterine activity. Both systems were found to function equally well in the display of abnormal uterine activity.

Sciscione et al. (2005) found in a study of 249 women that the transducer-tipped catheters were significantly more likely to have an extra-ovular placement, where the catheter is inadvertently placed outside the amniotic membranes and between the chorion and the decidua in the extramembranous space of the lower uterine segment. Placement in this space (as opposed to the fluid-filled amniotic cavity) is believed to be due to the rigidity of this type of catheter, which may increase the risk for abruption, especially in the presence of an amnioinfusion. Although

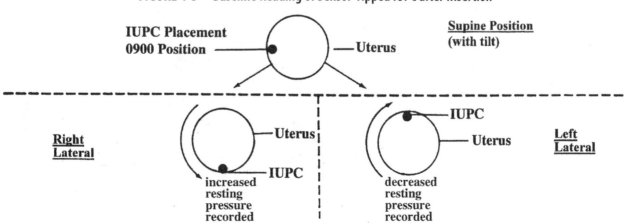

FIGURE 4-8   Baseline Reading of Sensor-Tipped IUPC after Insertion

Adapted from Utah Medical Products. (2006). Intran® Plus User Guidelines. Midvale, UT: Author.

Sciscione et al. report that IUPCs may function normally if placed in the extramembranous space, the true rate of these extraovular placements is unknown. Clear catheter lumens, now available in both types of catheters, assist in determining proper placement in addition to assessing for the presence of meconium-stained amniotic fluid.

MONITOR TRACING ISSUES

Although the focus of this section of the chapter is FHM techniques, it is important to address tracing and paper speed technology when EFM is used. Changes in paper speed can substantially alter the appearance of the tracing (Freeman et al., 2003), which could inherently provide for differences in interpretation of FHR data.

Fetal monitor technology provides the capacity to set the tracing paper speed as well as the visual tracing display at specific settings. In the United States, markings on the vertical scale range from 30 to 240 bpm, with dividing lines at 10-bpm intervals. On the European-scaled paper, which is also used in South America and certain centers in the United States, markings range from 50 to 210 bpm, with dividing lines at 5-bpm intervals. Paper speeds also vary throughout the United States, Canada, and Europe. Paper speed in the United States and Canada commonly runs at 3 cm per minute on the horizontal scale, whereas paper speed in Europe, South America, and some centers in the United States and Canada runs at a range of 1 or 2 cm/minute.

Despite these apparent differences, one recommendation is constant across professional practice organizations: standardization of paper speed within and across practice settings is essential for optimal interpretation by professional care providers (RCOG, 2001; SOGC, 2007), and switching of paper speeds during individual labors is *not* recommended. Overall, the pattern at a slower speed will appear compressed with variability accentuated and periodic/episodic changes appearing more abrupt in nature (Freeman et al., 2003). Despite the recommendations for a consistent paper speed, there are geographic differences regarding paper speed practices even across North American and Canadian centers. These differences may be related to historical tradition, the country or location in which particular nurses and physicians previously trained and practiced, and/or the argument that slower paper speeds save paper and maximize storage efficiency.

Lack of consistency in paper speed settings may make interpretation and communication more challenging; and such inconsistency may set the stage for misinterpretation of EFM data or miscommunication of those data. Because team communication is a key issue in cases with poor outcomes as discussed in the Joint Commission Sentinel Event Alert (2004), each institution should define uniform paper speed standards, and individual clinicians should use the defined paper speed consistently. Clinicians should also know where the paper speed switch is located on the monitors where she/he works and document changes in paper speed if they occur. To date, scientific study of possible clinical influences of differences in paper speed has not been published.

Intrapartum Fetal Surveillance Technology and the Nurse's Role
Patient Education

Patient education regarding methods of fetal assessment and options is essential for women to make fully informed decisions about their health care. Advances in technological capabilities and the technological society within which we live and practice may influence patients' preferences for IA or EFM. More current studies regarding patient preferences or feelings about monitoring methods are warranted, although patients have reported that they prefer to have a supportive professional present during labor (Hodnett et al., 2002; Killien & Shy, 1989). Wood (2003) discusses the ethical decision-making models used to assist nurses to better delineate their role as patient advocates, in this case, with the use of IA versus EFM in labor.

Labor Support

All women benefit from receiving labor support. Hodnett, Gates, Hofmeyr, and Sakala's (2003) systematic review of 15 RCTs ($n = 12,791$) found that continuous labor support was associated with increased spontaneous vaginal births and decreased operative births (both vaginal and cesarean), as well as reduction in the use of intrapartum pain medications and regional analgesia/anesthesia, and reduced likelihood of reports of negative birth experiences. The authors concluded that all women should have support throughout the labor and birth process. Support that began earlier in labor also seemed to be more effective than when it was initiated later in labor (Hodnett et al.).

It is unclear, however, which type of caregiver is most efficacious in achieving labor support outcomes because 13 of the 15 studies in the review included support persons other than nurses. Although they conclude that continuous labor support appears to be more effective if provided by support persons other than nurses, Hodnett and colleagues also note that constraints and other responsibilities placed on nurses by institutional policies, and routine practices may have influenced these results (Hodnett et al, 2003). A randomized clinical trial of nurse-provided labor support in North America concluded that nursing care per se was not associated with reductions in cesarean birth rates or psychosocial outcomes for laboring women giving birth in environments characterized by high rates of routine intervention (Hodnett et al, 2002). Despite these findings, every effort should be made to provide women in labor with continuous support, because the birth experience can have a lifelong impact and affect women's psychological well-being (Goodman, Mackey, & Tavakoli, 2004; Simkin, 1991). Many organizations advocate that ideally women should receive one-to-one nursing care and support in labor (AWHONN, 2000; Health Canada, 2000; SOGC, 2007).

Providing supportive care during labor is not dependent on the method of fetal surveillance used but rather on the philosophy, attitudes, and values of care providers. Although women undergoing EFM during labor can definitely benefit from all aspects of supportive care practices, women being monitored using IA may be more likely to receive close continuous presence of a caregiver because of the constant need for hands-on touch and palpation.

Clinicians and researchers have cautioned against nursing activities becoming more heavily focused on monitors and other machinery, rather than on the woman in labor (Hoerst & Fairman, 2000; McNiven, Hodnett, & O'Brien-Pallas, 1992; Sandelowski, 1998). EFM technology does not replace the need for care by experienced providers (AWHONN, 2009). The Royal College of Obstetricians and Gynaecologists stated that "Women should have the same level of care and support regardless of the mode of monitoring," (RCOG, 2001, p. 9) and SOGC strongly supports 1:1 nurse-patient ratios in labor so that patients may receive adequate supportive care (SOGC, 2007). In summary, women desire and deserve supportive care regardless of the method of monitoring being used.

Institutional Policies

Individual facilities should develop interdisciplinary policies and procedures for IA, uterine palpation, and EFM that are consistent with their appropriate state, provincial, or national guidelines or regulations. Inclusion of key nursing and obstetric providers and development of collaborative teams are suggested for planning and implementing evidence-based practices (AWHONN, 2006; Simpson, 2008; Smith & Onstad, 2005). Policies should address when it is appropriate to use IA and EFM, the frequency of assessment, and documentation of findings (AAP/ACOG, 2007).

Professional Education Regarding Monitoring Methods

It is important for professionals to receive preparation for implementing fetal monitoring that includes the physiologic interpretation of data and its implications for care (AWHONN,

2009; SOGC, 2007). Facilitators to implementing evidence-based practice include education preparation, resources, and support (Davies et al., 2002). Whether new skills are being taught or existing skills reinforced, the level of the learner (novice to expert) should be considered (Benner, 1984). Educational programs that employ adult learning principles with attention to the levels of learners can assist care providers in increasing their skills in IA and EFM and aid in building their skill and confidence.

According to The Joint Commission Sentinel Event Alert (2004), many risk-reduction strategies have been identified, based on the examination of multiple root cause analyses. Included in these strategy recommendations are the development of clear guidelines for fetal monitoring interpretation, interdisciplinary FHM education for nurses, residents, nurse midwives and physicians, and the use of standardized terminology to communicate fetal heart rate findings. The Joint Commission also recommends team training in perinatal areas to teach staff to work together and communicate more effectively. In order to successfully accomplish this goal, joint education programs with nurses, residents, nurse midwives, and physicians and discontinuation of long-practiced segregated educational models must be a priority.

Future Research

Additional research on methods of monitoring will continue to inform us regarding our use of alternative monitoring methods, including identifying which women may be appropriately monitored with EFM or IA, as well as how frequently assessments should occur.

SUMMARY

Fetal surveillance methods allow data to be gathered for assessment of fetal well-being and uterine activity. High-quality data are vital for accurate interpretation, diagnosis, and subsequent interventions. As labor progresses, depending on the quality of information received for interpretation, the need for a change in methods may be required for adequate assessment, interpretation, clinical interventions, and evaluation. Understanding the methods, benefits, limitations, and troubleshooting measures for fetal surveillance is critical for informed decision-making and skill in the use of these methodologies.

REFERENCES

Alexander, J. M., Sharma, S. K., McIntire, D. D., & Leveno, K. J. (2002). Epidural analgesia lengthens the Friedman active phase of labor. *Obstetrics and Gynecology, 100*(1), 46–50.

American Academy of Pediatrics, & American College of Obstetricians & Gynecologists. (2007). *Guidelines for perinatal care* (6th ed.). Elk Grove Village, IL: Authors.

American College of Nurse Midwives. (2007). Intermittent auscultation for intrapartum fetal heart rate surveillance (Clinical Bulletin No. 9, March 2007). *Journal of Nurse Midwifery & Women's Health, 52,* 314-319.

American College of Obstetricians and Gynecologists. (1995). *Fetal heart rate patterns: Monitoring, interpretation, and management* (Technical Bulletin No. 207). Washington, DC: Author (withdrawn).

American College of Obstetricians and Gynecologists. (2003). *Dystocia and augmentation of labor* (Practice Bulletin No. 49). Washington, DC: Author.

American College of Obstetricians and Gynecologists. (2005). *Intrapartum fetal heart rate monitoring* (Practice Bulletin No. 70). Washington, DC: Author.

American Nurses Association. (2005). *ANA principles on safe staffing.* Silver Spring, MD: Author.

Amer-Wåhlin, I., Bördahl, P., Eikeland, T., Hellsten, C., Norén, H., Sörnes, T., et al. (2002). ST analysis of the fetal electrocardiogram during labor: Nordic observational multicenter study. *The Journal of Maternal-Fetal and Neonatal Medicine, 12,* 260–266.

Amer-Wåhlin, I., Ingemarsson, I., Marsal, K., & Herbst, A. (2005). Fetal heart rate patterns and ECG ST segment changes preceding metabolic academia at birth. *BJOG: An International Journal of Obstetrics and Gynaecology, 112,* 160–165.

Association of Women's Health, Obstetric and Neonatal Nurses. (2000). *Professional nursing support of laboring women* (Clinical Position Statement). Washington, DC: Author.

Association of Women's Health, Obstetric and Neonatal Nurses. (2006). *Antepartum and intrapartum fetal* heart monitoring: Clinical competencies and education guide (4th ed.). Washington, DC: Author.

Association of Women's Health, Obstetric and Neonatal Nurses. (2009). *Fetal heart monitoring* (Position Statement). Washington, DC: Author.

Banta, D. H., & Thacker, S. B. (2001). Historical controversy in health technology assessment: The case of electronic fetal monitoring. *Obstetrics and Gynecology Survey, 56,* 707–719.

Beeson, J., & Martens, M. (2005). Variable intrauterine pressure catheter (IUPC) tracings with two catheters. Data presented at the Society of Maternal-Fetal Medicine annual meeting.

Benner, P. (1984). *From novice to expert. Excellence and power in clinical nursing practice.* Menlo Park: Addison-Wesley.

Boehm, F. H., Fields, L. M., Hutchison, J. M., Bowen, A. W., & Vaughn, W. K. (1986). The indirectly obtained fetal heart rate: Comparison of first and second generation electronic fetal monitors. *American Journal of Obstetrics and Gynecology, 155,* 10–14.

Caldeyro-Barcia, R., Pose, S., & Alvarez, H. (1957). Uterine contractility in polyhydramnios and the effects of withdrawal of the excess of amniotic fluid. *American Journal of Obstetrics and Gynecology, 73,* 1238–1254.

Caldeyro-Barcia, R., & Poseiro, J. (1959). Oxytocin and contractility of the pregnant human uterus. *Annals of the New York Academy of Science, 72,* 813–830.

Caldeyro-Barcia, R., & Poseiro, J. (1960). Physiology of the uterine contraction. *Clinics in Obstetrics and Gynecology, 3,* 386.

Canadian Perinatal Regionalization Coalition, Society of Obstetricians & Gynaecologists of Canada, & Perinatal Educator Program. (2002). *Fundamentals of fetal health surveillance in labour: A self-learning manual.* Ottawa, Canada: Author.

Cesario, S. K. (2004). Reevaluation of Friedman's labor curve: A pilot study. *Journal of Obstetric, Gynecologic, & Neonatal Nursing, 33,* 713–722.

Clinical Innovations. (2001). Koala® IPC 5000, What is soft, sensitive, and great for measuring intrauterine pressure? [Brochure]. Murray, UT: Author.

Davies, B., Hodnett, E., Hannah, M., O'Brien-Pallas, L., Pringle, D., Wells, G., et al. (2002). Fetal health surveillance: A community-wide approach versus a tailored intervention for the implementation of clinical practice guidelines. *Canadian Medical Association Journal, 167,* 469–474.

Davies, B. L., Niday, P. A., Nimrod, C. A., Drake, E. R., Sprague, A. E., & Trépanier, M. J. (1993). Electronic fetal monitoring: A Canadian survey. *Canadian Medical Association Journal, 148,* 1737–1742.

Devoe, L. D., Smith, R. P., & Stoker, R. (1993). Intrauterine pressure catheter performance in an in vitro

uterine model: A stimulation of problems for intrapartum monitoring. *Obstetrics and Gynecology, 82,* 285–289.

Declercq, E.R., Sakala, C., Corry, M. P., & Applebaum, S. (2006), *Listenting to mothers II: Report of the second national U.S. survey of women's childbearing experiences.* New York: Childbirth Conection.

Dowdle, M. (2003). Comparison of two intrauterine pressure catheters during labor. *The Journal of Reproductive Medicine, 48,* 501–505.

Feinstein, N. F., Sprague, A., & Trepanier, M. J. (2008). *Fetal heart rate auscultation* (2nd ed.). Washington, DC: Association of Women's Health, Obstetric and Neonatal Nurses.

Freeman, R. K., Garite, T. J., & Nageotte, M. P. (2003). *Fetal heart rate monitoring.* Philadelphia: Lippincott Williams & Wilkins.

Goodman, P. Mackey, M. C, Tavakoli, A. S. (2004). Factors related to childbirth satisfaction. *Journal of Advanced Nursing, 46*(2), 212–219.

Goodwin, L. (2000). Intermittent auscultation of the fetal heart rate: A review of general principles. *Journal of Perinatal and Neonatal Nursing, 14*(3), 53–61.

Haggerty, L. A. (1999). Continuous electronic fetal monitoring: Contradictions between practice and research. *Journal of Obstetric, Gynecologic, and Neonatal Nursing, 28,* 409–416.

Health Canada. (2000). Family-centered maternity and newborn care: National guidelines (4th ed.). Ottawa: Minister of Public Works and Government Services.

Hodnett, E. D., Gates, S., Hofmeyr, G. J., & Sakala, C. (2003). Continuous support for women during childbirth. *Cochrane Database of Systematic Reviews, Vol. 3.*

Hodnett, E. D., Lowe, N. K., Hannah, M. E., Willan, A. R., Stevens, B., Weston, J. A., et al. (2002). Effectiveness of nurses as providers of birth labor support in North American hospitals: A randomized controlled trial. *Journal of the American Medical Association, 288*(11), 1373–1381.

Hoerst, B. J., & Fairman, J. (2000). Social and professional influences of the technology of electronic fetal monitoring on obstetrical nursing. *Western Journal of Nursing Research, 22*(4), 475–491.

Hutson, J. M., & Petrie, R. H. (1986). Possible limitations of fetal monitoring. *Clinical Obstetrics and Gynecology, 29*(1), 104–113.

Joint Commission. (2004, July 21). *Preventing infant death and injury during delivery* (Sentinel Event Alert, Issue 30). Chicago: Author.

Killien, M. G., & Shy, K. (1989). A randomized clinical trial of electronic fetal monitoring in preterm labor: Mother's views. *Birth, 16*(1), 7–12.

Klapholz, H. (1978). Techniques of fetal heart monitoring. *Seminars in Perinatology, 2,* 119–129.

Kwee, A., Dekkers, A. H., van Wijk, H. P., van der Hoorn-van den Beld, C. W., & Visser, G. (2007). Occurrence of ST-changes recorded with STAN® S21-monitor during normal and abnormal fetal heart rate patterns during labour. *European Journal of Obstetrics, Gynecology and Reproductive Biology, 135,* 28–34.

LaCroix, G. E. (1968). Monitoring labor by an external tocodynamometer. *American Journal of Obstetrics and Gynecology, 101,* 111–119.

Levitt, C., Hanvey, L., Avard, D., Chance, G., & Kaczorowski, J. (1995). *Survey of routine maternity care and practices in Canadian hospitals.* Ottawa: Health Canada and Canadian Institute of Child Health.

Macones, G. A., Hankins, G. D., Spong, C. Y., Hauth, J. D., & Moore, T. (2008). The 2008 National Institute of Child Health Human Development workshop report on electronic fetal monitoring: Update on definitions, interpretations, and research guidelines. *Obstetrics & Gynecology, 112,* 661–666; and *Journal of Obstetric, Gynecologic and Neonatal Nursing, 37,* 510–515.

Malinowski, J., Pedigo, C., & Phillips, C. (1989). *Nursing care during the labor process* (3rd ed.). Philadelphia: F.A. Davis.

Martin, J. A., Hamilton, B. E., Sutton, P. D., Ventura, S. J., Menacker, F., & Munson, M. L. (2003). Birth: Final data for 2002. *National Vital Statistics Reports, 52*(10), 1–113.

McNiven, P., Hodnett, E., & O'Brien-Pallas, L. L. (1992). Supporting women in labor: A work sampling study of the activities of labor and delivery nurses. *Birth, 19*(1), 3–8.

Murray, M. (2007). *Antepartum and intrapartum fetal monitoring* (3rd ed.). New York: Springer Publishing.

Murray, M. L. (2004). Maternal or fetal heart rate? Avoiding intrapartum misidentification. *Journal of Obstetric, Gynecologic & Neonatal Nursing, 33*(1), 93–104.

National Institute of Child Health and Human Development Research Planning Workshop (NICHD). (1997). Electronic fetal heart rate monitoring: Research guidelines for interpretation. *American Journal of Obstetrics and Gynecology, 177,* 1385–1390 and *Journal of Obstetric, Gynecologic, and Neonatal Nursing, 26,* 635–640.

Neilson, J. P. (2006). Fetal electrocardiogram (ECG) for fetal monitoring during labour. *Cochrane Database of Systems Reviews, The Cochrane Collaboration Vol. (4). Accession No.: 00075320-100000000-00782.*

Norén, H., Amer-Wåhlin, I., Hagberg, H., Herbst, A., Kjellmer, I., Marsál, K., et al. (2003). Fetal electrocardiography in labor and neonatal outcome: Data from the Swedish randomized controlled trial on intrapartum fetal monitoring. *American Journal of Obstetrics and Gynecology, 188,* 183–192.

Olofsson, P. (2003). Current status of intrapartum fetal monitoring: Cardiotocography versus cardiotocography + ST analysis of the fetal ECG. *European Journal of Obstetrics, Gynecology and Reproductive Biology, 110,* S113–S118.

Parer, J. T. (1997). *Handbook of fetal heart rate monitoring* (2nd ed.). Philadelphia: W.B. Saunders.

Parer, J. T. (2003). Electronic fetal heart rate monitoring: A story of survival. *Obstetrical and Gynecological Survey, 58,* 561–563.

Rosén, K. G. (2005). Fetal electrocardiogram waveform analysis in labour. *Current Opinion in Obstetrics and Gynecology, 17,* 147–150.

Rosén, K. G., Amer-Wåhlin, I., Luzietti, R., & Norén, H. (2004). Fetal ECG waveform analysis. *Best Practice & Research Clinical Obstetrics & Gynaecology, 18,* 485–514.

Ross, M. G., Devoe, L. D., & Rosén, K. G. (2004). ST-segment analysis of the fetal electrocardiogram improves fetal heart rate tracing interpretation and clinical decision making. *The Journal of Maternal-Fetal and Neonatal Medicine, 15,* 181–185.

Rouse, D.J., Owen, J., & Hauth, J.C. (1999). Active phase labor arrest: Oxytocin augmentation for at least four hours. *Obstetrics and Gynecology, 93,* 323–328.

Rouse, D. J., Owen, J., Savage, K. G., & Hauth, J. C. (2001). Active phase labor arrest: Revisiting the 2-hour minimum. *Obstetrics and Gynecology, 98,* 550–554.

Royal College of Obstetricians and Gynaecologists. (2001). *The use of electronic fetal monitoring: The use and interpretation of cardiotocography in intrapartum fetal surveillance.* (Evidence-based Clinical Guideline No. 8). London: Author.

Sandelowski, M. (1998). Looking to care or caring to look? Technology and the rise of spectacular nursing. *Holistic Nursing Practice, 12*(4), 1–11.

Schifrin, B., Harwell, R., Rubinstein, T., & Visser, G. (2001). Maternal heart rate pattern: A confounding factor in intrapartum fetal surveillance. *Prenatal and Neonatal Medicine, 6,* 75–82.

Schofield, L.M. (2003). *Perinatal staffing and the nursing shortage: Challenges and Principle based strategies.* Washington, DC: Association of Women's Health, Obstetric and Neonatal Nurses.

Schwartz, N., & Young, B. K. (2006). Intrapartum fetal monitoring today. *Journal of Perinatal Medicine, 34,* 99–107.

Sciscione, A. C., Duhl, A., Pollock, M. A., Hoffman, M. K., Rhee, A., & Colmorgen, G. H. (2005). Extramembranous placement of an air-coupled vs. transducer-tipped intrauterine pressure catheter. *The Journal of Reproductive Medicine, 50,* 578–584.

Sherman, D. J., Frenkel, E., Kurzweil, Y., Padua, A., Arieli, S., & Bahar, M. (2002). Characteristics of maternal heart rate patterns during labor and delivery. *Obstetrics and Gynecology, 99,* 542–547.

Simkin, P. (1991). Just another day in a woman's life? Women's long-term perceptions of their first birth experience. Part I. *Birth, 18,* 203–210.

Simpson, K. R. (2008). Perinatal patient safety and professional liability issues. In K.R. Simpson & P. Creehan (Eds). *Perinatal nursing* (3rd ed., pp. 1–28). Philadelphia: Lippincott Williams & Wilkins.

Smith, J., & Onstad, J. (2005). Assessment of the fetus: Intermittent auscultation, electronic fetal heart rate tracing, and fetal pulse oximetry. *Obstetrics and Gynecology Clinics of North America, 32,* 245–254.

Society of Obstetricians and Gynaecologists of Canada. (2007). Fetal health surveillance: Antepartum and intrapartum consensus guideline (No 197, Replaces No. 90 and No. 112). *Journal of Obstetrics and Gynaecology in Canada, 29*(4), Suppl. 4, S1–S56.

Strong, T. H., Jr., & Paul, R. H. (1989). Intrapartum uterine activity evaluation of an intrauterine pressure catheter. *Obstetrics and Gynecology, 73,* 432–434.

Utah Medical Products Inc. (2006). Intrans® plus user guidelines. [Brochure]. Midvale, UT: Author.

Vahratian, A., Zhang, J., Troendle, J., Sciscione, A. C., & Hoffman, M. K. (2005). Labor progression and risk of cesarean delivery in electively induced nulliparas. *Obstetrics and Gynecology, 105,* 698–704.

Wood, S. H. (2003). Should women be given a choice about fetal assessment in labor? *MCN: American Journal of Maternal Child Nursing, 28,* 292–298.

Zhang, J., Troendle, J., & Yancey, M. K. (2002). Reassessing the labor curve in nulliparous women. *American Journal of Obstetrics and Gynecology, 187,* 824–828.

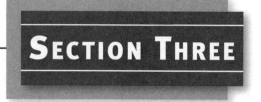

SECTION THREE

Fetal Monitoring: Diagnosis and Intervention

1. Read This Book
2. Take the On-Line Test
3. Earn Continuing Nursing Education Credit

www.awhonn.org/fhm

AWHONN is accredited as a provider of continuing nursing education by the American Nurses Credentialing Center's Commission on Accreditation.

CHAPTER 5

Fetal Heart Rate Interpretation

Audrey Lyndon
Nancy O'Brien-Abel
Kathleen Rice Simpson

INTRODUCTION

The purpose of this chapter is to discuss current concepts in fetal heart rate (FHR) interpretation, including points of both consensus and dissent about interpretation in the FHR monitoring literature. A review of the assumptions of the 2008 National Institute of Child Health and Human Development (NICHD) framework and definitions is followed by discussion of parameters for interpretation of FHR characteristics. The interpretation, presumed physiology and clinical significance, and general management of various FHR findings are discussed in this chapter. The underlying physiologic basis for fetal monitoring was discussed in Chapter 2. Physiologic goals and more detail on interventions for management of FHR tracings are discussed in Chapter 6. For a detailed discussion of the development of fetal monitoring techniques and the historical research base for fetal monitoring, refer to the first chapter of this book as well as the comprehensive summaries presented by Freeman, Garite, and Nageotte (2003) and Parer (1997).

Synthesis of the literature on FHR monitoring is challenging because of the lack of comparability of variables and outcome measures across documents. Comparison is hindered by both inconsistent definitions of FHR characteristics across studies [which NICHD (Macones, Hankins, Spong, Hauth, & Moore, 2008; NICHD, 1997) attempts to remedy] and lack of consistent definition of "acidemia" across studies and guidelines.

Clinically significant acidemia is associated with an arterial umbilical blood pH value of less than 7.00 and a base excess below -12 mmol/L (American College of Obstetricians and Gynecologists [ACOG], 2006; Andres et al., 1999; Low, Lindsay, & Derrick, 1997; MacLennan, 1999). However, studies of relationships between FHR characteristics and fetal or newborn acidemia use values ranging from 7.00 to 7.20 to define "acidemia." For the purposes of the Association of Women's Health, Obstetric and Neonatal Nurses (AWHONN) Fetal Heart Monitoring Program (FHMP) courses and this chapter, the physiologic threshold for avoiding significant acidemia at birth is an umbilical artery pH greater than 7.10 and a base excess greater than or equal to -12 mmol/L (i.e. between 0 and -12) (Andres et al.; Fox, Kilpatrick, King, & Parer, 2000; Low et al.). The absence of significant acidemia at birth may also be inferred by the presence of a 5-minute Apgar score of 7 or greater (Parer, King, Flanders, Fox, & Kilpatrick, 2006).

Fetal heart monitoring is a complex skill requiring knowledge of maternal-fetal physiology, clinical judgment, and specialized education in the use of intermittent auscultation (IA) and electronic fetal monitoring (EFM) techniques. Professional registered nurses are the primary bedside provider of intrapartum FHM in most settings in the United States and Canada and are qualified to perform this ongoing assessment independently as well as in collaboration with a physician or midwife. It is inappropriate to delegate auscultation of the FHR, application of FHR transducers, or initial and ongoing assessment of maternal-fetal status, including interpretation of auscultation and electronic FHR findings to unlicensed assistive personnel (AWHONN, 2000; 2009).

Registered nurses, physicians, and midwives should work together using a problem-solving framework such as the nursing process to achieve an effective, integrated, patient-centered plan for ongoing maternal-fetal assessment and intervention in support of a family-centered birth. Within this framework, interpretation of FHR findings flows directly from the systematic anal-

ysis of maternal and fetal assessment data for the independent and collaborative diagnosis of patient problems, as indicated in Figure 5-1. Systematic use of a standardized language for interpreting and discussing FHR findings promotes understanding among clinicians, thereby promoting safe and effective care of laboring women.

Assumptions of the NICHD Terminology

The consensus reached by the Research Planning Workshop on Electronic Fetal Monitoring included the following set of assumptions about

FIGURE 5-1   The Nursing Process and FHR Interpretation

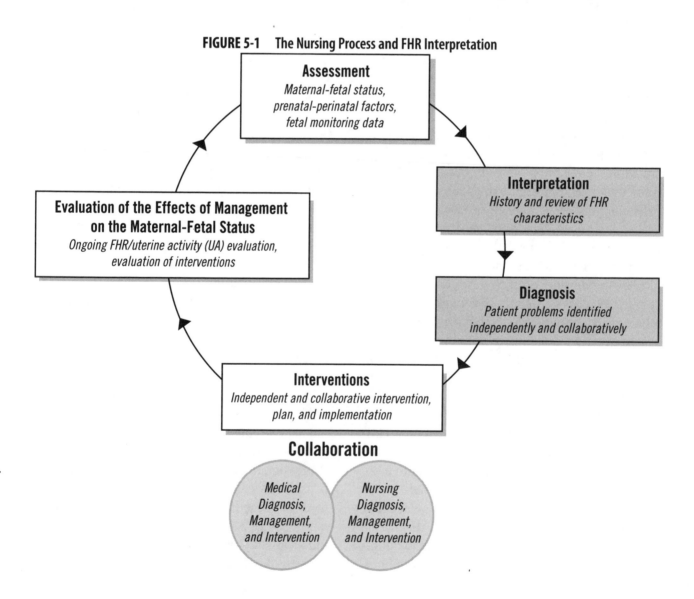

BOX 5-1   NICHD Consensus Assumptions about the Interpretation of Electronic Fetal Monitoring Data

A. The definitions are primarily developed for visual interpretation of FHR patterns. However, it is recognized that computerized interpretation is being developed and the definitions must also be adaptable to such applications.

B. The definitions apply to the interpretations of patterns produced from either a direct fetal electrode detecting the fetal electrocardiogram or an external Doppler device detecting the FHR events with use of the autocorrelation technique.

C. The record of both the FHR and uterine activity should be of adequate quality for visual interpretation.

D. The prime emphasis in [the 2008 NICHD] report is on intrapartum patterns. The definitions may also be applicable to antepartum observations.

E. The characteristics to be defined are those commonly used in clinical practice and research communications.

F. The features of FHR patterns are categorized as either baseline, periodic, or episodic. Periodic patterns are those associated with uterine contractions, and episodic patterns are those not associated with uterine contractions.

G. The periodic patterns are distinguished on the basis of waveform, currently accepted as either "abrupt" or "gradual" onset.

H. Accelerations and decelerations are generally determined in reference to the adjacent baseline FHR.

I. No distinction is made between short-term variability (or beat-to-beat variability or R–R wave period differences in the electrocardiogram) and long-term variability, because in actual practice they are visually determined as a unit. Hence, the definition of variability is based visually on the amplitude of the complexes, with exclusion of the sinusoidal pattern.

J. There is good evidence that a number of characteristics of FHR patterns are dependent upon fetal gestational age and physiologic status as well as maternal physiologic status. Thus, FHR tracings should be evaluated in the context of many clinical conditions including gestational age, prior results of fetal assessment, medications, maternal medical conditions, and fetal conditions (e.g., growth restriction, known congenital anomalies, fetal anemia, arrhythmia, etc).

K. The individual components of defined FHR patterns do not occur independently and generally evolve over time.

L. A full description of the EFM tracing requires a qualitative and quantitative description of
   1. Uterine contractions
   2. Baseline FHR
   3. Baseline FHR variability
   4. Presence of accelerations
   5. Periodic or episodic decelerations
   6. Changes or trends of FHR patterns over time.

Note From: "The 2008 National Institute of Child Health Human Development Workshop Report on Electronic Fetal Monitoring: Update on Definitions, Interpretations, and Research Guidelines," by G. A. Macones, G. D. Hankins, C. Y. Spong, J. D. Hauth, & T. Moore, 2008, *Journal of Obstetric, Gynecologic and Neonatal Nursing, 37,* 510-515; *Obstetrics & Gynecology, 112,* p. 662. Copyright 2008 by the American College of Obstetricians and Gynecologists. Reprinted with permission.

the interpretation of fetal monitoring data (NICHD, 1997) which were reaffirmed and updated at the 2008 meeting (Box 5-1) (Macones et al., 2008).

Definitions of Terms

The definitions of the FHR characteristics discussed in this chapter are presented in Table 5-1. Clinicians should be familiar with these definitions and use them consistently in the AWHONN FHM courses and in clinical practice.

Systematic Assessment of FHR Data

Appropriate interventions require an accurate interpretation of the characteristics of both the FHR and uterine activity. Although there may be disagreement among experts about the interpretation of some combinations of FHR characteristics, there is consensus on what constitutes a normal FHR tracing as illustrated in Figure 5-2: normal baseline rate, moderate variability, and the absence of late or variable decelerations. Accelerations and early decelerations may or may not be present in a normal (category I) FHR tracing (Macones et al., 2008). Tracings exhibiting these normal characteristics are highly predictive of a well-oxygenated, nonacidotic fetus (Berkus, Langer, Samueloff, Xernaxis, & Field, 1999; Krebs, Petres, & Dunn, 1981; Krebs, Petres, Dunn, Jordaan, & Segreti, 1979; Low, Victory, & Derrick, 1999; Macones et al., 2008). Likewise, normal IA findings (normal baseline rate and rhythm, presence of increases in FHR, absence of decreases in FHR) are predictive of fetal well-being (Paine, Zanardi, Johnson, Rorie, & Barger, 2001; Paine, Benedict, Strobino, Gregor, & Larson, 1992).

Attention should be given to the overall clinical picture and stability of, or changes in, FHR characteristics over time. Although the experienced clinician may assess individual characteristics such as rate and rhythm of the FHR simultaneously, a detailed and thorough evaluation of each component may be useful when planning appropriate interventions. Developing a structured approach to assessment and analysis of FHR findings is also helpful in developing skill in interpretation. A systematic fetal monitoring assessment includes the following data:

- Baseline FHR characteristics
  - Baseline rate
    - Is the rate normal, tachycardic, or bradycardic?
  - Rhythm in intermittent auscultation (IA)
    - Is the rhythm regular or irregular?
  - Variability (EFM)
    - Is the FHR variability moderate, or is it absent, minimal, marked or unclassifiable?
- Periodic and episodic changes
  - Presence or absence of increases in FHR (IA) or accelerations (EFM)
  - Presence or absence of decreases in FHR (IA) or decelerations (EFM)
  - Are decelerations early, late, variable, or prolonged? (EFM)
  - Are there other unusual characteristics such as sinusoidal or arrhythmic FHR? (EFM)
- Uterine activity
  - What are the frequency, duration, and intensity of contractions?
  - What is the uterine resting tone?
- Evolution of the FHR over time
  - How has the FHR changed over time? What features of the FHR are stable?
- Integration of findings with the overall clinical picture
  - How do the FHR findings fit with the overall clinical picture, including maternal medical history, current pregnancy history and fetal condition, gestational age, and other physical and laboratory findings?
  - How does the overall clinical history guide interpretation of the fetal monitoring findings?
  - What does the team need to prepare for?
  - Are there potential complications the team needs to be especially vigilant for?
  - Who needs to be aware of current maternal-fetal status?

Table 5-1	2008 NICHD Descriptive Terms for FHR Characteristics
TERM	**DEFINITION**
Baseline Rate	Approximate mean FHR rounded to increments of 5 bpm during a 10-minute window excluding accelerations and decelerations and periods of marked variability. There must be $\geq$2 minutes of identifiable baseline segments (not necessarily contiguous) in any 10-minute window, or the baseline for that period is indeterminate. In such cases, one may need to refer to the previous 10-minute window for determination of the baseline.
Bradycardia	Baseline rate of < 110 bpm.
Tachycardia	Baseline rate of > 160 bpm.
Baseline Variability	Determined in a 10-minute window, excluding accelerations and decelerations. Fluctuations in the baseline FHR that are irregular in amplitude and frequency and are visually quantified as the amplitude of the peak-to-trough in bpm.
- Absent variability	Amplitude range undetectable.
- Minimal variability	Amplitude range visually detectable but $\leq$ 5 bpm. (Greater than undetectable but $\leq$ 5 bpm)
- Moderate variability	Amplitude range 6–25 bpm.
- Marked variability	Amplitude range > 25 bpm.
Acceleration	Visually apparent **abrupt** increase in FHR. *Abrupt* increase is defined as an increase from onset of acceleration to peak in < 30 seconds. Peak must be $\geq$15 bpm, and the acceleration must last $\geq$15 seconds from the onset to return. Acceleration lasting $\geq$10 minutes is defined as a baseline change. Before 32 weeks of gestation, accelerations are defined as having a peak $\geq$10 bpm and a duration of $\geq$ 10 seconds.
Prolonged acceleration	Acceleration $\geq$ 2 minutes but < 10 minutes in duration.
Early deceleration	Visually apparent, usually symmetrical, **gradual** decrease and return of the FHR associated with a uterine contraction. A *gradual* FHR decrease is defined as one from the onset to the FHR nadir of $\geq$30 seconds. The decrease in FHR is calculated from the onset to the nadir of the deceleration. The nadir of the deceleration occurs at the same time as the peak of the contraction. In most cases, the onset, nadir, and recovery of the deceleration are coincident with the beginning, peak, and ending of the contraction, respectively.
Late deceleration	Visually apparent, usually symmetrical, **gradual** decrease and return of the FHR associated with a uterine contraction. A *gradual* FHR decrease is defined as from the onset to the FHR nadir of $\geq$30 seconds. The decrease in FHR is calculated from the onset to the nadir of the deceleration. The deceleration is delayed in timing, with nadir of the deceleration occurring after the peak of the contraction. In most cases, the onset, nadir, and recovery of the deceleration occur after the beginning, peak, and ending of the contraction, respectively.
Variable deceleration	Visually apparent **abrupt** decrease in FHR. An *abrupt* FHR decrease is defined as from the onset of the deceleration to the beginning of the FHR nadir of < 30 seconds. The decrease in FHR is calculated from the onset to the nadir of the deceleration. The decrease in FHR is $\geq$15 bpm, lasting $\geq$15 seconds, and < 2 minutes in duration. When variable decelerations are associated with uterine contractions, their onset, depth, and duration commonly vary with successive uterine contractions.
Prolonged deceleration	Visually apparent decrease in FHR from the baseline that is $\geq$15 bpm, lasting $\geq$ 2 minutes, but < 10 minutes. A deceleration that lasts $\geq$ 10 minutes is baseline change.
Recurrent	Occurring with $\geq$ 50% of contractions in any 20 minute window.
Intermittent	Occurring with < 50% of contractions in any 20 minute window.
Sinusoidal pattern	Visually apparent, smooth, sine wave-like undulating pattern in FHR baseline with cycle frequency of 3-5/minute that persists for $\geq$ 20 minutes.

Adapted from Macones, G. A., Hankins, G. D., Spong, C. Y., Hauth, J. D., & Moore, T. (2008). The 2008 National Institute of Child Health Human Development workshop report on electronic fetal monitoring: Update on definitions, interpretations, and research guidelines. *Obstetrics & Gynecology, 112*, 661–666; and *Journal of Obstetric, Gynecologic and Neonatal Nursing, 37*, 510–515.

FIGURE 5-2 Visual Representation of Normal (Category I) FHR Characteristics by EFM

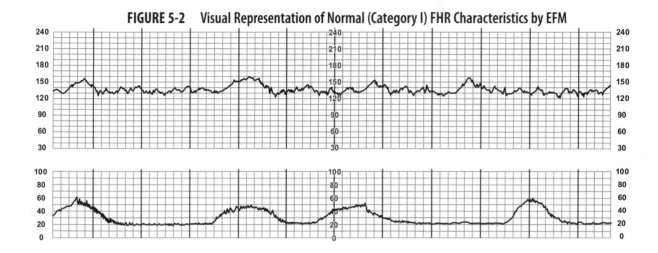

CHARACTERISTICS OF THE FHR AND UTERINE ACTIVITY

Baseline Fetal Heart Rate

The normal range for the baseline is 110 to 160 beats per minute (bpm) (Macones et al., 2008). With IA the baseline is established by counting the FHR at repeated intervals for at least 30 to 60 seconds after uterine contractions (Feinstein, Sprague, & Trepanier, 2008) (see also Chapter 4). With EFM the baseline is determined by evaluating the tracing over a time frame of at least 10 minutes to determine the approximate mean rate rounded to the closest 5-bpm interval. Thus, if the FHR varies between 120 and 130 bpm over a 10-minute period, the baseline is reported at 125 bpm. Determination of the baseline by EFM requires at least 2 minutes of interpretable FHR data in any 10-minute period and excludes areas recording periodic or episodic changes and marked variability. The sections of tracing used to determine the baseline do not necessarily need to be contiguous, but if there are not at least two minutes of interpretable baseline within a 10-minute period, the baseline is classified as indeterminate. When this occurs, the clinician may need to review other recent sections of the tracing to deter-mine the baseline. Regardless of monitoring method, a baseline rate less than 110 bpm for 10 minutes or longer is a bradycardia, and a baseline greater than 160 bpm for 10 minutes or longer is a tachycardia.

The baseline rate reflects integration of the many physiologic influences on the FHR but is predominantly controlled by the autonomic nervous system. The baseline rate is generated by the sinoatrial node of the fetal heart, which has an intrinsic pacemaker. The intrinsic rate in early gestation is under primary influence of the sympathetic nervous system and is there-fore slightly higher in the preterm fetus. As the fetus matures, parasympathetic influence becomes stronger, and the intrinsic rate decreases incrementally (Nageotte & Gilstrap, 2009). However, the difference in baseline FHR between 28 to 30 weeks gestation and term is approximately 10 bpm. Therefore, any preterm fetus with a baseline FHR greater than 160 bpm should be evaluated further to rule out fetal compromise, rather than assuming that the tachycardia is secondary to prematurity (Freeman et al., 2003).

Further discussion of the physiologic influences on the FHR, the fetal cardiac conduction system, and aberrations in conduction may be found in Chapters 2 and 12.

Tachycardia

Tachycardia represents increased sympathetic or decreased parasympathetic autonomic tone. Physiologic conditions that cause tachycardia may originate from the mother or the fetus, as illustrated in Table 5-2. A number of causes of tachycardia do not reflect a risk of acidemia, including the most common causes of fetal tachycardia in labor: maternal fever and medications affecting the heart rate (Garite, 2007; Parer & Nageotte, 2004). Maternal fever raises core temperature, and fetal tachycardia in the setting of maternal fever is believed to be a response to an increase in the fetal metabolic rate rather than an indicator of sepsis. The FHR is estimated to increase by 10 bpm for every 1° increase in maternal temperature and may also be mildly elevated in response to beta-sympathomimetics, atropine, scopolamine, and phenothiazines (Garite). Other maternal causes of tachycardia include hyperthyroidism (Garite) and dehydration. Premature fetuses may have baseline heart rates at or near the upper limits of the normal range (Freeman et al., 2003). Fetal tachyarrhythmias are discussed in Chapter 12.

Fetal tachycardia is not believed to indicate fetal hypoxia when it occurs in the absence of decelerations (Garite, 2007; Parer & Nageotte, 2004). However, tachycardia does increase myocardial oxygen demand, potentially taxing fetal reserve. Fetal tachycardia is sometimes seen as a normal fetal compensatory or recovery response from acute hypoxia or acidosis (Blackburn, 2007; Parer & Nageotte). This response is probably due to a rise in catecholamine levels following sympathetic nervous or adrenal stimulation and reduction in vagal activity when the hypoxia is relieved (Parer & Nageotte). In contrast, when fetal tachycardia is seen without FHR variability, it is difficult to determine whether the diminution in variability is a result of the rapid rate and sympathetic dominance versus a reflection of fetal central nervous system depression (Garite).

As with other FHR characteristics, assessment and management of fetal tachycardia is based on the associated baseline FHR variability and the presence or absence of accelerations and decelerations. Efforts should be taken to determine the underlying etiology, including evaluation of maternal temperature, hydration status, and medication history. Maximizing uteroplacental perfusion and avoiding excessive uterine activity are appropriate. The primary provider should be notified of fetal tachycardia. If tachycardia is observed in combination with recurrent late or variable decelerations or in combination with absent variability, a bedside evaluation by a physician is indicated. When tachycardia is observed in preterm fetuses, a bedside evaluation by a physician may also be indicated because preterm fetuses appear to have lower tolerance for stress as a result of the immaturity of their compensatory responses (Freeman et al., 2003).

Bradycardia

Fetal bradycardia may be due to normal physiologic variation, a change in maternal-fetal condition interrupting blood flow or gas exchange (e.g., a prolapsed cord, uterine rupture, abruptio placentae, maternal hypotension), or medication, hypoglycemia, hypothermia, and fetal bradyarrhythmias. One of the key issues in assessment of bradycardia is distinguishing it from a prolonged deceleration, which lasts at least 2 minutes but less than 10 minutes. This is important clinically

Table 5-2	Potential Causes of Fetal Tachycardia	
MATERNAL	**FETAL**	
Fever	Anemia	
Chorioamnionitis	Heart failure	
Dehydration	Hypoxia	
Hyperthyroidism	Infection or sepsis	
Illicit substance use	Tachyarrhythmia	
Medications:		
Beta-sympathomimetics		
Parasympatholytics		

Source: Freeman, Garite, & Nageotte, 2003; Garite, 2007.

because although baseline bradycardia above 90 bpm is usually innocuous, an acute prolonged deceleration may indicate significant fetal hypoxia (Garite, 2007).

When bradycardia is observed in the range of 90 to 110 bpm with moderate variability, it may represent normal physiologic variation in the rate of the intrinsic pacemaker in the sinoatrial node (Garite, 2007). Bradycardias in this range are not associated with hypoxemia when moderate variability is maintained (Freeman et al., 2003; Garite; Parer & Nageotte, 2004). Rarely, conditions such as heart block result in bradycardia and require further evaluation, but these do not represent an acute hypoxic insult to the fetus (Garite; Parer & Nageotte). Heart block is discussed in Chapter 12.

When a bradycardia is observed on admission, differentiation of maternal and fetal heart rates is essential to rule out the possibility that the maternal rate is being recorded with a dead fetus. This can occur with both Doppler and fetal spiral electrode recordings (Garite, 2007). It could also occur if maternal sounds are mistaken for fetal heart sounds on auscultation.

Sudden profound bradycardia is a medical emergency and may result from an acute drop in maternal oxygenation (maternal respiratory depression, apnea, or seizure), acute impairment of uteroplacental exchange (maternal hypotension, excessive uterine activity, or loss of placental area with uterine rupture or abruptio placentae), prolonged occlusion of the umbilical cord, or profound vagal stimulation (Parer & Nageotte, 2004). In clinical practice, intervention is often necessary before the distinction can be made between a new onset of true bradycardia and a prolonged deceleration (see Table 5-1). These terms are therefore often used interchangeably when discussing emergent response to a profound drop in the FHR in the clinical setting. Immediate vaginal examination to rule-out cord prolapse and rapid descent as causes of the bradycardia is indicated, as is mobilization of the team in preparation to expedite birth, if necessary. The clinical picture at the onset of the bradycardia and the depth, duration, and FHR variability are critical factors in assessing fetal condition and determining the need to proceed with emergent cesarean birth.

Several clinical factors affect the potential impact of bradycardia on fetal outcome. Studies comparing decision-to-incision times for emergency cesarean birth have shown that there is a time-dependent relationship between the onset of the bradycardia, the depth of the bradycardia, the presence or absence of variability, and the development of metabolic acidosis (Korhonen & Kariniemi, 1994). Because the fetus has minimal capacity to increase stroke volume, very low heart rates result in inadequate cardiac output for sustaining oxygenation and fetal life. Bradycardias with rates of less than 60 bpm, those accompanied by late or variable decelerations, and those with minimal or absent variability are most often associated with adverse outcome (Berkus et al., 1999; Low et al., 1999; Parer 1997).

The onset of a fetal bradycardia when a woman is laboring after a prior cesarean birth should cause concern for the onset of uterine rupture, signaling provider attendance at the bedside and preparation for an emergent cesarean birth. Bradycardia is the most common FHR pattern that develops during uterine rupture (Leung, Leung, & Paul, 1993; Ridgeway, Weyrich, & Benedetti, 2004). Leung et al. evaluated the fetal consequences of catastrophic uterine rupture when the diagnosis was made at the onset of a fetal bradycardia. All infants with a previously normal FHR pattern born within 17 minutes following the onset of a prolonged deceleration that progressed to bradycardia survived without significant perinatal morbidity. However, perinatal asphyxia could occur as early as 10 minutes after the onset of such bradycardias when these events were preceded by other signs of fetal stress, specifically "severe" late and variable decelerations.

Bradycardias occurring during the second stage of labor following a previously normal FHR pattern may be less concerning. These may be due to increased vagal tone related to head compression during descent (Parer & Nageotte, 2004) or, occasionally, umbilical cord occlusion. Prolonged deceleration or bradycardia may reflect a progressive decrease in fetal oxygenation. Fetal cardiac output is presumed to fail at rates below 60 bpm (Ball & Parer, 1992; Parer, 1997). However, if the variability remains moderate or minimal and the FHR does not fall below 90 to 100 bpm, expediting birth may not be warranted (Ball & Parer; Gull et al., 1996; Parer & Nageotte). In this situation, efforts to alleviate the bradycardia should be taken and maternal pushing should be modified to allow the fetus to recover (see Chapter 6 for discussion of physiologic management of the second stage of labor).

Baseline Fetal Heart Rate Variability

The term "variability" refers to the fluctuations in the FHR over time and is considered the most important predictor of adequate fetal oxygenation during labor (Dellinger, Boehm, & Crane, 2000; Martin, 1982; Parer et al., 2006). Variability is present when there are irregular fluctuations in the baseline FHR. Because the fluctuations in FHR are irregular in both amplitude and frequency, they are quantified by visual assessment of the amplitude of variation in the FHR, as described in Table 5-1 and illustrated in Figure 5-3. Clinically, variability is visually determined as a unit (Macones et al., 2008). This single visual assessment captures both the long-term cycling (long-term variability) and short term R-R interval changes in the fetal QRS cycle (short-term variability) that contribute to overall variability in the FHR. Variability by definition is a baseline FHR characteristic and therefore is assessed during baseline FHR, not during decelerations or accelerations. The sinusoidal FHR pattern does not fall into the standard classification of variability (Macones et al.).

Moderate Variability

The normal FHR tracing demonstrates moderate variability with an amplitude range of 6 to 25 bpm (Macones et al., 2008). Moderate variability pre-

sents visually as a rough line that is jagged and unpredictable (Fox et al., 2000). As discussed in Chapter 2, the presence of FHR variability represents an intact nervous pathway through the cerebral cortex, the midbrain, the vagus nerve, and the normal cardiac conduction system. The parasympathetic influence is the predominant determinant of variability. When the fetus is alert and active, the central nervous system responds with moderate FHR variability. The presence of moderate variability is one of the FHR characteristics that predict adequate fetal oxygenation; another is the presence of accelerations (Berkus et al., 1999). However, decreases in variability and absence of accelerations are not necessarily predictive of fetal hypoxemia. Fetal sleep states, some maternal medications or substance use, congenital neurologic abnormalities, and cardiac conduction defects can also depress FHR variability (Garite, 2007; Parer & Nageotte, 2004; Nageotte & Gilstrap, 2009).

Alterations in Fetal Heart Rate Variability
Minimal Variability

Minimal variability without concurrent decelerations is almost always unrelated to fetal acidemia (Parer & Livingston, 1990). When found in isolation, a decrease in FHR variability may be the result of a fetal sleep cycle or other nonhypoxic central nervous system depression such as maternal medication or substance use, and these possible causes should be ruled out prior to invasive intervention. The most common causes of a decrease in variability not associated with a risk for acidemia are centrally acting medications such as opioids, tranquilizers, magnesium sulfate, general anesthetics, and other analgesics administered to women during labor. Minimal variability is visually detectable, with an amplitude of 5 bpm or less (Macones et al., 2008). Visually, minimal variability may still display some jagged and unpredictable qualities or it may be more smooth and blunted in appearance (Fox et al., 2000).

Minimal (but not absent) variability is also seen during fetal sleep cycles. During quiet sleep, a fetus may demonstrate minimal FHR

FIGURE 5-3　Visual Variability Scale

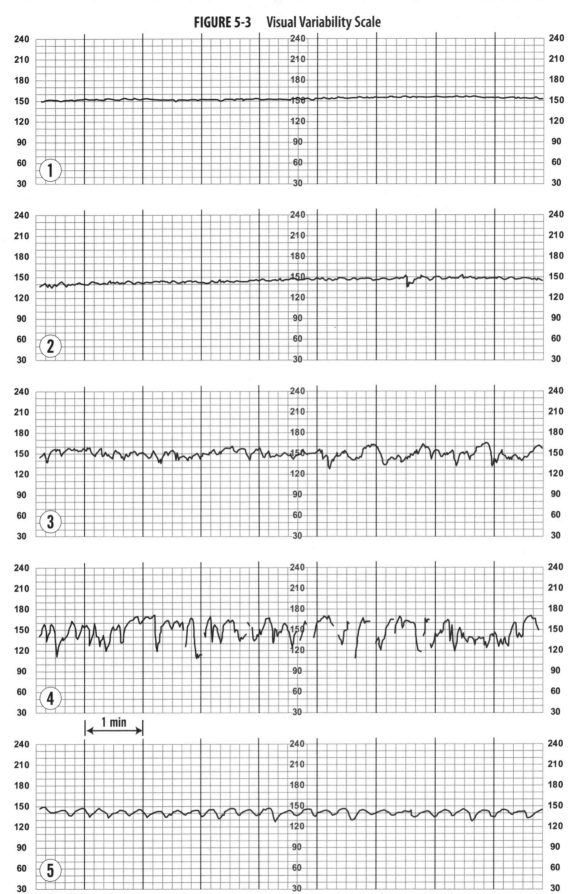

NOTE: Varying degrees of FHR variability. 1. undetectable; 2. minimal; 3. moderate; 4. marked; and 5. sinusoidal pattern. Original scaling, 30 bmp per cm vertical axis, and paper speed 3 cm-min^{-1} horizontal axis.

From: "Electronic Fetal Heart Rate Monitoring: Research Guidelines for Interpretation," National Institutes of Child Health and Human Development Research Planning Workshop, 1997, *Journal of Obstetric, Gynecologic and Neonatal Nursing, 26,* 635-640.

variability and no accelerations (Parer & Nageotte, 2004). At term, studies suggest that the mean length of the fetal quiet sleep is 23 minutes, but this behavioral state may persist for as long as 75 minutes (Patrick, Campbell, Carmichael, Natale, & Richardson, 1982; Timor-Tritsch, Dierker, Hertz, Deagan, & Rosen, 1978). In this situation, the clinician should review the preceding hour or two of FHR tracing for the presence of accelerations and FHR variability and absence of late or variable decelerations and bradycardia. However, when a woman first presents to the birth suite with minimal or absent FHR variability, there is no prior tracing to review. Therefore, prompt assessment of fetal well-being is indicated because it is not known whether the decrease in variability was preceded by other FHR changes indicative of hypoxic stress. Interviewing the mother about perceived fetal movement over the past several hours and days or performing vibroacoustic stimulation per unit protocol may provide additional information to differentiate between normal quiet and active sleep cycles versus insufficient fetal oxygenation. FHR tracings presenting minimal or absent variability without other FHR abnormalities may reflect a preexisting fetal neurologic insult or the presence of a major neurologic or cardiac congenital abnormality (MacLennan, 1999).

Absent Variability

Absent variability in conjunction with variable or late decelerations or bradycardia is presumed to reflect a significant risk for fetal acidemia (Parer et al., 2006; Paul, Suidan, Yeh, Schifrin, & Hon, 1975) and requires prompt evaluation (Macones et al., 2008). Despite low positive predictive value, this combination of characteristics is the most sensitive indicator of metabolic acidemia in a fetus (Beard et al., 1971; Clark et al., 1984; Low et al., 1999; Parer et al., 2006). Intrauterine resuscitation and interventions to expedite birth are warranted if fetal well-being cannot be rapidly confirmed (Parer & Ikeda, 2007). As mentioned previously, a tracing with absent FHR

variability in the context of a normal baseline rate and the absence of decelerations may represent a preexisting neurologic insult to the fetus (MacLennan, 1999). Absent variability has an amplitude change that is undetectable. The FHR tracing with absent variability is smooth, blunted, and flat in appearance.

Marked Variability

Marked variability is relatively uncommon, occurring in approximately 2% of FHR tracings (O'Brien-Abel & Benedetti, 1992). The etiology of marked variability is unclear; the increase in variability is presumed to result from an increase in alpha-adrenergic activity, which causes selective vasoconstriction of certain vascular beds. Marked variability was first described by Hammacher, Huter, Bokelmann, and Werners (1968), who found the pattern associated with low Apgar scores and poor neonatal outcome; however, it is unclear whether the pattern was present immediately before birth or whether it preceded an evolution to a more serious pattern (Hammacher et al.).

In fetal sheep and monkeys, marked variability has been observed with episodes of acute hypoxemia or hypoxia (Dalton, Dawes, & Patrick, 1977; Martin, 1978; Parer et al., 1980). Other studies of human fetuses have associated marked variability with prolonged pregnancies (Cibils, 1975; O'Brien-Abel & Benedetti, 1992), maternal ephedrine administration (O'Brien-Abel & Benedetti; Wright, Shnider, Levinson, Rolbin, & Parer, 1981), fetal breathing (Dawes, Visser, Goodman, & Levine, 1981), and decreased uteroplacental perfusion or umbilical cord compression (Leveno et al., 1984; O'Brien-Abel & Benedetti). Marked variability has an amplitude range greater than 25 bpm and a chaotic appearance.

Interventions to eliminate marked variability may include maternal lateral positioning and correcting any maternal hypotension or excessive uterine activity (Parer & Nageotte, 2004). In the absence of abnormal FHR heart rate changes, marked variability is not associated with acidemia as judged by fetal blood pH or Apgar scores (O'Brien-Abel & Benedetti, 1992; Wright et al., 1981).

Periodic and Episodic Changes

Characteristic changes from the FHR baseline are classified as either periodic (occurring in association with uterine contractions) or episodic (not associated with uterine contractions). These changes include accelerations and decelerations, both of which may occur in an episodic or periodic fashion. In EFM, periodic and episodic changes are classified by the shape of the onset of the waveform, which is described as either "abrupt" or "gradual." The difference between abrupt and gradual onset is quantified by whether the onset to nadir or peak of the FHR change occurs in less than 30 seconds (abrupt) or takes 30 seconds or longer (gradual) (Macones et al.,

2008). The onset, offset, and waveform shape of periodic and episodic changes are generally determined in reference to the adjacent baseline FHR. With both IA and EFM, any FHR change with a duration 10 minutes or longer is classified as a change in baseline rate rather than a periodic or episodic change (Macones et al.), although in practice clinicians do not necessarily wait to make this differentiation, especially in the case of prolonged decelerations.

Accelerations

Accelerations are audible (IA) or visually apparent (EFM) abrupt increases in the FHR above baseline (see Table 5-1 and Figure 5-4). With EFM in term fetuses, accelerations peak at least 15 bpm above baseline and last at least 15 seconds from their onset to the point at which the FHR returns to baseline. Before 32 weeks gestation, accelerations are defined as peaking at least 10

FIGURE 5-4 Accelerations

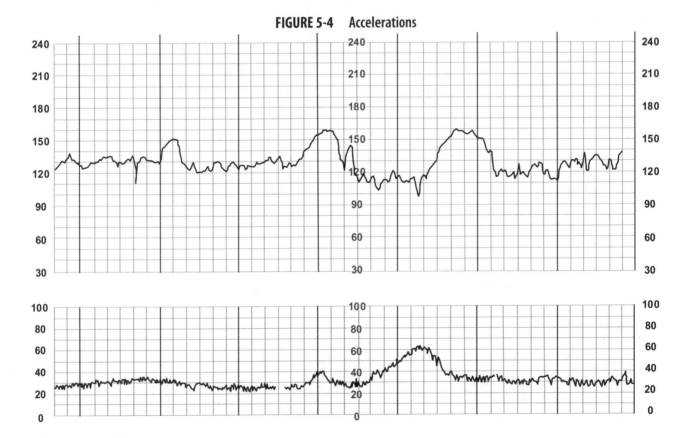

bpm above baseline and lasting at least 10 seconds (Macones et al., 2008). Accelerations, whether spontaneous or induced, are predictive of adequate central fetal oxygenation (Nageotte & Gilstrap, 2009), and a pH of at least 7.19, therefore, they rule out acidemia at the time they are observed (Porter & Clark, 1999; Williams & Galerneau, 2003). Accelerations lasting 2 to 10 minutes are termed prolonged.

Decreases in Fetal Heart Rate

When auscultation is used to monitor the FHR, audible decreases in rate may be noted, and these are interpreted in the context of the overall clinical picture. There is no established nomenclature for describing FHR decreases noted with IA. When decreases in FHR are auscultated, interventions to promote maternal-fetal oxygenation are indicated, as is ongoing or additional assessment to clarify

FHR findings and establish fetal well-being (Feinstein et al., 2008).

Decelerations

With the NICHD terminology, four types of decelerations are used to describe decreases in FHR recorded via EFM: early, late, variable, and prolonged (see Table 5-1). Decelerations are defined as *recurrent* when they occur with at least 50% of the contractions in a 20-minute period, and *intermittent* when they occur with less than 50% of contractions in a 20-minute period (Macones et al., 2008).

Early Decelerations

Early decelerations are visually apparent gradual decreases in the FHR (Figure 5-5). The onset, nadir, and recovery of early decelerations generally occur coincident with the onset, peak, and recovery of uterine contractions. Early de-

FIGURE 5-5   Early Decelerations

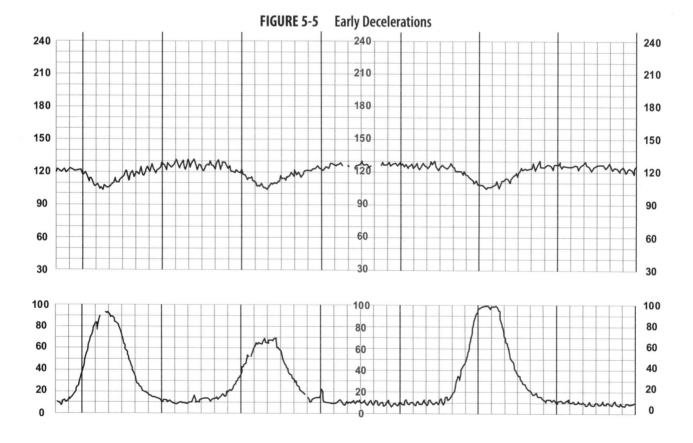

celerations are typically symmetrical in shape (Macones et al., 2008).

These decelerations are believed to represent a vagal response to a cerebral redistribution of blood flow caused by compression of the fetal head (Freeman et al., 2003). When the contraction occurs, the fetal head is subjected to pressure, which stimulates the vagus nerve. The heart rate begins to drop at the onset of the contraction when the head compression begins and returns to the baseline rate at the end of the contraction when the head is no longer compressed. Early decelerations are often said to "mirror" the contraction causing them. They can be present in a normal FHR pattern (Macones et al., 2008), are considered benign, and no intervention is needed.

Late Decelerations

Late decelerations are visually apparent gradual decreases in the FHR that are associated with uterine contractions (Figure 5-6). Late decelera-

tions are delayed in timing, meaning the deceleration reaches its nadir (lowest point) after the peak of the contraction. In most cases the onset, nadir, and recovery of the deceleration occur after the respective onset, peak, and resolution of the contraction. Late decelerations are typically symmetrical in shape (Macones et al., 2008).

Late decelerations occur on a continuum from those seen in conjunction with moderate baseline variability to those presenting with minimal and absent variability. They are believed to reflect the fetal response to transient or chronic uteroplacental insufficiency (Freeman et al., 2003; Martin, 1978; Nageotte & Gilstrap, 2009). When late decelerations are accompanied by moderate variability, this is believed to reflect a chemoreceptor-mediated response to a transient hypoxemic event (i.e., reversible reduction in uterine blood flow). In this situation, the decelerations are thought to occur when uterine blood flow decreases from baseline, resulting in decreased oxygenation of the fetal blood. The resulting hypoxemia is de-

FIGURE 5-6   Late Decelerations

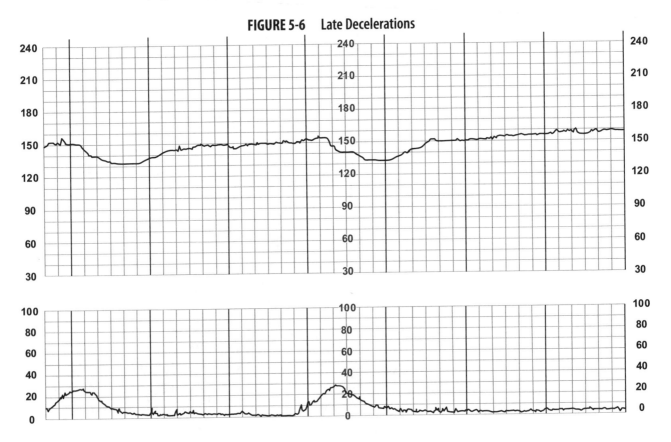

tected by chemoreceptors and ultimately results in firing of the vagus nerve and slowing of the fetal heart. Because the detection of hypoxemia by the chemoreceptors takes time, the deceleration is delayed in timing relative to the uterine contraction (Nageotte & Gilstrap). Potential causes of both transient and chronic uteroplacental insufficiency are listed in Table 5-3.

It is important to remember that moderate variability is predictive of adequate fetal oxygenation *at that moment in time* (Macones et al., 2008; Garite, 2007; Low et al., 1999; Nageotte & Gilstrap, 2009; Parer et al., 2006; Williams & Galerneau, 2003). Thus, tracings with moderate variability and recurrent late decelerations reflect a compensatory response to stress, and such patterns are not associated with significant acidemia (Parer et al.). In the context of moderate variability, late decelerations are considered neurogenic in origin and are typically amenable to intrauterine resuscitation techniques directed toward maximizing uterine blood flow (see Chapter 6). Such decelerations are likely to resolve when the source of hypoxemia (e.g., maternal hypotension or excessive uterine activity) is resolved (Parer, 1997; Parer & Nageotte, 2004), as illustrated in the Dynamic Physiologic Response Model (Figure 5-7). Efforts should therefore be taken to eliminate the cause and prevent progression to patterns that are associated with significant acidemia. Some experts also recommend repeated assessments of fetal acid-base status whenever recurrent late decelerations are present (Freeman et al., 2003). (See Chapter 7 for a discussion of fetal acid-base assessment.)

When recurrent late decelerations occur in the context of absent or minimal variability they are believed to reflect direct myocardial hypoxic depression and presumed to represent a risk of significant acidemia (Berkus et al., 1999; Cibils, 1975; Martin, 1978; Parer, 1997; Parer et al., 2006). Therefore, late decelerations in the context of minimal or absent variability warrant intervention to expedite birth if fetal well-being cannot be

Table 5-3	Maternal Factors Potentially Related to Uteroplacental Insufficiency
FACTOR	**RELATED CAUSES OR CHARACTERISTICS**
Hypotension	• Supine positioning • Regional anesthesia (sympathetic blockade) • Maternal trauma or hemorrhage
Hypertension	• Gestational or chronic hypertension • Medications or substances such as cocaine and methamphetamine
Placental changes affecting gas exchange	• Postmaturity • Premature aging of the placenta • Placental infarctions • Placenta previa • Small or malformed placenta
Decreased maternal hemoglobin or decreased oxygen saturation	• Hyperventilation or hypoventilation • Cardiopulmonary disease • Severe anemia
Tachysystole	• Oxytocin, misoprostol, or prostaglandin administration
Other high risk conditions of pregnancy	• Preexisting chronic disease • Maternal smoking • Poor maternal nutrition • Multiple gestation

positively and rapidly ascertained (Garite, 2007; Parer & Ikeda, 2007; Parer & Nageotte, 2004). A bedside evaluation by the primary provider should be obtained simultaneously with intrauterine resuscitation measures, and appropriate personnel should be mobilized so that the team will be ready if a decision is made to proceed with an operative birth (Fox et al., 2000; Parer & Ikeda). Implementation of intrauterine resuscitation techniques should not delay team activation to expedite birth (Fox et al.; Simpson, 2008b).

FIGURE 5-7 Dynamic Physiologic Response Model

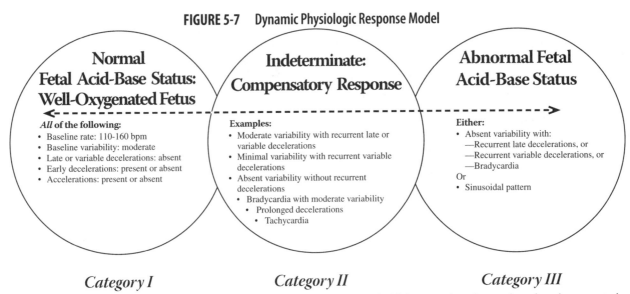

NOTE: This diagram is not intended to be all inclusive. All patterns must be treated with interventions that are based on the suspected underlying physiologic causes and ongoing evaluation of individual patient presentation.

Variable Decelerations

Variable decelerations are visually apparent, abrupt decreases in the FHR that may occur with or without relationship to uterine contractions (Figure 5-8). Variable decelerations decrease at least 15 bpm below baseline and last for at least 15 seconds but less than 2 minutes (Macones et al., 2008). They tend to vary in shape, depth, and duration and in their timing in relation to uterine contractions. Variable decelerations are the most frequently seen FHR deceleration pattern in labor (Freeman et al.). The clinical significance of features such as slow return to baseline, variations in rate during the deceleration, and associated accelerations ("shoulders" and "overshoots") accompanying variable decelerations has not been established (Macones et al., 2008).

The abrupt FHR change characteristic of variable decelerations is most commonly caused by occlusion of umbilical blood flow. When the umbilical cord is compressed, the cessation of blood flow generates an increase in systemic vascular resistance and an increase in blood pressure that is detected by the fetal baroreceptors, triggering a vagal response and protective slowing of the FHR. Because the primary response is baroreceptor mediated rather than chemoreceptor mediated, the change in the heart rate is rapid (Freeman et al., 2003; Garite, 2007), although chemoreceptors are also believed to have a role in variable decelerations (Freeman et al.).

Lee, Di Loreto, and O'Lane's (1975) classic illustration of a variable deceleration (Figure 5-9) depicts the relationship between the variable deceleration, uterine contraction, umbilical cord compression, and fetal blood pressure. As a contraction begins, partial umbilical cord compression causes occlusion of the low-pressure vein and decreased return of blood to the fetal heart, resulting in decreased cardiac output, hypotension, and a compensatory FHR acceleration (Freeman et al., 2003; James et al., 1976; Lee et al.). With complete umbilical cord occlusion, the two umbilical arteries also become occluded, resulting in sudden fetal hypertension, stimulation of the baroreceptors, and a sudden drop in FHR (Freeman et al.; Lee & Hon, 1963).

As the contraction begins to dissipate, the umbilical arteries open first, and a transient increase in FHR (a "secondary acceleration") may

FIGURE 5-8   Variable Decelerations

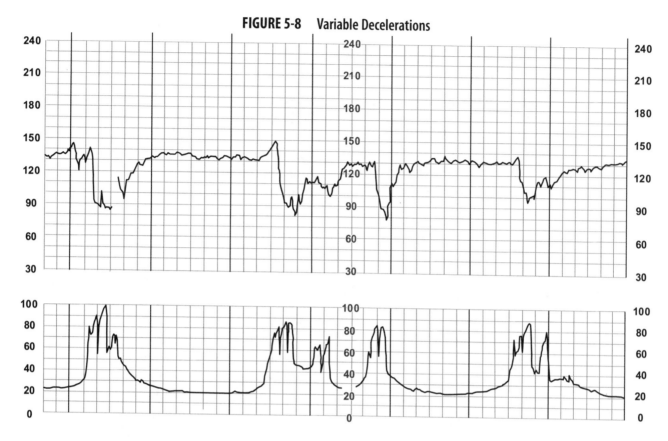

be seen. Finally, the contraction subsides and all three umbilical vessels are open, returning the FHR to predeceleration values. When variable decelerations occur during the second stage of labor, they may also be caused by the marked head compression and resultant intense vagal stimulation that occurs during rapid descent (Ball & Parer, 1992; Parer & Nageotte, 2004). Variable decelerations vary in all aspects of their appearance except one: the initial FHR change is abrupt.

As with late decelerations, interpretation of tracings with recurrent variable decelerations hinges on the assessment of the accompanying baseline FHR variability and the evolution of the tracing over time in the context of the overall clinical picture. When moderate variability is present, the fetus is adequately oxygenated at that moment in time. In this context the decelerations represent a physiologic response to intermittent fetal stress (see Figure 5-7) and can be followed as long as the baseline FHR is

within normal range, moderate variability is maintained (Freeman et al., 2003; Garite, 2007; Parer & Ikeda, 2007; Parer et al., 2006), and there is adequate recovery time for fetal oxygenation between contractions (Bakker, Kurver, Kuik, & Van Geijn, 2007). It is important to keep in mind that although variable decelerations are common in labor and especially in the second stage, the underlying conditions producing the decelerations can tax fetal reserve. It is appropriate to modify or eliminate these stressors whenever possible with measures such as position changes, amnioinfusion (ACOG, 2005b), decreasing or discontinuing oxytocin infusion, and modified pushing (Simpson & James, 2005) (see Chapter 6 for further discussion of interventions).

Prolonged Decelerations

Prolonged decelerations are visually apparent decreases in the FHR that drop at least 15 bpm below baseline and last at least 2 minutes but less than 10 minutes from their onset to the return to baseline (Macones et al., 2008) (Figure 5-10).

Prolonged decelerations can be caused by more sustained instances of any of the previously

FIGURE 5-9   Fetal Heart Rate (FHR) and Fetal Systemic Blood Pressure (FSBP) Occurring during a Uterine Contraction (UC) with Compression of Umbilical Vein (UV) and Umbilical Artery (UA)

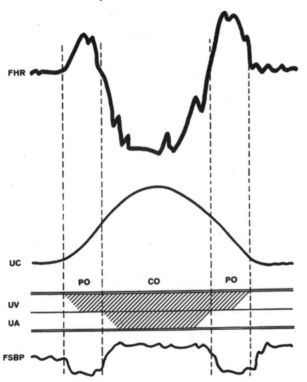

NOTE: From "A study of fetal heart rate acceleration patterns," by C. V. Lee, P. C. Di Loreto, and J. M. O'Lane, *Obstetrics and Gynecology, 50*, p. 142. Copyright 1975 by the American College of Obstetricians and Gynecologists. Reprinted with permission.

discussed deceleration mechanisms (uteroplacental insufficiency, umbilical cord compression, or head compression), resulting in a profound response of a more sustained deceleration. FHR recovery from a prolonged deceleration may be abrupt or gradual. Prolonged decelerations may occur in association with factors affecting uteroplacental perfusion or gas exchange, umbilical perfusion, or stimulation of the vagus nerve, as illustrated in Table 5-4.

Key factors in assessing prolonged decelerations include the baseline variability immediately preceding and following the decelerations, frequency of occurrence, duration of decelerations, and the individual characteristics of the overall clinical picture as well as institutional capacity to expedite birth should variability decrease or a prolonged deceleration evolve to frank bradycardia. Prolonged decelerations that are not recurrent and are preceded and followed by an FHR with a normal baseline and moderate variability are not associated with fetal hypoxemia of clinical significance. Management considerations are similar to those discussed previously in relation to fetal bradycardia, and in clinical practice clinicians may not wait to differentiate between the two before initiating intrauterine resuscitation measures and mobilizing a team response.

Quantification of Decelerations

For documentation purposes it is sufficient to report the type of decelerations observed and the clinician's overall assessment of fetal status with-

Table 5-4	Potential Causes of Prolonged Decelerations		
INTERRUPTION OF UTEROPLACENTAL PERFUSION OR EXCHANGE		**INTERRUPTION OF UMBILICAL BLOOD FLOW**	**VAGAL STIMULATION**
Tachysystole Acute maternal hypotension Acute maternal hypoxia (e.g., seizure, respiratory, or cardiac arrest) Abruptio placentae Uterine rupture		Cord compression Cord prolapse Ruptured vasa previa	Profound head compression Rapid fetal descent

Source: Parer & Nageotte, 2004; Simpson, 2008.

FIGURE 5-10   Prolonged Deceleration

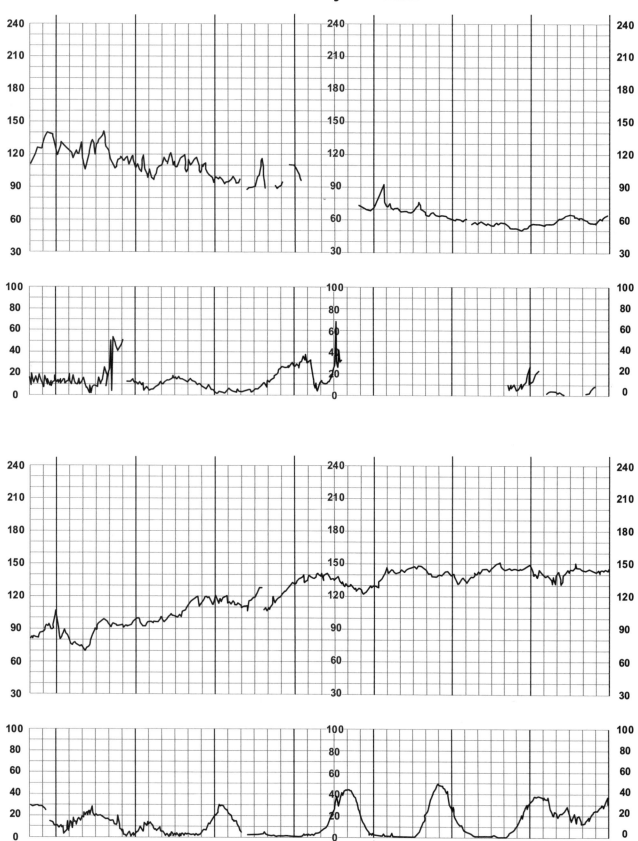

out a written description of depth or duration of decelerations when this information is already recorded by an EFM tracing (see Chapter 8 for further discussion of documentation issues). In verbal communication regarding FHR findings, inclusion of more detail regarding depth and duration may be needed. Although the NICHD report discusses quantification of decelerations, it does not specify how depth and duration of decelerations should be interpreted (Macones et al., 2008).

Uterine Activity

During the intrapartum period, the FHR is interpreted in relation to uterine activity, and the degree of uterine activity is a central component of the overall clinical picture. Therefore, interpretation of FHR patterns cannot occur in isolation of evaluation of uterine activity, which includes a complete assessment of four components of the uterine contractions: (1) frequency, (2) duration, (3) intensity, and (4) uterine resting tone between contractions. These assessments can be made by either palpation alone, or by palpation in conjunction with an external tocodynamometer or intrauterine pressure catheter (IUPC), as discussed in Chapter 4.

Contraction frequency is measured from the beginning of one contraction to the beginning of the next and is described in minutes. Duration is the length of the contraction and is described in seconds. Intensity refers to the strength of the contraction. Intensity is described as mild, moderate, or strong by palpation or in millimeters of mercury (mm Hg) if an IUPC is used. Uterine resting tone is assessed in the absence of contractions or between contractions. By direct palpation, resting tone is described as soft or hard, and via IUPC it is measured in mm Hg. As with any procedure, the least invasive approach is preferred unless there is a clear maternal-fetal indication for internal monitoring.

After the frequency, duration, intensity, and resting tone have been determined, one can as-

sess the adequacy of the uterine activity. Normal contraction frequency in the active phase of labor is every 2 to 3 minutes (ACOG, 2003). Some uterine activity patterns are dysfunctional or inadequate for generating progress in labor (Figure 5-11). Assessments of maternal pain, coping, and uterine tenderness also contribute to the interpretation of uterine activity, labor progress, and the overall clinical picture.

Uterine activity is classified by the number of contractions present in a 10 minute period, averaged over 30 minutes (Macones et al., 2008):

- Normal: ≤5 contractions in 10 minutes.
- Tachysystole: >5 contractions in 10 minutes. Tachysystole is further qualified by the presence or absence of associated FHR decelerations.

This definition of tachysystole is primarily based on expert opinion, as there are only a few published studies in the literature evaluating the affects of uterine activity on fetal well-being. Emerging evidence (Bakker, Kurver, Kuik, & Van Geijn, 2007; Simpson & James, 2008) suggests that less than five contractions in 10 minutes may be optimal for supporting fetal well-being. Although tachysystole (Figure 5-12) can be spontaneous as a result of endogenous maternal oxytocin or prostaglandins, it is more often seen during exogenous stimulation with agents used in cervical ripening and induction and augmentation of labor (Crane, Young, Butt, Bennett, & Hutchens, 2001). The 2008 NICHD recommendations indicate that hyperstimulation and hypercontractility are not defined and both terms should be abandoned (Macones et al., 2008).

It is important to recognize that tachsystole increases the amount of time that blood in the intervillous spaces is in stasis, reducing the potential for maternal-fetal exchange of respiratory gases. These conditions result in physiologic stress for the fetus, whether or not associated FHR decelerations are present, and should be avoided. Although data on the effects of uterine activity are limited, increased uterine

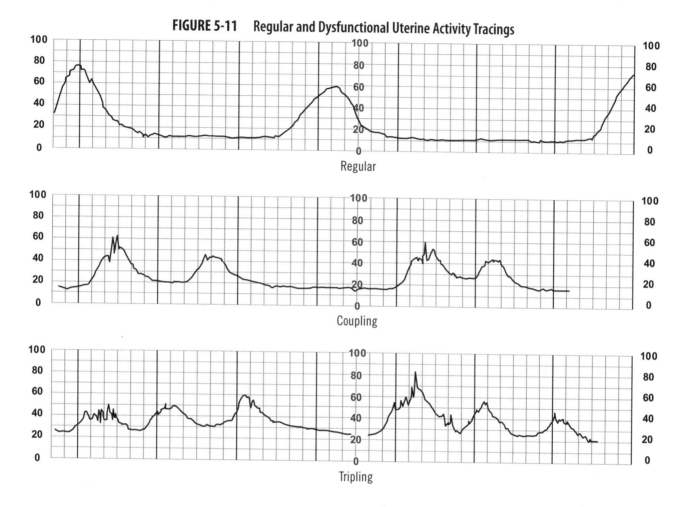

FIGURE 5-11   Regular and Dysfunctional Uterine Activity Tracings

Regular

Coupling

Tripling

activity in labor has been linked to an increased risk for umbilical artery acidemia at birth (Bakker et al., 2007). If tachysystole occurs during oxytocin administration and the FHR is normal, the infusion should be managed as suggested in the protocol discussed in Chapter 6. If the FHR is not normal during oxytocin administration, the infusion should be discontinued until the FHR and uterine contraction pattern return to normal. Similarly, in the event of excessive uterine activity, additional doses of other uterotonic agents (e.g., dinoprostone [Cervidil, Prepidil] or misoprostol) should be delayed until the FHR is normal and the uterine contraction pattern returns to normal frequency, duration, and resting tone. A comprehensive protocol for the management of oxytocin-induced tachysystole is presented in Chapter 6.

"Coupling" or "tripling" refers to a pattern of two or three contractions with little or no interval followed by a regular interval of approximately 2 to 5 minutes (see Figure 5-11). This pattern may be indicative of a dysfunctional labor process and saturation or down regulation of uterine oxytocin receptor sites in response to excess exposure to oxytocin (Dawood, 1995; Phaneuf, Rodriguez-Linares, TambyRaja, MacKenzie, & Lopez-Bernal, 2000; Zeeman, Khan-Dawood, & Dawood, 1997). Therefore, interventions to resolve the dysfunctional labor pattern do not include further increases in the oxytocin rate. Instead, an oxytocin rate decrease or discontinuation along with an intravenous fluid bolus may be therapeutic in creating conditions in which oxytocin receptor sites are again responsive to exogenous oxytocin for labor induction or augmentation.

FIGURE 5-12 Tachysystole

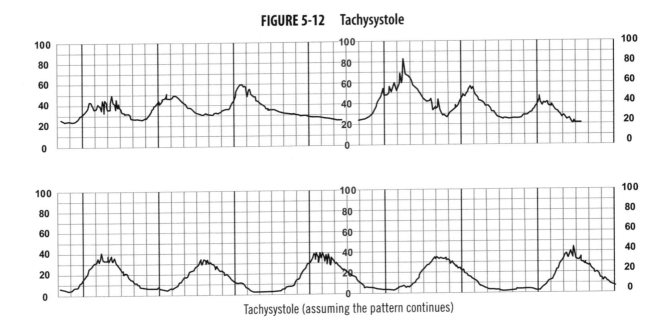

Tachysystole (assuming the pattern continues)

Unusual Fetal Heart Rate Characteristics

Whenever an unusual tracing is observed from the beginning of EFM, the possibility of a previously unobserved hypoxic insult or the presence of a congenital fetal anomaly should be considered. An initial tracing with minimal or absent variability without accelerations or with other unusual characteristics should prompt an urgent assessment of fetal well-being. This may include fetal stimulation, an ultrasound evaluation, or other assessments as indicated by the overall clinical picture. Although most fetuses with congenital anomalies have normal FHR tracings (Nageotte & Gilstrap, 2009), hydrocephalic and anencephalic fetuses may present with an unusual FHR patterns that do not fit any category or definition (Freeman et al., 2003). If possible, an ultrasound examination may be performed to rule out gross anomalies as the cause of the pattern, although results may be inconclusive. An anomaly that affects the fetal central nervous system most likely will have an impact on FHR variability or on the ability of the fetal cardiac system to accelerate and decelerate. Unusual decelerations with a flat, fixed rate may be seen.

Sinusoidal Heart Rate Pattern

A sinusoidal fetal heart rate pattern is a visually apparent undulating smooth sine wave-like pattern in the FHR baseline with a cycle frequency of 3-5 per minute which persists for *at least* 20 minutes (Macones et al., 2008) (Figure 5-13). There are no accelerations and no response to uterine contractions, fetal movement, or stimulation (Modanlou & Freeman, 1982).

The sinusoidal FHR pattern is a rare occurrence (Modanlou & Murata, 2004). First identified in 1972, the sinusoidal FHR pattern was described as an undulating wave alternating with a flat or smooth baseline FHR in severely affected, Rh-sensitized and dying fetuses (Manseau, Vaquier, Chavinié, & Sureau, 1972). The FHR pattern was named "sinusoidal" because of its sine waveform. The etiology of the sinusoidal heart rate includes severe fetal anemia as a result of Rh isoimmunization, massive fetomaternal hemorrhage, twin-to-twin transfusion syndrome, ruptured vasa previa, and fetal intracranial hemorrhage (Modanlou & Murata). Other fetal conditions that have been reported to be associated with sinusoidal heart rate patterns include fetal hypoxia or asphyxia,

FIGURE 5-13   Sinusoidal Fetal Heart Rate Pattern

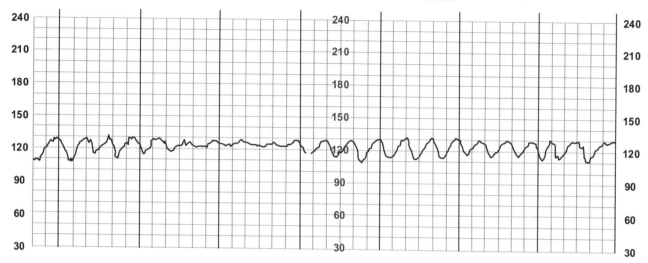

FIGURE 5-13   Sinusoidal Fetal Heart Rate Pattern

fetal infection, fetal cardiac anomalies, and gastroschisis. Whatever the pathogenesis, a true sinusoidal heart rate pattern is an extremely significant finding that implies fetal jeopardy and impending fetal death (Modanlou & Murata).

A sinusoidal-appearing FHR pattern has been noted to follow the maternal administration of some opioids (especially butorphanol and fentanyl), fetal sleep cycles, and thumb sucking or rhythmic movements of the fetal mouth (Modanlou & Murata, 2004). As the medication is excreted or the fetus awakens or stops sucking, the sinusoidal-appearing FHR resolves, thus giving it the name of "pseudosinusoidal" or "medication-induced sinusoidal." Usually this undulating FHR pattern is of short duration and is both preceded and followed by an FHR with normal characteristics (Modanlou & Murata). No treatment is indicated for these sinusoidal-appearing patterns when history of maternal opioid administration is clearly related to the subsequent FHR pattern.

Fetal Arrhythmias

During the past decade, fetal cardiac arrhythmias have been recognized with increasing frequency at routine prenatal visits (Kleinman & Nehgme, 2004). The most common finding is the impression that the fetal heart is intermittently "skipping" beats. In most cases, this rep-

resents either a pause following an extrasystole that has not reset the sinus node pacemaker or an extrasystole occurring early in the cardiac cycle with a stroke volume that is inadequate to produce a detectable Doppler signal (Kleinman & Nehgme; Kleinman, Nehgme, & Copel, 2004). Although the extrasystoles may be a source of anxiety for the parents, they usually resolve spontaneously later during pregnancy or during the first few days after birth.

Sustained fetal tachyarrhythmias or bradyarrhythmias are rare. However, when detected during routine prenatal visits, they require multidisciplinary evaluation. The most common tachyarrhythmia is supraventricular tachycardia (Kleinman et al., 2004). Typically, supraventricular tachycardia occurs at a rate of about 240 to 260 bpm with minimal or absent variability (Copel, Friedman, & Kleinman, 1997; Kleinman & Nehgme, 2004; Kleinman et al.). The most important sustained bradyarrhythmia is complete heart block, or atrioventricular dissociation, in which the ventricular rate ranges from 40 to 80 bpm (Kleinman & Nehgme). Assessment of fetal well-being may be difficult in the presence of an arrhythmia because of the inability to see a consistent baseline or evaluate variability. Evaluation of fetal arrhythmias is discussed further in Chapter 12.

INTERPRETATION OF ELECTRONIC FETAL MONITORING FINDINGS ACROSS THE CONTINUUM

FHR patterns present on a continuum from those displaying the classic characteristics of a normal tracing predictive of a normally oxygenated fetus, through tracings that suggest some degree of relative hypoxemia or hypoxia, to those tracings that experts agree are predictive of significant risk for fetal compromise resulting from inadequate tissue oxygenation and metabolic acidosis.

The 2008 NICHD guidelines suggest a three-tiered system for interpretation of FHR patterns: category I (normal), category II (indeterminate), and category III (abnormal) (Box 5-2).

A normal (category I) FHR tracing exhibits a baseline rate of 110-160 bpm, moderate baseline FHR variability, and no late or variable decelerations. Normal tracings may or may not exhibit accelerations or early decelerations. Experts generally agree that this type of FHR tracing is strongly predictive of normal fetal acid-base status at the time of observation (Macones et al., 2008). Normal FHR tracings may be followed with routine measures to support labor progress, maternal coping, and fetal oxygenation (see Chapter 6). At the other end of the continuum from a completely normal tracing are abnormal (category III) FHR patterns predictive of abnormal fetal acid-base status at the time of observation. Category III FHR tracings are those exhibiting a sinusoidal pattern or exhibiting *absent variability* in conjunction with bradycardia or recurrent late or variable decelerations (Macones et al.). These patterns require prompt evaluation in conjunction with attempts to expeditiously resolve the abnormal findings.

A majority of intrapartum FHR tracings may be classified as category II (indeterminate), which includes all FHR tracings that do not meet criteria for category I or III classification (Macones et al., 2008). Category II includes (but is not limited to) tracings with *moderate or minimal variability* and recurrent late or variable decelerations, baseline tachycardia, marked

variability, prolonged decelerations, and the absence of an acceleration response to fetal stimulation. Indeterminate tracings minimally require heightened surveillance and ongoing reevaluation. In most cases supportive actions to promote maternal and fetal adaptation to labor are also indicated, as described in Chapter 6.

Electronic FHR Patterns and Fetal Acid-Base Status

A review of the published literature to date on the association between FHR patterns and fetal acidemia found moderate FHR variability was strongly (98%) associated with an umbilical pH greater than 7.15 or newborn vigor (5-minute Apgar score of 7 or higher) (Parer, et al., 2006). In this review the most consistent predictor of newborn acidemia was absent or minimal FHR variability with recurrent late or variable decelerations (although the association was only 23%), and there was a positive relationship between the degree of acidemia and the depth of decelerations or bradycardia. The authors therefore conclude that in the absence of a catastrophic event or a sudden profound bradycardia, newborn acidemia (expressed as decreasing variability in combination with decelerations) develops over a period of time approximating one hour (Parer et al.), suggesting that there is usually time for attempting to improve fetal oxygenation through intrauterine resuscitation measures.

Many fetuses have FHR findings that are somewhere on the continuum between normal (normal baseline rate with moderate variability and no late or variable decelerations) and abnormal (absent variability with recurrent late or variable decelerations or bradycardia), but there has not been general agreement among experts on clinical management of these tracings (Macones et al., 2008; NICHD, 1997). Parer and colleagues (Fox et al., 2000; Parer & Nageotte, 2004; Nageotte & Gilstrap, 2009) have suggested that when moderate variability is present, these tracings are not associated with fetal morbidity because although they reflect the presence of fetal stress, the maintenance of moderate variability

BOX 5-2 2008 Three-Tier Fetal Heart Rate Interpretation System

CATEGORY I
*Category I fetal heart rate (FHR) tracings include **all** of the following:*
- Baseline rate: 110–160 beats per minute (bpm)
- Baseline FHR variability: moderate
- Late or variable decelerations: absent
- Early decelerations: present or absent
- Accelerations: present or absent

CATEGORY II
Category II FHR tracings include all FHR tracings not categorized as Category I or Category III. Category II tracings may represent an appreciable fraction of those encountered in clinical care. Examples of Category II FHR tracings include any of the following:

Baseline rate
- Bradycardia not accompanied by absent baseline variability
- Tachycardia

Baseline FHR variability
- Minimal baseline variability
- Absent baseline variability not accompanied by recurrent decelerations
- Marked baseline variability

Accelerations
- Absence of induced accelerations after fetal stimulation

Periodic or episodic decelerations
- Recurrent variable decelerations accompanied by minimal or moderate baseline variability
- Prolonged deceleration $\geq$ 2 minutes but $<$ 10 minutes
- Recurrent late decelerations with moderate baseline variability
- Variable decelerations with other characteristics, such as slow return to baseline, "overshoots," or "shoulders"

CATEGORY III
Category III FHR tracings include either
- Absent baseline FHR variability and any of the following:
  - Recurrent late decelerations
  - Recurrent variable decelerations
  - Bradycardia
- Sinusoidal Pattern

Note From: "The 2008 National Institute of Child Health Human Development Workshop Report on Electronic Fetal Monitoring: Update on Definitions, Interpretations, and Research Guidelines," by G. A. Macones, G. D. Hankins, C. Y. Spong, J. D. Hauth, & T. Moore, 2008, *Journal of Obstetric, Gynecologic and Neonatal Nursing, 37,* 510-515; *Obstetrics & Gynecology, 112,* p. 665. Copyright 2008 by the American College of Obstetricians and Gynecologists. Reprinted with permission.

indicates appropriate mobilization of compensatory mechanism and maintenance of adequate central oxygenation. Other experts similarly describe a variety of specific types of tracings that vary from normal characteristics but are not considered to represent an immediate risk for hypoxic injury to the fetus (Dellinger et al., 2000; Garite, 2007; Royal Australian and New Zealand College of Obstetricians and Gynecologists [RANZCOG], 2006; Royal College of Obstetricians and Gynecologiests [RCOG], 2001; Society of Obstetricians and Gynaecologists of Canada [SOGC], 2007). Some experts also classify additional characteristics as suggestive of significant risk for acidemia (Freeman, et al., 2003; RANZCOG; RCOG; SOGC). Thus, experts continue to grapple with classification of FHR characteristics as they present along a continuum and have yet to reach consensus regarding management of FHR tracings that exhibit neither the classic characteristics of normal FHR tracings nor the characteristics believed to be frankly abnormal (Fox et al.; Macones et al.). Several published frameworks for fetal heart monitoring interpretation are presented in Table 5-5.

Evolution of FHR Patterns over Time

The most important factors in interpreting FHR patterns are the degree of FHR variability and the evolution of the tracing over time in the context of the entire clinical picture (Fox et al., 2000; Macones et al., 2008; Parer et al., 2006). In interpreting indeterminate tracings, it is also essential to take into account the estimated proximity to birth, any maternal or fetal factors presenting threats to fetal reserve, and the specific logistics of the birth setting. In the absence of catastrophic events, the gradual nature of pattern evolution and the reliability of moderate FHR variability as a predictor of adequacy of fetal oxygenation indicate that there is usually a period of time, in the range of approximately 60 minutes, when observing the evolution of many FHR patterns can be safe practice. Naturally, the presence of concerning factors in a given patient may warrant more prompt intervention. During this observation period the bedside provider can do the following:

- Arrange for consultation
- Request in-house, bedside evaluation of FHR tracings
- Initiate interventions aimed at resolution of FHR changes
- Initiate preparations for operative or surgical birth when birth rather than continued observation appears warranted
- Secure the presence of anesthesia providers and the neonatal resuscitation team (Fox, et al., 2000; Simpson, 2008b).

Overall interpretation of the urgency of FHR findings will take into account the specific current FHR characteristics in combination with other factors such as maternal medical and obstetric history, gestational age, labor progress, and proximity or remoteness from birth as well as institutional factors such as availability and response time of anesthesia, surgical personnel, and pediatric support for birth should the pattern progress. Suggested general guidelines for management of selected tracings are presented in Figure 5-14.

The challenge in assessing pattern evolution is the potential for loss of situation awareness with resulting lack of recognition or appreciation of an increased threat to fetal well-being. This rarely occurs when there is an acute event such as severe maternal hypotension, cord prolapse, or uterine rupture. Acute events typically present dramatic and recognizable FHR changes that prompt a rapid response from the perinatal team. Acute events differ from close observation of FHR characteristics over time. Although intrauterine resuscitation techniques supporting improvement of maternal-fetal exchange are often the most appropriate approach to concerning characteristics of the FHR, clinicians also need to be aware of the risk of failure to recognize more subtle signs of progressive fetal deterioration over longer periods or when they are focused on a perceived imminent endpoint such as vaginal birth "in just a few more pushes."

Table 5-5	Selected Interpretive Frameworks across the Continuum of FHR Presentations

NICHD (2008)

CATEGORY I (NORMAL)	CATEGORY II (INDETERMINATE)	CATEGORY III (ABNORMAL)
Baseline 110–160 bpm Moderate baseline FHR variability Accelerations present or absent Early decelerations present or absent Late and variable decelerations absent	All FHR patterns not categorized as normal or abnormal. Examples include but are not limited to: alterations in FHR variability without recurrent decelerations, minimal or moderate variability with recurrent late or variable decelerations, and absence of acceleration response to fetal stimulation	Absent baseline FHR variability and bradycardia or recurrent late or variable decelerations or Sinusoidal pattern

SOGC (2007)

NORMAL	ATYPICAL	ABNORMAL
Baseline 110–160 bpm Moderate variability Minimal variability for < 40 min Accelerations: spontaneous or stimulated No decelerations or "occasional uncomplicated variable or early decelerations"	Bradycardia 100–110 bpm Tachycardia > 160 bpm > 30 min Minimal variability for 40–80 min Absence of acceleration in response to stimulation Single prolonged deceleration < 3 min duration Repetitive (≥3) "uncomplicated" variable decelerations	Bradycardia < 100 bpm Tachycardia > 60 min Erratic baseline Minimal variability > 80 min Marked variability > 25 min Sinusoidal FHR Recurrent late decelerations Repetitive "complicated" variable decelerations Single prolonged deceleration > 3 min

RCOG (2001)

Tracings are categorized as normal, suspicious, or pathological on the basis of the number of FHR features classified as reassuring, nonreassuring, or abnormal.
Normal tracings: All four features fall into the reassuring category.
Suspicious tracings: Features fall into *one* nonreassuring category and remainder of features are reassuring.
Pathological tracings: Features fall into *two or more* nonreassuring categories and one or more abnormal categories.

FEATURE	BASELINE (BPM)	VARIABILITY (BPM)	DECELERATIONS	ACCELERATIONS
Reassuring	110–160	≥5	None	Present
Nonreassuring	100–109 161–180	<5 for ≥ 40 but < 90 min	Early deceleration Variable deceleration Single prolonged deceleration ≤ 3 min	The absence of accelerations on an otherwise normal tracing is of uncertain significance
Abnormal	<100 >180 Sinusoidal pattern ≥ 10 min	<5 for ≥ 90 min	"Atypical" variable decelerations Late decelerations Single prolonged deceleration >3 min	

EFM = Electronic fetal monitoring; FHR = fetal heart rate

FIGURE 5-14   Fetal Monitoring Decision Tree

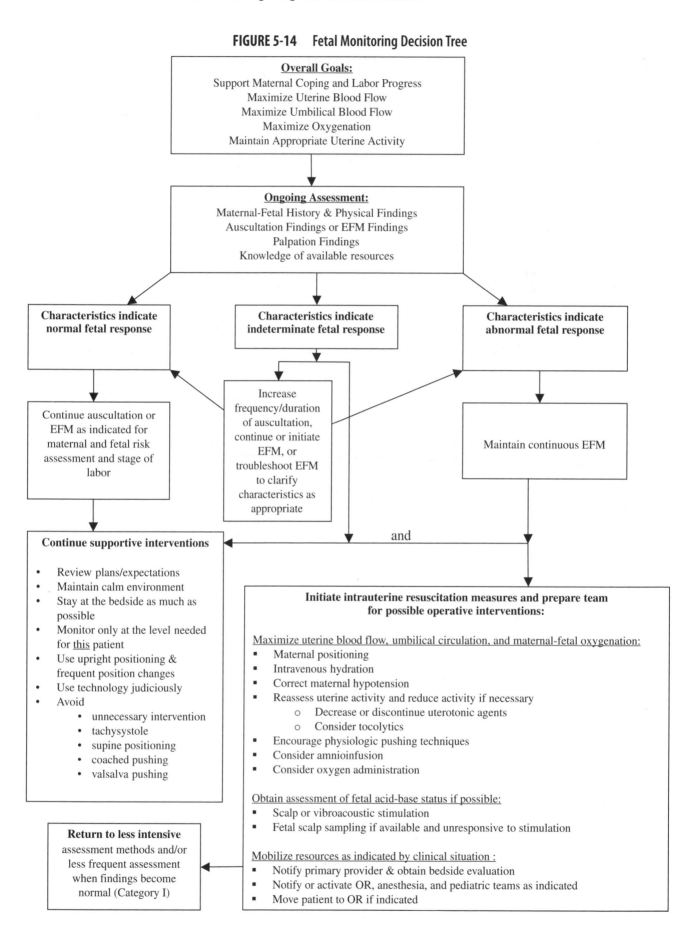

When the FHR evolves from a baseline within normal limits with moderate variability and accelerations to tachycardia, minimal to absent variability and recurrent late, variable, or prolonged decelerations, risk of fetal deterioration to hypoxemia and eventually acidemia is significant (Freeman et al., 2003). Oxytocin-induced tachysystole can exacerbate the situation, so it is important to carefully titrate the oxytocin infusion based on contraction frequency and the fetal response (Freeman et al.; Bakker et al., 2007). If the usual intrauterine resuscitation techniques do not result in pattern resolution, expeditious birth should be considered. A request for bedside evaluation by the primary provider is warranted so that plans can be made and implemented for fetal rescue in a timely manner.

There is consensus on interpretation of tracings at the end of the continuum: tracings with absent FHR variability and recurrent late or variable decelerations or bradycardia are believed by most experts to be associated with a significant risk for fetal acidemia. Birth should be expedited in these cases unless evidence of fetal well-being can be ascertained without

delay (Parer & Ikeda, 2007). Intrauterine resuscitation techniques are appropriate while preparing for birth, but they must not delay such preparations.

INTERPRETATION OF INTERMITTENT AUSCULTATION FINDINGS ACROSS THE CONTINUUM

The three-tiered EFM interpretation system also has implications for the interpretation and communication of FHR data obtained using IA. Using a common language for discussion of fetal status is a key principle for effective clinical communication and has the potential to decrease communication errors. For the purposes of interpreting auscultation findings, two categories are presented herein; Category I and Category II (Box 5-3). The definitions of these categories are consistent with the terminology used to interpret EFM patterns, but refer only to auscultation.

Category I auscultated FHR characteristics are normal (Box 5-3). Normal IA findings include all of the following characteristics: FHR baseline between 110 and 160 bpm, regular rhythm, the presence of FHR increases or accelerations, and the absence of FHR decreases or decelerations. Normal FHR characteristics are predictive of fetal well-being at the time they are observed and may be followed with routine supportive measures.

Category II auscultated FHR characteristics include all findings that are not classified as normal (Box 5-3). Irregular rhythm, presence of decreases or decelerations from baseline, tachycardia and bradycardia are all indeterminate IA findings. They cannot be classified as abnormal without information about FHR variability, as the patterns identified in Category III all include assessment of variability. Category II FHR characteristics require evaluation, ongoing surveillance, and re-evaluation, consistent with the assessment of the overall clinical circumstances. This may include, but is not limited to: continuous electronic fetal monitoring, use of intrauterine resuscitation techniques, ruling out maternal

---

BOX 5-3   Interpretation of Auscultation Findings

CATEGORY I
Category I FHR characteristics by auscultation include **all** of the following:
- Normal FHR baseline between 110 and 160 bpm
- Regular rhythm
- Presence of FHR increases or accelerations from the baseline rate
- Absence of FHR decreases or decelerations from the baseline

CATEGORY II
Category II FHR characteristics by auscultation include any of the following:
- Irregular rhythm
- Presence of FHR decreases or decelerations from the baseline
- Tachycardia (baseline >160 bpm > 10 minutes in duration)
- Bradycardia (baseline <110 bpm > 10 minutes in duration)

heart rate, and assessment of the continuation of indeterminate findings. As with EFM, auscultation findings and management needs are interpreted in the context of the overall clinical picture. Preparations to expedite birth in emergent situations (e.g. apparent significant fetal bradycardia) should be undertaken simultaneously with efforts to ameliorate, verify and determine the precise nature of the FHR findings.

⌐ SUMMARY

Fetal heart monitoring is a complex psychomotor and interpretative skill that requires specialized education and practice. The care of childbearing women is enhanced when registered nurses, physicians, and midwives use standardized language for communicating FHR findings and engage in ongoing collaborative dialogue regarding FHR interpretation in the context of specific clinical cases. Timely identification and communication of FHR findings is essential to optimal maternal-fetal care. Systematic assessment, accurate interpretation, and effective teamwork will lead to selection of the most appropriate physiologic interventions for the condition of a given mother and fetus. These interventions and their physiologic rationales are discussed in Chapter 6.

REFERENCES

American College of Nurse Midwives. (2007). Intermittent auscultation for intrapartum fetal heart rate surveillance. (Clinical Bulletin No. 9). *Journal of Midwifery & Women's Health, 52,* 314–319.

American College of Obstetricians and Gynecologists. (1999). *Induction of labor* (Practice Bulletin No.10). Washington, DC: Author.

American College of Obstetricians and Gynecologists. (2003). *Dystocia and augmentation of labor* (Practice Bulletin No. 49). Washington, DC: Author.

American College of Obstetricians and Gynecologists. (2005a). *Inappropriate use of the terms fetal distress and birth asphyxia* (Committee Opinion No. 326). Washington, DC: Author.

American College of Obstetricians and Gynecologists. (2005b). *Intrapartum fetal heart rate monitoring* (Practice Bulletin No. 70). Washington, DC: Author.

American College of Obstetricians and Gynecologists. (2006). *Umbilical cord blood gas and acid-base analysis* (Committee Opinion No. 368). Washington, DC: Author.

Andres, R. L., Saade, G., Gilstrap, L. C., Wilkins, I., Witlin, A., Zlatnik, F., et al. (1999). Association between umbilical blood gas parameters and neonatal morbidity and death in neonates with pathologic fetal acidemia. *American Journal of Obstetrics and Gynecology, 181,* 867–871.

Association of Women's Health, Obstetric and Neonatal Nurses. (2000). *The role of unlicensed assistive personnel in the nursing care for women and newborns* (Position Statement). Retrieved January 29, 2008 from http://www.awhonn.org/awhonn/content.do?name=05_HealthPolicyLegislation/5H_PositionStatements.htm

Association of Women's Health, Obstetric and Neonatal Nurses. (2009). *Fetal heart monitoring* (Position Statement). Washington, DC: Author.

Bakker, P. C., Kurver, P. H., Kuik, D. J., & Van Geijn, H. P. (2007). Elevated uterine activity increases the risk of fetal acidosis at birth. *American Journal of Obstetrics and Gynecology, 196,* e311–e316.

Ball, R. H., & Parer, J. T. (1992). The physiologic mechanisms of variable decelerations. *American Journal of Obstetrics and Gynecology, 166,* 1683–1688; discussion 1688–1689.

Beard, R. W., Filshie, G. M., Knight, C. A., & Roberts, G. M. (1971). The significance of the changes in the continuous fetal heart rate in the first stage of labour. *Journal of Obstetrics and Gynaecology of the British Commonwealth, 78,* 865–881.

Berkus, M. D., Langer, O., Samueloff, A., Xenakis, E. M., & Field, N. T. (1999). Electronic fetal monitoring: What's reassuring? *Acta Obstetricia et Gynecologica Scandinavica, 78*(1), 15–21.

Blackburn, S. T. (2007). *Maternal, fetal, and neonatal physiology: A clinical perspective* (3rd ed.). St. Louis: Saunders.

Cibils, L. A. (1975). Clinical significance of fetal heart rate patterns during labor. II. Late decelerations. *American Journal of Obstetrics and Gynecology, 123,* 473–494.

Clark, S. L., Gimovsky, M. L., & Miller, F. C. (1984). The scalp stimulation test: A clinical alternative to fetal scalp blood sampling. *American Journal of Obstetrics and Gynecology, 148,* 274–277.

Copel, J. A., Friedman, A. H., & Kleinman, C. S. (1997). Management of fetal cardiac arrhythmias. *Obstetrics and Gynecology Clinics of North America, 24,* 201–211.

Crane, J. M., Young, D. C., Butt, K. D., Bennett, K. A., & Hutchens, D. (2001). Excessive uterine activity accompanying induced labor. *Obstetrics & Gynecology, 97,* 926–931.

Dalton, K. J., Dawes, G. S., & Patrick, J. E. (1977). Diurnal, respiratory, and other rhythms of fetal heart rate in lambs. *American Journal of Obstetrics and Gynecology, 127*, 414–424.

Dawes, G. S., Visser, G. H., Goodman, J. D., & Levine, D. H. (1981). Numerical analysis of the human fetal heart rate: Modulation by breathing and movement. *American Journal of Obstetrics and Gynecology, 140*, 535–544.

Dawood, M. Y. (1995). Pharmacologic stimulation of uterine contraction. *Seminars in Perinatology, 19*(1), 73–83.

Dellinger, E. H., Boehm, F. H., & Crane, M. M. (2000). Electronic fetal heart rate monitoring: Early neonatal outcomes associated with normal rate, fetal stress, and fetal distress. *American Journal of Obstetrics and Gynecology, 182*, 214–220.

Feinstein, N. F., Sprague, A., & Trepanier, M. J. (2008). *Fetal heart rate auscultation* (2nd ed.). Washington, DC: Association of Women's Health, Obstetrics, and Neonatal Nurses.

Fox, M., Kilpatrick, S., King, T., & Parer, J. T. (2000). Fetal heart rate monitoring: Interpretation and collaborative management. *Journal of Midwifery & Women's Health, 4*, 498–507.

Freeman, R. K., Garite, T. J., & Nageotte, M. P. (2003). *Fetal heart rate monitoring* (3rd ed.). Philadelphia: Lippincott Williams & Wilkins.

Garite, T. J. (2007). Intrapartum evaluation. In S. G. Gabbe, J. R. Neibyl, & J. L. Simpson (Eds.), *Obstetrics: Normal and problem pregnancies* (5th ed., pp. 364–395). Philadelphia: Churchill Livingstone.

Gull, I., Jaffa, A. J., Oren, M., Grisaru, D., Peyser, M. R., & Lessing, J. B. (1996). Acid accumulation during end-stage bradycardia in term fetuses: How long is too long? *British Journal of Obstetrics and Gynaecology, 103*, 1096–1101.

Hammacher, K., Huter, K. A., Bokelmann, J., & Werners, P. H. (1968). Foetal heart frequency and perinatal condition of the foetus and newborn. *Gynaecologia, 166*, 349–360.

James, L. S., Yeh, M. N., Morishima, H. O., Daniel, S. S., Caritis, S. N., Niemann, W. H., et al. (1976). Umbilical vein occlusion and transient acceleration of the fetal heart rate. Experimental observations in subhuman primates. *American Journal of Obstetrics and Gynecology, 126*, 276–283.

Kleinman, C. S., & Nehgme, R. A. (2004). Cardiac arrhythmias in the human fetus. *Pediatric Cardiology, 25*, 234–251.

Kleinman, C. S., Nehgme, R. A., & Copel, J. A. (2004). Fetal cardiac arrhythmias. In R. K. Creasy, R. Resnik, & J. D. Iams (Eds.), *Maternal-fetal medicine: Principles and practice* (5th ed., pp. 465–482). Philadelphia: W.B. Saunders.

Korhonen, J., & Kariniemi, V. (1994). Emergency cesarean section: The effect of delay on umbilical arterial gas balance and Apgar scores. *Acta Obstetricia et Gynecologica Scandinavica, 73*, 782–786.

Krebs, H. B., Petres, R. E., & Dunn, L. J. (1981). Intrapartum fetal heart rate monitoring. V. Fetal heart rate patterns in the second stage of labor. *American Journal of Obstetrics and Gynecology, 140*, 435–439.

Krebs, H. B., Petres, R. E., Dunn, L. J., Jordaan, H. V., & Segreti, A. (1979). Intrapartum fetal heart rate monitoring I: Classification and prognosis of fetal heart rate patterns. *American Journal of Obstetrics and Gynecology, 133*, 762–772.

Lee, C. Y., Di Loreto, P. C., & O'Lane, J. M. (1975). A study of fetal heart rate acceleration patterns. *Obstetrics & Gynecology, 45*, 142–146.

Lee, S. T., & Hon, E. H. (1963). Fetal hemodynamic response to umbilical cord compression. *Obstetrics & Gynecology, 22*, 553–562.

Leung, A. S., Leung, E. K., & Paul, R. H. (1993). Uterine rupture after previous cesarean delivery: Maternal and fetal consequences. *American Journal of Obstetrics and Gynecology, 169*, 945–950.

Leveno, K. J., Quirk, J. G., Jr., Cunningham, F. G., Nelson, S. D., Santos-Ramos, R., Toofanian, A., et al. (1984). Prolonged pregnancy I: Observations concerning the causes of fetal distress. *American Journal of Obstetrics and Gynecology, 150*, 465–473.

Low, J. A., Lindsay, B. G., & Derrick, E. J. (1997). Threshold of metabolic acidosis associated with newborn complications. *American Journal of Obstetrics and Gynecology, 177*, 1391–1394.

Low, J. A., Victory, R., & Derrick, E. J. (1999). Predictive value of electronic fetal monitoring for intrapartum fetal asphyxia with metabolic acidosis. *Obstetrics & Gynecology, 93*, 285–291.

MacLennan, A. (1999). A template for defining a causal relation between acute intrapartum events and cerebral palsy: International consensus statement. *British Medical Journal, 319*, 1054–1059.

Macones, G. A., Hankins, G. D., Spong, C. Y., Hauth, J. D., & Moore, T. (2008). The 2008 National Institute of Child Health Human Development workshop report on electronic fetal monitoring: Update on definitions, interpretations, and research guidelines. *Obstetrics & Gynecology, 112*, 661–666; and *Journal of Obstetric, Gynecologic and Neonatal Nursing, 37*, 510–515.

Manseau, P., Vaquier, J., Chavinié, J., & Sureau, C. (1972). Le rythme cardiaque foetal "sinusoidal" aspect evocateur de souffrance fortale au cours de a grossesse. *Journal de Gynécologie, Obstétrique et Biologie de la Reproduction, 1*, 343–52.

Martin, C. B., Jr. (1978). Regulation of the fetal heart rate and genesis of FHR patterns. *Seminars in Perinatology, 2*(2), 131–146.

Martin, C. B., Jr. (1982). Physiology and clinical use of fetal heart rate variability. *Clinics in Perinatology, 9,* 339–352.

Modanlou, H. D., & Freeman, R. K. (1982). Sinusoidal fetal heart rate pattern: Its definition and clinical significance. *American Journal of Obstetrics and Gynecology, 142,* 1033–1038.

Modanlou, H. D., & Murata, Y. (2004). Sinusoidal heart rate pattern: Reappraisal of its definition and clinical significance. *Journal of Obstetrics & Gynaecology Research, 30*(3), 169–180.

Nageotte, M. P., & Gilstrap, L. C. (2009). Intrapartum fetal surveillance. In R. K. Creasy, R. Resnik, J. D. Iams, C. J. Lockwood, & T. R. Moore (Eds.) Creasy & Resnik's *Maternal-fetal medicine: Principles and practice,* (6th ed., pp. 397-417). Philadelphia: Saunders.

National Institute of Child Health and Human Development Research Planning Workshop. (1997). Electronic fetal heart rate monitoring: Research guidelines for interpretation. *American Journal of Obstetrics and Gynecology, 177,* 1385–1390, and *Journal of Obstetric, Gynecologic, and Neonatal Nursing, 26,* 635–640.

O'Brien-Abel, N. E., & Benedetti, T. J. (1992). Saltatory fetal heart rate pattern. *Journal of Perinatology, 12*(1), 13–17.

Paine, L. L., Benedict, M. I., Strobino, D. M., Gregor, C. L., & Larson, E. L. (1992). A comparison of the auscultated acceleration test and the nonstress test as predictors of perinatal outcomes. *Nursing Research, 41,* 87–91.

Paine, L. L., Zanardi, L. R., Johnson, T. R., Rorie, J. L., & Barger, M. K. (2001). A comparison of two time intervals for the auscultated acceleration test. *Journal of Midwifery & Women's Health, 46,* 98–102.

Parer, J. T. (1997). *Handbook of fetal heart monitoring* (2nd ed.). Philadelphia: W.B. Saunders.

Parer, J. T., Dijkstra, H. R., Vredebregt, P. P., Harris, J. L., Krueger, T. R., & Reuss, M. L. (1980). Increased fetal heart rate variability with acute hypoxia in chronically instrumented sheep. *European Journal of Obstetrics, Gynecology, and Reproductive Biology, 10,* 393–399.

Parer, J. T., & Ikeda, T. (2007). A framework for standardized management of intrapartum fetal heart rate patterns. *American Journal of Obstetrics and Gynecology, 197,* 26 e21–e26.

Parer, J. T., King, T., Flanders, S., Fox, M., & Kilpatrick, S. J. (2006). Fetal acidemia and electronic fetal heart rate patterns: Is there evidence of an association? *Journal of Maternal, Fetal, and Neonatal Medicine, 19,* 289–294.

Parer, J. T., & Livingston, E. G. (1990). What is fetal distress? *American Journal of Obstetrics and Gynecology, 162,* 1421–1425; discussion 1425–1427.

Parer, J. T., & Nageotte, M. P. (2004). Intrapartum fetal surveillance. In R. K. Creasy, R. Resnik, & J. D. Iams (Eds.), *Maternal-fetal medicine: Principles and practice* (5th ed., pp. 403–427). Philadelphia: W.B. Saunders.

Patrick, J., Campbell, K., Carmichael, L., Natale, R., & Richardson, B. (1982). Patterns of gross fetal body movements over 24-hour observation intervals during the last 10 weeks of pregnancy. *American Journal of Obstetrics and Gynecology, 142,* 363–371.

Paul, R. H., Suidan, A. K., Yeh, S., Schifrin, B. S., & Hon, E. H. (1975). Clinical fetal monitoring VII: The evaluation and significance of intrapartum baseline FHR variability. *American Journal of Obstetrics and Gynecology, 123,* 206–210.

Phaneuf, S., Rodriguez Linares, B., TambyRaja, R. L., MacKenzie, I. Z., & Lopez Bernal, A. (2000). Loss of myometrial oxytocin receptors during oxytocin-induced and oxytocin-augmented labour. *Journal of Reproduction and Fertility, 120*(1), 91–97.

Porter, T. F., & Clark, S. L. (1999). Vibroacoustic and scalp stimulation. *Obstetrics and Gynecology Clinics of North America, 26,* 657–669.

Ridgeway, J. J., Weyrich, D. L., & Benedetti, T. J. (2004). Fetal heart rate changes associated with uterine rupture. *Obstetrics & Gynecology, 103,* 506–512.

Royal Australian and New Zealand College of Obstetricians and Gynecologists (RANZCOG). (2006). Intrapartum fetal surveillance: Clinical Guidelines (2nd ed.). Retrieved November 13, 2007 from http://www.ranzcog.edu.au/publications/pdfs/ClinicalGuidelines-IFSSecEd.pdf

Royal College of Obstetricians and Gynecologists (RCOG). (2001). The use of electronic fetal monitoring: The use and interpretation of cardiotocography in intrapartum fetal surveillance. Evidence-based clinical practice guideline No. 8. Retrieved November 13, 2007 from http://www.rcog.org.uk/index.asp?PageID=695

Simpson, K. R. (2008a). *Cervical ripening and induction and augmentation of labor* (3rd ed.). Washington, DC: Association of Women's Health, Obstetric, and Neonatal Nurses.

Simpson, K. R. (2008b). Fetal assessment during labor. In K. R. Simpson & P. A. Creehan (Eds.), *Perinatal nursing* (3rd ed., pp. 399–442). Philadelphia: Lippincott.

Simpson, K. R., & James, D. C. (2005). Effects of immediate versus delayed pushing during second-stage labor on fetal well-being: A randomized clinical trial. *Nursing Research, 54*(3), 149–157.

Society of Obstetricians and Gynaecologists of Canada. (2007). Fetal health surveillance: Antepartum and intrapartum consensus guideline. *Journal of Obstetrics and Gynaecology Canada, 29,* S1–S56.

Timor-Tritsch, I. E., Dierker, L. J., Hertz, R. H., Deagan, N. C., & Rosen, M. G. (1978). Studies of antepartum behavioral state in the human fetus at term. *American Journal of Obstetrics and Gynecology, 132,* 524–528.

Williams, K. P., & Galerneau, F. (2003). Intrapartum fetal heart rate patterns in the prediction of neonatal acidemia. *American Journal of Obstetrics and Gynecology, 188,* 820–823.

Wright, R. G., Shnider, S. M., Levinson, G., Rolbin, S. H., & Parer, J. T. (1981). The effect of maternal administration of ephedrine on fetal heart rate and variability. *Obstetrics & Gynecology, 57,* 734–738.

Zeeman, G. G., Khan-Dawood, F. S., & Dawood, M. Y. (1997). Oxytocin and its receptor in pregnancy and parturition: Current concepts and clinical implications. *Obstetrics & Gynecology, 89,* 873–883.

CHAPTER 6

Physiologic Interventions for Fetal Heart Rate Patterns

Kathleen Rice Simpson

The goal of fetal monitoring is ongoing assessment of fetal oxygenation to promote fetal safety. The clinician can best develop an understanding of fetal physiologic status by thoroughly assessing the maternal medical and obstetric history; current risk factors; and physical assessment findings, including fetal heart rate (FHR) characteristics and uterine activity. Selection of appropriate interventions to maximize fetal oxygenation is based on these assessment data and other relevant clinical information. This chapter reviews concepts for collaborative diagnosis and interventions based on assessment and interpretation of FHR characteristics in the context of the ongoing clinical condition of the mother and fetus (Figure 6-1). The Dynamic Physiologic Response Model is used to conceptualize fetal status as the basis for interventions (Figure 6-2). Independent and collaborative interventions are discussed, with emphasis on the goal of supporting or improving fetal oxygenation.

PROMOTING FETAL WELL-BEING

Fetal well-being requires a hemodynamically stable, well-oxygenated mother and a well-oxygenated fetus. The mother's condition is a significant determinant of fetal well-being. To promote fetal oxygenation, essential clinical criteria must be met, including adequate maternal cardiac output, blood pressure, hemoglobin levels, and oxygen saturation; adequate blood flow to the uterus and placenta; adequate placental function; normal uterine activity; and uninterrupted umbili-

cal blood flow to fetus (e.g., absence of umbilical cord compression). Perinatal clinicians have limited ability to influence some of these criteria, such as adequacy of placental function. However, clinicians can support fetal well-being by implementing interventions based on the specific physiologic goals of supporting maternal coping and labor progress and maintaining appropriate uterine activity. Upright positioning and frequent position changes can promote labor progress. Maintaining a calm environment; minimizing fear, anxiety, and pain; and assisting a woman to cope with labor may decrease her catecholamine production, thereby promoting adequate blood flow and fetal oxygenation. Likewise, maintaining appropriate levels of uterine activity, avoiding tachysystole, and using a physiologic approach to pushing support optimal fetal oxygenation and maternal-fetal adaptation to the labor process.

CLASSIFICATION OF ELECTRONICALLY OBTAINED FETAL HEART RATE PATTERNS

The 2008 NICHD Workshop guidelines propose a three-tiered system for classification of intrapartum EFM findings: category I (normal), category II (indeterminate), and category III (abnormal) (Macones et al., 2008). The Society of Obstetricians and Gynaecologists of Canada (SOGC, 2007) uses the terms "normal," "atypical," and "abnormal" in their *Fetal Health Surveillance: Antepartum and Intrapartum Consensus Guideline* (See Table 5-6 in Chapter 5).

FIGURE 6-1   The Nursing Process and Fetal Heart Monitoring: Interventions

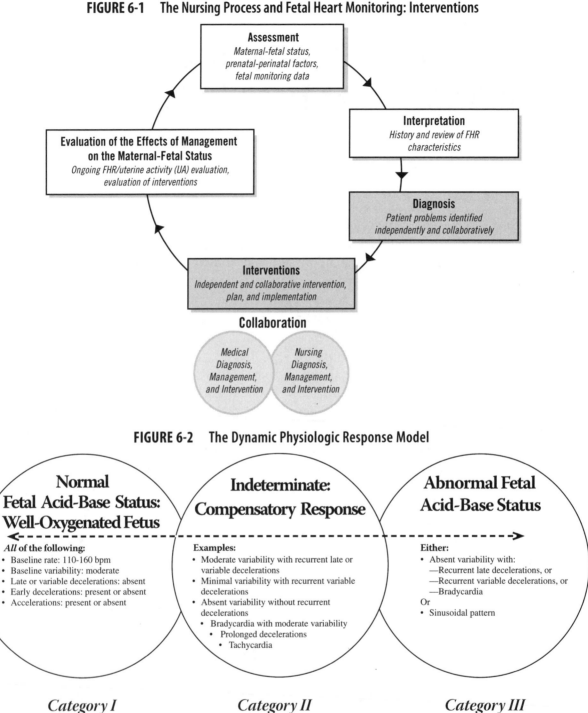

FIGURE 6-2   The Dynamic Physiologic Response Model

Category I   *Category II*   *Category III*

NOTE: This diagram is not meant to be all inclusive. All patterns must be treated with interventions that are based on suspected underlying physiologic causes and evaluation of individual patient presentation.

A normal (category I) FHR tracing exhibits a baseline rate of 110-160 bpm, moderate baseline FHR variability, and no late or variable decelerations. Normal tracings may or may not exhibit accelerations or early decelerations. Experts generally agree that this type of FHR tracing confers an extremely high predictability of a normally oxygenated fetus (Macones et al., 2008). Normal FHR tracings may be followed with routine measures to support labor progress, maternal coping, and fetal oxygenation. At the other end of the continuum from completely normal tracings are abnormal (category III) FHR patterns requiring prompt evaluation and attempts to expeditiously resolve the abnormal findings. Category III FHR tracings are those exhibiting a sinusoidal pattern or exhibiting *absent variability* in conjunction with bradycardia or recurrent late or variable decelerations (Macones et al.).

A majority of intrapartum FHR tracings may be interpreted as indeterminate (category II), which includes all FHR tracings that do not meet criteria for category I or III classification. This includes (but is not limited to) tracings with *moderate or minimal variability* and recurrent late or variable decelerations, baseline tachycardia, marked variability, prolonged decelerations, and the absence of an acceleration response to fetal stimulation. Category II tracings require, at a minimum, heightened surveillance and ongoing reevaluation (Macones et al., 2008). In most cases supportive actions to promote maternal and fetal adaptation to labor are also indicated.

The Parer et al. (2006) review of the published literature to date on the association between FHR patterns and fetal acidemia found moderate FHR variability was strongly (98%) associated with an umbilical pH of greater than 7.15 or newborn vigor (5-minute Apgar score ≥7). Absent or minimal FHR variability with late or variable decelerations was the most consistent predictor of newborn acidemia (although the association was only 23%); there was a positive relationship between the degree of acidemia and the depth of decelerations or bradycardia; and, except for a sudden profound bradycardia, newborn acidemia with decreasing variability in combination with decelerations develops over a period of time approaching 1 hour (Parer et al., 2006). These findings are consistent with the results of a systematic review by the Royal College of Obstetricians and Gynaecologists (RCOG, 2001b) on both specific and overall features of FHR patterns as they relate to neonatal outcomes. Thus, there is supportive evidence for associations between category III patterns and some category II patterns and risk for significant fetal acidemia. The predictive value of grading schemes for the depth, duration, and/or absolute

nadir of decelerations requires further research (Macones et al., 2008).

Interventions aimed at improving fetal oxygenation via one or more intrauterine resuscitation techniques should be used when category II or III FHR patterns are present. Ideally, members of the perinatal team have a shared method of interpreting FHR patterns and an agreed-on management guideline for specific FHR patterns.

SYSTEMATIC INTERPRETATION OF THE FETAL HEART RATE TRACING

Appropriate interventions require an accurate interpretation of the characteristics of both the FHR and uterine activity and their relationship with each other. Attention should be given to the overall clinical picture and to the trends in the FHR pattern over time. Although the experienced clinician may assess the individual characteristics of the FHR simultaneously, a detailed and thorough evaluation of each component may be useful when planning appropriate interventions. The method of monitoring used determines which characteristics can be assessed.

A systematic fetal monitoring assessment includes, but is not limited to, the following data:

Baseline FHR Characteristics
- Baseline rate
- Rhythm (with auscultation)
- Variability
- Sinusoidal

Baseline Changes
- Presence or absence of accelerations
- Presence or absence of decelerations
  - Early
  - Late
  - Variable
  - Prolonged

Uterine Activity
- Frequency
- Duration
- Intensity
- Resting Tone

The clinician may review these physiologic data through the following process:

- What is the baseline FHR?
- Is it within normal limits for this fetus?
- If not, what clinical factors could be contributing to this baseline rate?
- Is there evidence of moderate baseline variability?
- If not, does fetal stimulation elicit an acceleration of the FHR appropriate for gestational age?
- What clinical factors could be contributing to this baseline variability?
- Are there periodic or episodic FHR patterns?
- If so, what are they and what are the appropriate interventions (if any)?
- Does the FHR pattern suggest a chronic or acute maternal-fetal condition?
- Is uterine activity normal in frequency, duration, intensity, and resting tone?
- What is the relationship between the FHR and uterine activity?
- What is the relationship between the FHR and maternal vital signs?
- If the FHR pattern is not normal, what types of interventions would be appropriate to maximize fetal oxygenation?
- Do these appropriate interventions resolve the situation?
- If not, are further interventions needed?
- Is the FHR pattern such that notification of the physician or midwife is warranted?
- Is the FHR pattern such that actions should be initiated for expeditious birth?
- What steps should be taken in the case of clinical disagreement between caregivers regarding FHR interpretation and/or appropriate response to the FHR patterns?

Adapted from: Simpson, K. R. (2006). *Critical Care Nursing Quarterly, 29*(1), 20–31.

INTERVENTIONS FOR CATEGORY II AND III FETAL HEART RATE PATTERNS
Intrauterine Resuscitation Techniques

When an indeterminate or abnormal FHR pattern is identified, initial assessment may include a cervical exam to rule out umbilical cord prolapse, rapid cervical dilation or rapid descent of the fetal head; review of uterine activity to rule out tachysystole; and evaluation of maternal vital signs, in particular temperature and blood pressure, to rule out maternal fever or maternal hypotension (ACOG, 2005b). These assessment data can guide appropriate interventions to attempt to resolve the pattern. The physiologic goals for intrauterine resuscitation include the following:

- Support maternal coping and labor progress.
- Maximize uterine blood flow.
- Maximize umbilical circulation.
- Maximize oxygenation.
- Maintain appropriate uterine activity.

Intrauterine resuscitation refers to a series of techniques that include but may not be limited to the following:

- Maternal repositioning
- Reduction of uterine activity
- An intravenous (IV) fluid bolus
- Correction of maternal hypotension
- Oxygen administration
- Amnioinfusion
- Modification of maternal pushing efforts during second stage labor

The type of resuscitative technique is based on the specific characteristics of the FHR pattern. In some cases, a combination of techniques will be required to resolve the pattern. A summary of the goals and techniques for intrauterine resuscitation are presented in Table 6-1.

Although intrauterine resuscitation techniques are commonly used (ACOG, 2005b; SOGC, 2007), supportive data for their effectiveness could be more robust (Simpson, 2007). It is generally believed that these interventions improve maternal blood flow to the placental intervillous space and oxygen delivery to the fetus. There are data to suggest that these techniques can improve fetal oxygen status, but it is important to remember that there is no evidence that any of these techniques individually or collectively will reverse fetal acidemia. If the clinical characteristics of the FHR patterns are such that they represent a serious, immediate risk to the fetus (e.g., bradycardia unresponsive to other inter-

Table 6-1	Intrauterine Resuscitation
GOAL	**TECHNIQUES/METHODS**
Promote fetal oxygenation	Lateral positioning (either left or right) IV fluid bolus of at least 500 mL of lactated Ringer's solution Discontinuation of oxytocin/removal of dinoprostone insert (prostaglandin E_2) /withholding of next dose of misoprostol Discontinuation of pushing temporarily or pushing with every other or every third contraction (during second stage labor) Oxygen administration at 10 L/min via nonrebreather face mask (discontinue as soon as possible based on the fetal response)
Reduce uterine activity	Discontinuation of oxytocin/removal of dinoprostone insert (prostaglandin E_2)/withholding of next dose of misoprostol IV fluid bolus of at least 500 mL of lactated Ringer's solution Lateral positioning (either left or right) If no response, terbutaline 0.25 mg subcutaneously may be considered
Alleviate umbilical cord compression	Repositioning Amnioinfusion (during first stage labor) Discontinuation of pushing temporarily or pushing with every other or every third contraction (during second stage labor) If prolapse umbilical cord is noted, elevation of the presenting fetal part as preparations are underway for expeditious birth may be effective
Correct maternal hypotension	Lateral positioning (either left or right) IV fluid bolus of at least 500 mL of lactated Ringer's solution If no response, ephedrine 5 to 10 mg IV push may be considered

IV, Intravenous.
Adapted from: Simpson, K. R. (2008c). Labor and birth. In K. R. Simpson & P. A. Creehan (Eds.). *AWHONN's perinatal nursing* (3rd ed., pp. 300–398). Philadelphia: Lippincott Williams and Wilkins.

vention), these techniques should be initiated only if doing so does not delay expeditious birth (Simpson, 2007).

Lateral Positioning or Change in Position

Lateral positioning alters the relationship between the umbilical cord and fetal parts or the uterine wall and is usually performed to minimize or correct umbilical cord compression and decrease the frequency of uterine contractions. In a lateral position, the uterus does not compress the vena cava or aorta; thus, maternal cardiac return and cardiac output are maximized, and blood flow to the uterus is optimal (ACOG, 2005b; Clark et al., 1991; Freeman, Garite, & Nageotte, 2003). Several studies have compared the effects of right lateral, left lateral, and supine maternal positions on fetal oxygen status; the findings of each suggest that lateral positioning on either side is more favorable for enhancing fetal oxygenation when compared

with a supine position (Aldrich et al., 1995; Carbonne et al., 1996; Simpson & James, 2005b). When compared with supine positioning, upright and lateral positions are associated with fewer "nonreassuring" FHR characteristics (Abitbol, 1985; Gupta & Hofmeyr, 2004). A lateral position or a change in position can resolve or decrease the severity of late, variable, and/or prolonged decelerations (Abitbol; Freeman et al., 2003). Lateral positioning may also modify or eliminate late decelerations if the etiology is decreased uterine blood flow (usually secondary to supine positioning and inferior vena caval compression) (Abitbol; Freeman et al.). The supine position should be avoided in general to prevent compression of the vena cava and supine hypotensive syndrome. When indeterminate or abnormal FHR patterns are occurring, changing maternal position to where the FHR pattern is most improved is typically an effective therapeutic strategy (Freeman et al.).

Reduction of Uterine Activity

Care should be taken to maintain appropriate intervals between contractions by avoiding tachysystole and using timely measures to reduce uterine activity when it occurs. Normal contraction frequency in the active phase of labor is every 2 to 3 minutes (ACOG, 2003). Assessments of maternal pain, coping, and uterine tenderness also contribute to the interpretation of uterine activity but are not required to make a determination of excessive uterine activity or tachysystole. *Hypertonus* generally refers to uterine resting tone above 20 to 25 mm Hg.

Uterine activity is determined by the number of contractions present in a 10 minute period, averaged over 30 minutes (Macones et al., 2008):

- Normal: ≤5 contractions in 10 minutes.
- Tachysystole: >5 contractions in 10 minutes. Tachysystole is further qualified by the presence or absence of associated FHR decelerations.

This definition is primarily based on expert opinion, as there are only a few published studies in the literature evaluating the affects of uterine activity on fetal well-being. Although fetal assessment during labor has been the subject of numerous research studies, uterine activity assessment has received much less attention in the literature. Quantification of uterine activity as it relates to labor progress and fetal status has not been well studied. This gap in knowledge presents a challenge for determining the level of appropriate uterine activity during labor to effect normal labor progress when using pharmacologic agents to stimulate uterine contractions, as well as the limits of uterine activity to ensure ongoing fetal well-being during labor.

Some authors and clinicians reserve the term *tachysystole* for a contraction frequency of five or more in 10 minutes with evidence that the fetus is not tolerating this contraction pattern, as demonstrated by late decelerations or fetal bradycardia (ACOG, 1999). Definitions of tachysystole that include evidence of category II or III FHR changes are not clinically appropriate because such definitions may delay interventions to

reduce uterine activity while fetal status is threatened. Some clinicians include the woman's perception of pain in their determination of tachysystole; however, this factor is not a reliable indicator of the potential physiologic implications of the frequency, duration, and intensity of uterine contractions (Simpson, 2008a).

Tachysystole can result in a progressive adverse effect on fetal oxygenation, and emerging evidence (Bakker, Kurver, Kuik, & Van Geijn, 2007; Simpson & James, 2008) suggests that *less than five* contractions in 10 minutes may be optimal for supporting fetal well-being. Uterine contractions cause an intermittent decrease in blood flow to the intervillous space where oxygen exchange occurs. If this intermittent interruption of blood flow reaches an abnormal level as a result of too-frequent contractions, the fetus is at risk for hypoxemia (ACOG & American Academy of Pediatrics [AAP], 2003). When fetal oxygenation is sufficiently impaired to produce metabolic acidosis from anaerobic glycolysis, direct myocardial depression occurs (ACOG & AAP). As fetal deterioration progresses, the fetus will likely respond with late decelerations and the FHR will lose variability and reactivity (ACOG & AAP). The more time between contractions, the more time there is to maximally perfuse the placenta and deliver oxygen to the fetus (Caldeyro-Barcia, 1992; Freeman et al., 2003).

As a contraction begins, the fetus uses the reservoir of oxygen (fetal reserve) in the intervillous space; restricted blood flow prevents complete recovery until some time after the contraction when full oxygenation has been restored (Paternoster et al., 2001). In most healthy fetuses, the physiologic effects of intermittent contractions of normal labor are well tolerated (Paternoster et al., 2001). Earlier research concerning the effects of uterine contractions on fetal oxygen saturation (FSpO$_2$) found that FSpO$_2$ decreased during contractions, reaching the lowest level 92 seconds after the peak of the contraction, with approximately 90 seconds required for FSpO$_2$ to return to normal levels (McNamara & Johnson, 1995). When contractions are occurring every 2 minutes or more, recovery of $FSpO_2$ to previous baseline levels is incomplete (Johnson et al., 1994). The $FSpO_2$ decreases incrementally after each contraction, and the fetus becomes hypoxemic, recovering only when oxytocin is discontinued (Johnson et al.). Comparable effects of too-frequent contractions on fetal oxygen levels were noted by Peebles et al. (1994). Contraction intervals of less than 2 to 3 minutes are less favorable on fetal cerebral oxygen saturation when compared with longer contraction intervals. Peebles et al. concluded that contractions occurring repeatedly at intervals less than 2 to 3 minutes were likely to result in progressive fetal cerebral desaturation.

Bakker et al. (2007) studied uterine activity involving 1,433 labors and births and found five or more contractions in 10 min during the last hour of the first stage of labor was significantly associated with a higher incidence of neonatal acidemia (umbilical arterial pH ≤ 7.11) at birth when compared to contractions that were less frequent. Simpson & James (2008) found five or more contractions in 10 minutes over a 30 minute period during first stage labor was associated with a 20% decrease in fetal oxygen saturation while six or more contractions in the same period was associated with a 29% decrease. When contractions were fewer than five in 10 minutes over a 30 minute period, there was no change in fetal oxygen saturation. Significantly more "nonreassuring" fetal heart rate (FHR) changes such as absent and minimal variability, no accelerations and late and recurrent decelerations were also noted when contractions were more than five in 10 minutes as compared to periods when contractions were less frequent (Simpson & James). These findings are consistent with the earlier studies suggesting contraction intervals closer than every two to three minutes are associated with progressive fetal oxygen desaturation. More research from well-designed studies with adequate sample sizes are needed to guide clinical practice with regard to safe and appropriate levels of uterine activity during labor induction and augmentation. While tachysystole can be the result of endogenous maternal oxytocin and prostaglandins, most tachy-

systole results from administration of exogenous pharmacologic agents. Tachysystole alone and tachysystole accompanied by FHR changes are more common during cervical ripening and labor induction than during spontaneous labor (Crane, Young, Butt, Bennett, & Hutchens, 2001).

Reduction of uterine activity can occur either by decreasing or discontinuing the oxytocin infusion, having the mother assume a lateral position, and/or administering an intravenous fluid bolus of lactated Ringer's solution (ACOG, 2005b; Freeman et al., 2003; SOGC, 2007). Simpson and James (2008) found that simultaneous initiation of all three interventions resolved oxytocin-induced tachysystole more rapidly than when used individually, as follows:

- Oxytocin discontinuation: resolution $= 14.2$ minutes
- Oxytocin discontinuation + an IV fluid bolus of at least 500 mL of lactated Ringer's solution: resolution $= 9.8$ minutes
- Oxytocin discontinuation + an IV fluid bolus of at least 500 mL of lactated Ringer's solution + change to lateral position: resolution $= 6.1$ minutes

From the perspective of fetal safety, interventions for tachysystole should not be delayed until the FHR exhibits indeterminate or abnormal findings (Simpson, 2008a). Late decelerations are a frequent result of excessive stimulation of contractions with oxytocin (Caldeyro-Barcia, 1992; Freeman et al., 2003; Shenker, 1973). If FHR decelerations occur with tachysystole, reduction of contraction activity will optimize fetal oxygenation (ACOG, 2005b; Freeman et al.). When the FHR pattern is abnormal or indeterminate with decelerations, oxytocin should be discontinued (ACOG, 2005b). The next dose of pharmacologic agents used to ripen the cervix or stimulate contractions should be delayed until uterine activity and FHR patterns return to normal (Simpson, 2008a).

Although tachysystole should be identified and treated in a timely manner, its effects on the fetus based on the FHR characteristics can be used to guide the interventions chosen. A suggested clinical protocol for interventions during tachysystole with and without a FHR changes is presented in Table 6-2. Each component of this suggested protocol is based on one or more of the following: the physiologic effects of oxytocin on maternal-fetal status, limited available evidence on interventions for tachysystole, promulgated professional practice guidelines, and the opinions of experts (ACOG & AAP, 2003; ACOG, 2005b; Arias, 2000; Bakker et al., 2007; Bakker & van Geijn, 2008; Caldeyro-Barcia, 1992; Freeman et al., 2003; Johnson et al., 1994; Peebles et al., 1994; Seitchik et al., 1984; SOGC, 2001; Simpson, 2008a, 2008c; Simpson & James, 2008). Thus, the components of the suggested protocol individually and collectively have not been rigorously evaluated in a prospective clinical trial and should be viewed as guidelines to be used in conjunction with independent professional judgment.

When tachysystole occurs or fetal status is such that oxytocin is discontinued, data are limited to guide the decision regarding the timing and dosage of subsequent IV oxytocin administration. Physiologic and pharmacologic principles may be used to determine the most appropriate dosage. If oxytocin has been discontinued for less than 20 to 30 minutes, the FHR is normal, and contraction frequency, intensity, and duration are normal, a suggested protocol may include restarting oxytocin at least at a lower rate of infusion than before the tachysystole occurred. In this clinical situation, many practitioners restart the

Table 6-2	Suggested Clinical Protocol for Oxytocin-Induced Tachysystole

Oxytocin-Induced Tachysystole (Normal FHR)

- Assist the mother to a lateral position.

- Give IV fluid bolus of at least 500 mL lactated Ringer's solution as indicated.

- If uterine activity has not returned to normal after 10–15 minutes, decrease oxytocin rate by at least half; if uterine activity has not returned to normal after 10–15 more minutes, discontinue oxytocin until uterine activity less than five contractions in 10 minutes.

- To resume oxytocin after resolution of tachsystole: If oxytocin has been discontinued for less than 20–30 minutes, the FHR is normal, and contraction frequency, intensity, and duration are normal, resume oxytocin at no more than half the rate that caused the tachysystole and gradually increase the rate as appropriate based on unit protocol and maternal-fetal status. If the oxytocin is discontinued for more than 30–40 minutes, resume oxytocin at the initial dose ordered.

Oxytocin-Induced Tachysystole (Indeterminate or Abnormal FHR)

- Discontinue oxytocin.

- Assist the mother to a lateral position.

- Give IV fluid bolus of at least 500 mL of lactated Ringer's solution as indicated.

- Consider oxygen at 10 L/min via nonrebreather face mask (discontinue as soon as possible based on the FHR pattern).

- If no response, consider 0.25 mg terbutaline SQ.

- To resume oxytocin after resolution of tachysystole: If oxytocin has been discontinued for less than 20–30 minutes, the FHR is normal, and contraction frequency, intensity, and duration are normal, resume oxytocin at no more than half the rate that caused the tachysystole and gradually increase the rate as appropriate based on unit protocol and maternal-fetal status. If the oxytocin is discontinued for more than 30–40 minutes, resume oxytocin at the initial dose ordered.

IV, Intravenous; SQ, subcutaneous.
Adapted from: Simpson, K. R. (2008c). Labor and birth. In K. R. Simpson & P. A. Creehan (Eds.). *AWHONN's Perinatal Nursing* (3rd ed., pp. 300–398). Philadelphia: Lippincott Williams and Wilkins.

infusion at half the rate that caused the tachystole and gradually increase the rate as appropriate based on unit protocol and maternal-fetal status. However, if the oxytocin is discontinued for more than 30 to 40 minutes, most of the exogenous oxytocin is metabolized and plasma levels are similar to that of a woman who has not received IV oxytocin (Seitchik et al., 1984). In this clinical situation, a suggested protocol may include restarting the oxytocin at or near the initial dose ordered. There are individual differences in myometrial sensitivity and the response to oxytocin during labor (Arias, 2000; Smith & Merrill, 2006; Ulstem, 1997). It may be necessary to use a lower dose and lengthen the interval between dosage increases when there is evidence of the patient's previous sensitivity to the drug.

Administration of tocolytics is another option that is occasionally used as a temporary measure to provide intrauterine resuscitation for a prolonged deceleration, or for other indeterminate or abnormal FHR patterns resulting from tachystole, by reducing uterine activity (ACOG, 2005b; Caldeyro-Barcia, 1992). It is presumed that the reduction in uterine activity as the result of tocolytic administration may improve uteroplacental blood flow, thereby improving fetal oxygenation (Pullen et al., 2007). A subcutaneous dose of terbutaline 0.25 mg is often used for this purpose; however, there are only limited supportive data regarding terbutaline or other tocolytics as an intervention for intrauterine resuscitation. Nitroglycerine is used in some institutions for intrauterine resuscitation; however, when compared with terbutaline, nitroglycerine results in a significant decrease in maternal mean arterial blood pressure and is less effective as a tocolytic in reducing uterine activity (Pullen et al., 2007). According to the latest Cochrane Review (three studies included), betamimetic therapy appears to be able to reduce the number of FHR abnormalities; however, there is not enough evidence based on clinically important outcomes to evaluate the use of these medications for suspected fetal compromise (Kulier & Hofmeyr, 2000).

One strategy to prevent tachysystole is to use a physiologic dosage regimen for oxytocin induc-tion and augmentation. Beginning at 1 milliunit per minute and increasing by 1 to 2 milliunits per minute no more frequently than every 30 to 40 minutes will minimize risk of oxytocin side effects. A meta-analysis of low-dose versus high-dose oxytocin for labor induction by Crane and Young (1998) found that this type of protocol resulted in fewer episodes of excessive uterine activity, fewer operative vaginal births, a higher rate of spontaneous vaginal birth, and a lower rate of cesarean birth.

Intravenous Fluid Administration

When a pregnant woman is hypovolemic or hypotensive, blood volume is shifted away from the uterus, decreasing uteroplacental perfusion and oxygen delivery to the fetus. It is believed that administration of fluids maximizes maternal intravascular volume and is therefore protective against decreases in uteroplacental perfusion. A reduction in uterine blood flow can occur following administration of regional anesthesia because the sympathectomy causes dilation of peripheral vessels, lower peripheral resistance, and a potential drop in uteroplacental blood flow. There are limited data to suggest that increasing IV fluids will positively affect uterine blood flow and thus fetal oxygenation, even in women who are normotensive and well hydrated. One study found that $FSpO_2$ was significantly increased after at least a 500-mL bolus of lactated Ringer's solution over 20 minutes in normotensive women who were otherwise receiving lactated Ringer's solution at 125 mL per hour (Simpson & James, 2005b). The increase in $FSpO_2$ was greatest with a 1000-mL IV fluid bolus. The positive effects on fetal oxygen status continued for more than 30 minutes after the IV fluid bolus (Simpson & James, 2005b). Thus, an IV fluid bolus of 500 to 1000 mL may be useful as an intrauterine resuscitation technique. However, caution should be exercised when increasing IV fluids or giving repeated IV fluid boluses. It is important to remember that some clinical situations such as preeclampsia, preterm labor treated with magnesium sulfate, or preterm labor treated with corticosteroids and beta-sympathomimetic medications carry an increased risk for pulmonary edema that might necessitate fluid restriction. Oxytocin has an antidiuretic effect, so prolonged use of oxytocin can also lead to fluid overload if IV fluids are used too liberally. An extreme effect of fluid overload related to excessive use of oxytocin is water intoxication.

Some clinicians believe that IV solutions containing glucose can improve FHR variability; however, there is no supportive evidence for this practice. Intravenous fluid boluses of glucose-containing solutions should generally be avoided because there is evidence to suggest that maternal IV administration of glucose can have potentially detrimental effects on fetal status, including increased fetal lactate and decreased fetal pH (Philipson et al., 1987; Wasserstrum, 1992). If the fetus is hypoxemic (a possibility when the FHR is indeterminate or abnormal), relatively small elevations in glucose can lead to lactic acidosis (Philipson et al.; Wasserstrum). IV solutions with glucose can cause fetal hyperglycemia and subsequent reactive hypoglycemia, hyperinsulinism, acidosis, jaundice, and transient tachypnea in the newborn after birth (Carmen, 1986; Grylack, Chu, & Scanlon, 1984; Mendiola, Grylack, & Scanlon, 1982; Singhi, 1988; Sleutel & Golden, 1999; Sommer, Norr, & Roberts, 2000). A bolus of IV solution containing glucose also can cause marked maternal hyperglycemia (Mendiola et al., 1982; Wasserstrum). Thus, when the clinical situation is such that a bolus of IV fluids may be necessary to rapidly expand plasma volume for the woman in labor, the research indicates that these IV fluids should not contain glucose, especially if birth is imminent (Cerri et al., 2000; Hawkins, 2003).

As a preventive measure, adequate hydration in labor should be maintained. Labor can be compared to sustained exercise during which participants do not ingest adequate amounts of fluid and become clinically dehydrated (Freeman et al., 2003). The increased insensible fluid loss associated with labor has the potential to lead to a decrease in intravascular volume if fluid replacement is inadequate, which can result in a decrease in uterine blood flow (Garite et al., 2000). Although oral hydration may be appropriate for most healthy women during labor, IV replacement fluids usually are provided simultaneously. Findings from two studies suggest that the usual amount of IV fluids of 125 mL per hour may not be not sufficient to support adequate labor hydration (Eslamian, Marsoosi, & Pakneeyat, 2006; Garite et al.). In these randomized clinical trials, women who received 250 mL per hour of IV fluids had shorter labors and were less likely to require oxytocin augmentation than women who received 125 mL per hour.

Oxygen Administration

Maternal oxygen therapy is commonly used for intrauterine resuscitation and appears to be beneficial in improving fetal oxygen status during labor. In a classic study of the effects of maternal oxygen administration on the fetus, 100% oxygen via face mask corrected "nonreassuring" FHR patterns by decreasing the baseline FHR during fetal tachycardia and reducing or eliminating late decelerations (Althabe et al., 1967). There is evidence that fetal oxygen levels will increase as a result of maternal oxygen administration of 10 L per minute via nonrebreather face mask (Aldrich et al., 1994; Bartnicki & Saling, 1994; Dildy, Clark, & Loucks, 1995; Haydon et al., 2006; McNamara, Johnson, & Lilford, 1993; Simpson & James, 2005b). Fetuses with lower oxygen saturation appear to benefit most, in terms of an increase in oxygen levels, from maternal oxygen administration (Haydon et al.; Simpson & James).

Although healthy women in labor have nearly 100% SpO_2 (usually between 96% and 99%), increasing inspired oxygen increases blood oxygen tension and results in more oxygen delivered to the fetus (McNamara et al., 1993). There is a more rapid increase in $FSpO_2$ when oxygen is given as compared with the decrease in $FSpO_2$ when it is discontinued, suggesting that the fetus responds to the new placental oxygen gradient by accepting oxygen more rapidly than it gives it up. In two studies, $FSpO_2$ levels higher than those preceding administration of oxygen to the mother persisted 30 minutes after the oxygen was discontinued (Dildy et al., 1995; Simpson & James, 2005b). Fetal hemoglobin has a higher affinity for oxygen than adult hemoglobin, and fetal hematocrit is higher than that of adults. These physiologic factors allow for a steeper increase in fetal oxygen concentration and $FSpO_2$ during maternal oxygen therapy.

The method that provides the highest fraction of inspired oxygen (FiO_2) should be used when oxygen is administered to the mother. The nonrebreather face mask works best because the FiO_2 at 10 L per minute is approximately 80% to 100%, as compared with a simple face mask (FiO_2 27%–40%) or nasal cannula (FiO_2 31%) (Simpson & James, 2005b).

There is scant evidence concerning how long maternal oxygen therapy should be continued and its effects on the mother and fetus (Simpson, 2008b). Both *hypo*xia and *hyper*oxia can result in production of oxygen-free radicals, which can cause oxidative stress and subsequent adverse effects such as damage to cell membranes, cell structures, and cellular lipoproteins and DNA (Klinger et al., 2005). These effects are more pronounced when oxygen is reintroduced after a period of hypoxia and are thought to be the genesis of reperfusion injuries in the newborn (Blackburn, 2006; Khaw & Ngan Kee, 2004; Klinger et al.). The newborn's brain is particularly vulnerable to oxidative stress because neuronal membranes are rich in polyunsaturated fatty acids and have a relative deficiency of several important antioxidant enzymes (Blackburn, 2006). Antioxidants are normal physiologic defense mechanisms that delay or prevent oxidative stress and formation of free radicals or damaging by-products; however, these defenses are limited in newborns, especially preterm babies, because of lowered intracellular antioxidant enzymes and other defense systems (Blackburn, 2005, 2006).

Data regarding the potential deleterious effects of hyperoxia on newborns during resuscitation at birth and in the first few hours of life (Vento et al., 2001, 2003; Klinger et al., 2005) prompted the neonatal experts who develop guidelines for neonatal resuscitation to make changes in their recommendations for care for depressed babies at birth (AAP & American Heart Association [AHA], 2006). Room air (21% FiO_2) is now considered an acceptable alternative to 100% oxygen for neonatal resuscitation in selected clinical situations and for preterm babies. Titration of FiO_2 to the resultant oxygen saturation of the baby is recommended when oxygen is administered for neonatal resuscitation. Damage to the baby from the oxidative stress produced by high levels of oxygen and associated oxygen-free radical activity and its by-products may be minimized by these techniques (AAP & AHA). However, it remains uncertain whether oxidative stress has a causal role or is merely a consequence of the physiologic sequelae associated with hypoxia and asphyxia (Blackburn, 2006; Higgins et al., 2007).

Although transfer of oxygen from the mother to the fetus via passive diffusion as well as placental equilibrium prevent fetal hyperoxia as a result of maternal oxygen administration (Khaw & Ngan Kee, 2004), even small increases in maternal and fetal PO_2 as a result of maternal oxygen administration can produce oxygen-free radical activity in mothers and their fetuses (Khaw et al., 2002). The potential long-term effects on the mother and fetus are unknown. Only one human study has involved measurement of by-products of oxygen-free radical activity in mothers and fetuses after mothers at term were given oxygen prior to birth (Khaw et al.). In this study, 22 women were randomized to receive oxygen at 60% FiO_2 prior to cesarean birth (mean oxygen exposure, 53 minutes; range, 33–150 minutes), compared with a control group of 22 women who did not receive oxygen. Levels of by-products of oxygen-free radical activity in the mothers were noted within 10 minutes of maternal oxygen administration, peaked at 30 minutes, and continued to be detected at abnormally high ranges throughout the 60 minutes of monitoring. Levels of oxygen-free radical activity also were noted in the umbilical arterial and venous cord blood at birth of fetuses whose mothers received 60% oxygen at levels significantly higher than the control group (Khaw et al.). There is evidence that some by-products of oxygen-free radical activity cross the placenta, whereas others do not (Rogers et al., 1999).

Conversely, fetal hypoxia and acidemia (umbilical artery pH < 7.15; base excess < −8) during labor also have been shown to cause abnormally elevated levels of by-products of oxygen-free radical activity (Rogers et al., 1997). Based on the research, withholding oxygen from mothers in labor when the FHR pattern is indeterminate or abnormal to prevent possible adverse effects of oxygen-free radicals is not recommended. The potential effects of progressive fetal hypoxemia and acidemia have been demonstrated (ACOG & AAP, 2003), so clinical interventions to avoid these conditions are warranted (Simpson, 2008b). Oxygen therapy via the mother to the fetus can be beneficial in increasing fetal oxygen levels (Aldrich et al., 1994; Dildy et al., 1995; Haydon et al., 2006; McNamara et al., 1993; Simpson & James, 2005b); however, prolonged use should be discouraged until more data are available regarding the potential risks to the mother and fetus (RCOG, 2001b). If other intrauterine resuscitation techniques have not resulted in resolution of the FHR pattern, maternal oxygen therapy has been shown to be reasonable (Dildy et al.; Haydon et al.; Simpson & James). However, oxygen should be discontinued as soon as possible based on the fetal response. Much more data are needed on the effects of longer periods of maternal oxygen administration on the mother and baby (Simpson, 2008b). When oxygen is chosen for intrauterine resuscitation, it is assumed that other sources of potential fetal physiologic stress have been minimized; thus, oxytocin should not be infusing concurrently with maternal oxygen administration.

Interventions for Anesthesia-Related Hypotension

Conduction anesthetics increase the risk of decreased placental blood flow secondary to maternal hypotension resulting from sympathetic blockade. If maternal repositioning and IV fluid bolus are not successful in resolving FHR changes, ephedrine may be given to increase vascular tone and thus maternal blood pressure (ACOG, 2005b). Ephedrine is the recommended agent because it is least likely to reduce uterine blood flow (Freeman et al., 2003).

Amnioinfusion

Amnioinfusion, the transcervical instillation of fluid into the amniotic cavity, is a reasonable therapeutic option to attempt to resolve variable FHR decelerations by correcting umbilical cord compression resulting from decreased amniotic fluid or oligohydramnios (ACOG, 2005b, 2006). Amnioinfusion has been found to significantly resolve patterns of "moderate to severe" variable decelerations but does not affect late decelerations or patterns with absent variability (Hofmeyr, 2007; Miño et al., 1999, Miyazaki & Nevarez, 1985).

Although amnioinfusion has been shown to dilute thick, meconium-stained amniotic fluid and decrease the incidence of meconium below the newborn's vocal cords (Klingner & Kruse, 1999; Pierce, Gaudier, & Sanchez-Ramos, 2000), in a large international study of 1998 women in term labor, amnioinfusion did not reduce risk of moderate or severe meconium aspiration syndrome or perinatal death (Fraser et al., 2005). Based on available evidence, amnioinfusion is no longer recommended as an intervention for meconium-stained fluid (ACOG, 2006).

Amnioinfusion does not seem to affect the length of labor (Strong, 1997) and appears to be safe for women who are attempting a vaginal birth after a previous cesarean birth (Hicks, 2005; Ouzounian, Miller, & Paul, 1996). Prophylactic amnioinfusion for oligohydramnios is not necessary and has not been shown to prevent the development of variable decelerations

(Hofmeyr, 2007). Because of its efficacy in resolving variable decelerations, risk of cesarean birth related to a "nonreassuring" FHR pattern may be decreased with amnioinfusion (Hofmeyr). Based on available evidence, amnioinfusion should be limited to the management of variable decelerations (ACOG, 2006). Contraindications may include vaginal bleeding, uterine anomalies, and active infection such as human immunodeficiency virus or herpes simplex virus. Careful monitoring and documentation of fluid infused is important to avoid iatrogenic polyhydramnios (Box 6-1).

Modification of Maternal Pushing Efforts during Second-Stage Labor

Indeterminate or abnormal FHR patterns may occur during the second stage of labor. The continuation of coached pushing in the presence of these FHR patterns can lead to iatrogenic fetal stress as evidenced by recurrent variable or prolonged decelerations, loss of normal baseline, minimal or absent variability, tachycardia, and bradycardia (Freeman et al., 2003). Although most fetuses tolerate decelerations during pushing, some fetuses enter the second stage of labor with less physiologic reserve than others. The active pushing phase of the second stage of labor is the most physiologically stressful part of labor for the fetus (Piquard et al., 1989; Roberts, 2002). When compared with the passive fetal descent phase, the active pushing phase results in more FHR decelerations (Hansen, Clark, & Foster, 2002; Piquard et al., 1988; Simpson & James, 2005a) and a progressive adverse effect on fetal acid-base status (Nordström et al., 2001) and FSpO$_2$ (Simpson & James, 2005a). Shortening the active pushing phase by delaying pushing until maternal urge to push can promote fetal well-being (Hansen et al.; Nordström et al.; Piquard et al.; Simpson & James). Prolonged active pushing may have a negative effect on fetal status and the condition of the baby at birth (Piquard et al.).

Fetal assessment data (either from electronic fetal monitoring or intermittent auscultation) should be used to guide maternal pushing efforts

and to minimize the risk of iatrogenic negative FHR changes. There is ample evidence that fetal status in the last 1 to 2 hours prior to birth has significant implications on neonatal well-being at birth. "Abnormal" FHR characteristics (variable and late decelerations and bradycardia) during second-stage labor are associated with higher rates of operative vaginal birth, Apgar scores lower than 7 at 1 minute, umbilical artery pH < 7.2, and admission to the neonatal intensive care unit (NICU) when compared with "normal" FHR patterns (Sheiner et al., 2001). "Abnormal" changes (a decrease) in FHR variability in the last hour prior to birth are associated with an increased risk of fetal acidemia (umbilical artery pH < 7.05) compared with normal variability (Siira et al., 2005). ("Abnormal" and "normal" were used by the researchers to describe FHR patterns in the Sheiner et al. (2001) and Siira et al. (2005) studies, but these descriptions may not correspond precisely with the 2008 NICHD definitions of these terms.) Variable and late decelerations occurring with every one to two contractions in the 30 minutes prior to birth are associated with lower 1-minute and 5-minute Apgar scores, more cases of umbilical artery pH < 7.2, and more admissions to the NICU when compared with decelerations occurring less frequently during this time period (Kazandi et al., 2003). Minimal to absent variability, bradycardia, prolonged decelerations, and late decelerations with absence of accelerations in the last hour prior to birth are associated with significant fetal acidemia (umbilical artery pH < 7.0) (Williams & Galerneau, 2002, 2003). Recurrent late or variable decelerations and minimal variability with absence of accelerations in the 2 hours prior to birth are associated with fetal acidemia (umbilical artery pH < 7.1) (Sameshima & Ikenoue, 2005).

Suggestions for care during second-stage labor to promote fetal well-being are presented in Box 6-2. Temporarily discontinuing pushing to allow the fetus to recover when the FHR is indeterminate or abnormal and limiting pushing to every other or every third contraction to

BOX 6-1   Amnioinfusion

Amnioinfusion is a reasonable therapeutic option when there are recurrent variable decelerations as a result of a decrease in amniotic fluid (ACOG, 2005b, 2006; Hofmeyr, 2007).

An institutional protocol may include the following:
- Contraindications (e.g., vaginal bleeding, uterine anomalies, active infections such as HIV or herpes, impending birth)
- Who can perform amnioinfusion
- Who can insert the intrauterine pressure catheter
- What type of fluid may be used (normal saline or lactated Ringer's solution)
- What instillation method may be used (gravity flow or infusion pump)
- What infusion techniques may be used (bolus, continuous, or a combination of both)
- When and why the procedure should be altered (e.g., loss of large amount of fluid resulting from position change or coughing, increased uterine resting tone, reappearance of variable decelerations, or no fluid return)

General guidelines for the procedure are as follows:
- The amnioinfusion procedure and the indication should be explained to the woman and her support persons prior to initiation.
- During amnioinfusion, room temperature normal saline or lactated Ringer's solution is infused into the uterus transcervically via an intrauterine pressure catheter.
- The initial bolus is usually 250 to 500 mL given over a 20- to 30-minute period using either an infusion pump or gravity flow. Both methods are appropriate and seem to be equally efficacious.
- Some protocols allow for a continuous infusion of 2 to 3 mL per minute (120–180 mL per hour) after the bolus until resolution of the variable decelerations (Tucker, Miller, & Miller, 2008). Usually the maximal amount of fluid infused is 1000 mL (Tucker et al.).
- If variable decelerations have not resolved after infusion of 800 to 1000 mL, the infusion may be discontinued and alternative approaches used (Tucker et al.).
- During bolus of the infusion and maintenance rate, approximate amount of fluid returning should be noted and recorded to avoid iatrogenic polyhydramnios.
- Assessment of fluid return can be accomplished by weighing the underpads (1 mL of fluid equals ≈ 1 gram of weight) (Tucker et al.).
- As a general consideration, if 250 mL has infused with no return, the amnioinfusion is discontinued until the fluid has returned.
- Overdistention is more likely when the presenting part obstructs flow, thus releasing the fluid by gently elevating the presenting part may be a successful intervention.
- A dual-lumen intrauterine catheter is preferred so that estimate of uterine resting tone can be assessed during the infusion.
- Uterine resting tone may appear higher than normal during the procedure (from 25 to 40 mm Hg). If there is a concern about an elevated uterine resting tone (>40 mm Hg), temporarily discontinue the infusion to attempt a more accurate assessment. If the uterine resting tone exceeds 25 mm Hg while the infusion is temporarily discontinued for assessment of uterine resting tone, consider discontinuing the infusion.
- Warming of the solution may not be necessary for full-term fetuses but may be appropriate for preterm or growth-restricted fetuses. Fetal bradycardia may occur if the solution is colder than room temperature and/or is infused too rapidly (Tucker et al.). Some providers prefer to warm the solution to body temperature. If the solution is warmed, acceptable temperatures are 93° to 96° F (34°–37° C). The safest method to warm the solution is by use of an electronic blood/fluid warmer. Microwaves and other types of warming techniques should not be used to heat the solution.
- Assessment and documentation:
  - Contraction intensity and frequency should be continually assessed during the procedure.
  - In addition to assessments appropriate for the first stage of labor, additional assessments may include the following:
    - Fundal height and leakage of fluids
    - Amount, color, and odor of fluid leaking from vagina
    - Fetal response such as resolution of the variable decelerations
- Documentation may include the maternal and fetal response; uterine resting tone; fluid output; and type, rate and amount of solution infused.

FHR, Fetal heart rate; HIV, human immunodeficiency virus.

BOX 6-2   Second-Stage Labor Care to Promote Fetal Well-Being

- For women with epidural anesthesia who do not feel the urge to push when they are completely dilated, consider delaying pushing until the urge to push is felt (up to 2 hours for nulliparous women and up to 1 hour for multiparous women).
- Discourage prolonged breath holding. Instead, instruct the woman to bear down and allow her to choose whether or not to hold her breath while pushing.
- Discourage more than three pushing efforts with each contraction and more than 6–8 seconds of each pushing effort.
- Avoid counting to ten to promote sustained breath-holding during pushing efforts.
- Take steps to maintain a normal FHR pattern while pushing. Push with every other or every third contraction if necessary to avoid recurrent FHR decelerations. Reposition as necessary for FHR decelerations.
- Avoid tachysystole during the second stage of labor

FHR, Fetal heart rate.
Adapted from: AWHONN. (2008). *Nursing care and management of the second stage of labor,* (Evidence-Based Clinical Practice Guideline, 2nd ed.), Washington, D. C.: Association of Women's Health, Obstetric and Neonatal Nurses.

maintain normal FHR characteristics can be effective methods to minimize risk of progressive fetal oxygen desaturation (Simpson & James, 2005a). Sustained coached closed-glottis pushing, that is, "take a deep breath and hold it for 10 to 15 seconds", and pushing more than four times with each contraction should be avoided (Association of Women's Health, Obstetric, and Neonatal Nurses [AWHONN], 2008; Barnett & Humenick, 1982; Caldyro-Barcia et al., 1981; Simpson & James). Instead, three to four pushing efforts per contraction lasting 6 to 8 seconds each is more appropriate for the mother and fetus (Figure 6-3) (AWHONN, 2008; Barnett & Humenick, 1982; Caldyro-Barcia et al., 1981; Roberts, 2002; Roberts & Hanson, 2007; Simpson & James). A baseline FHR should be identifiable between contractions. Some fetuses develop metabolic acidemia if recurrent variable or late decelerations continue over a long period, especially if accompanied by tachysystole (Bakker et al., 2007; Kazandi et al., 2003). As a potential preventive measure, shortening the active pushing phase by delaying active pushing until the woman feels the urge to push can minimize fetal stress (Hansen et al., 2002; Piquard et al., 1989; Roberts; Simpson & James). In the absence of an urge to push, delaying pushing for

FIGURE 6-3   Coached Closed-Glottis (Valsalva) Pushing during the Second Stage of Labor: Effect on Maternal Hemodynamics and Fetal Status

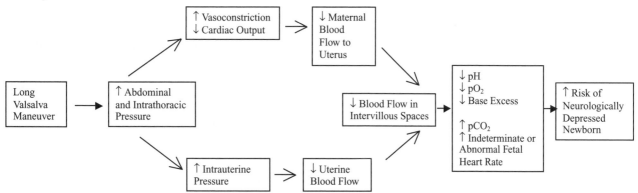

Note: From "Infant outcome in relation to second stage labor pushing method." by M. M. Barnett, and S. S. Humenick. 1982. *Birth and the Family Journal,* p.42. Copyright 1982 by Wiley Blackwell. Adapted with permission.

up to 2 hours for nulliparous women and up to 1 hour for multiparous women is suggested with regional analgesia/anesthesia (Fraser et al., 2000; Hansen et al., 2002; Mayberry et al., 1999; Simpson & James; Sprague et al., 2006).

Interventions to Support Coping and Labor Progress

In many modern labor and birth settings, nurses, physicians and midwives are often pressed for time and caring for more than one woman simultaneously. It is important to maintain a caring connection with each individual woman and her family and to assess and respond to each woman's needs, desires, and potential risk factors. Asking women about their expectations, providing accurate information, maintaining open communication, and staying engaged with women and their families increases the woman's trust and sense of control, therefore supporting her coping and improving her overall perception of her birth experience. The following aspects of care during labor and birth may promote coping, labor progress, and a positive childbirth experience:

- Review plans/expectations with the woman and her partner, friends, or family members.
- Maintain a calm environment whenever possible.
- Include family members as per the desires of the woman.
- Remain at the bedside as much as possible and per the desires of the woman.
- Assess maternal and fetal status at the level appropriate for this woman.
- Encourage frequent position changes, especially to an upright position.
- Minimize use of technology as appropriate to the woman's clinical condition.
- Avoid unnecessary interventions.

SUMMARY

All members of the perinatal team should ideally have a common understanding of the physiologic and pathophysiologic characteristics of common FHR patterns and shared expectations for how and when to intervene when the FHR characteristics are indeterminate or abnormal (Fox et al., 2000). Knowledge related to FHM is not exclusive to one discipline. Decisions regarding initial and subsequent interventions for indeterminate and abnormal FHR patterns should be individualized to each clinical situation on the basis of ongoing assessment and the maternal-fetal response. Although indeterminate or abnormal FHR patterns can develop at any time during labor despite excellent clinical care, in some cases, the need for intrauterine resuscitation may be the result of iatrogenic fetal compromise. Careful vigilance is required to avoid supine maternal positioning, hypotension, dehydration, oxytocin-induced tachysystole, elective amniotomy at high fetal station, and continued coached pushing when recurrent decelerations or abnormal FHR patterns are present. When the FHR characteristics are suggestive of acute or evolving fetal compromise, members of the interdisciplinary perinatal team should remain calm and provide clear directions to the woman as well as other team members to decrease patient anxiety and promote an effective and timely team response. While explaining the situation to the woman and her support persons, a calm, factual, concise statement regarding the concerns about fetal status and the need to provide interventions to potentially resolve the condition may be beneficial. Ideally, an ongoing explanation is provided concurrent with the team efforts to improve fetal status.

A decision tree that addresses the issues of intrapartum goals, physiologic interventions, and the use of additional measures such as monitoring equipment modifications is offered in Figure 6-4. This decision tree provides a general process outline, which must be interpreted and modified as appropriate, in light of the perinatal team's clinical assessment of the mother and fetus.

FIGURE 6-4   Decision Tree for Fetal Heart Monitoring

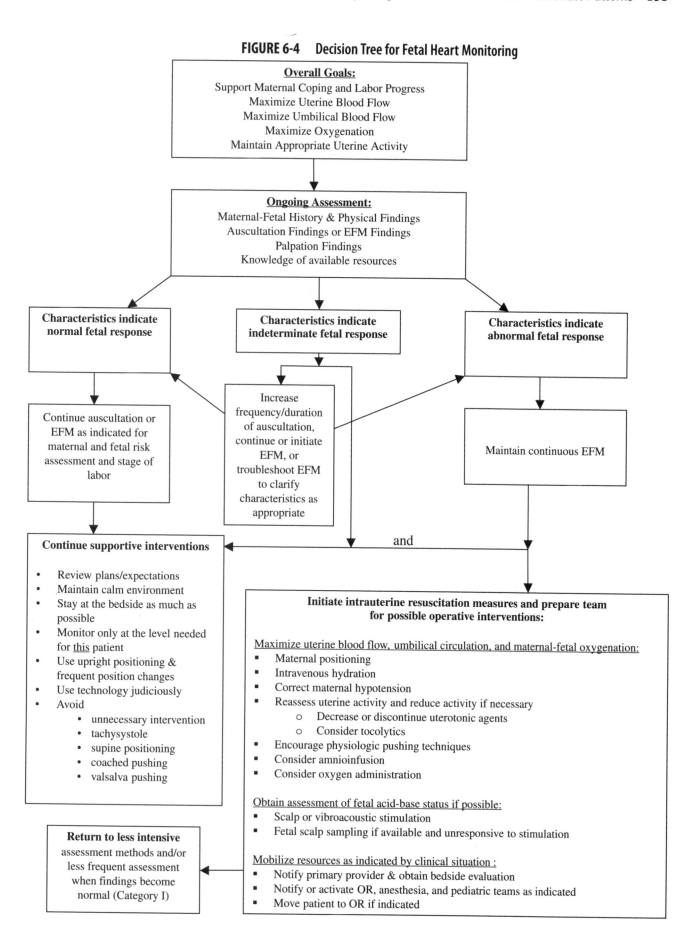

REFERENCES

Abitbol, M. M. (1985). Supine position in labor and associated fetal heart rate changes. *Obstetrics and Gynecology, 65*(4), 481–186.

Aldrich, C. J., D'Antona, D., Spencer, J. A., Wyatt, J. S., Peebles, D. M., Delpy, D. T., & Reynolds, E. O. (1995). The effect of maternal posture on fetal cerebral oxygenation during labour. *British Journal of Obstetrics and Gynaecology, 102*(1), 14–19.

Aldrich, C. J., Wyatt, J. S., Spencer, J. A., Reynolds, E. O., & Delpy, D. T. (1994). The effect of maternal oxygen administration on human fetal cerebral oxygenation measured during labour by near infrared spectroscopy. *British Journal of Obstetrics and Gynaecology, 101*(6), 509–513.

Althabe, O. Jr., Schwarcz, R. L., Pose, S.V., Escarcena, L., & Caldeyro-Barcia, R. (1967). Effects on fetal heart rate and fetal pO2 of oxygen administration to the mother. *American Journal of Obstetrics and Gynecology, 98,* 858–870.

American Academy of Pediatrics & American Heart Association. (2006). *Textbook of neonatal resuscitation* (5th ed.). Elk Grove Village, IL: Author.

American College of Obstetricians and Gynecologists. (1999). *Induction of labor* (Practice Bulletin No.10). Washington, DC: Author.

American College of Obstetricians and Gynecologists. (2003). *Dystocia and the augmentation of labor* (Practice Bulletin No. 49). Washington, DC: Author.

American College of Obstetricians and Gynecologists. (2005a). *Inappropriate use of the terms fetal distress and birth asphyxia* (Committee Opinion No. 326). Washington, DC: Author.

American College of Obstetricians and Gynecologists. (2005b). *Intrapartum fetal heart rate monitoring* (Practice Bulletin No. 70). Washington, DC: Author.

American College of Obstetricians and Gynecologists. (2006). *Amnioinfusion does not prevent meconium aspiration syndrome* (Committee Opinion No. 346). Washington, DC: Author.

American College of Obstetricians and Gynecologists, & American Academy of Pediatrics. (2003). *Neonatal encephalopathy and cerebral palsy: Defining the pathogenesis and pathophysiology.* Washington, DC: Author.

Arias, F. (2000). Pharmacology of oxytocin and prostaglandins. *Clinical Obstetrics and Gynecology, 43*(3), 455–468.

Association of Women's Health, Obstetric and Neonatal Nurses (2008). *Nursing management of the second stage of labor* (Evidence-Based Clinical Practice Guideline). Washington, DC. Author.

Bakker, P. C., Kurver, P. H., Kuik, D. J., & Van Geijn, H. P. (2007). Elevated uterine activity increases the risk of fetal acidosis at birth. *American Journal of Obstetrics and Gynecology, 196,* 313.e1–313.e6.

Bakker, P. C., & van Geijn, H. P. (2008). Uterine activity: Implications for the condition of the fetus. *Journal of Perinatal Medicine, 36,* 30-37.

Barnett, M. M., & Humenick, S. S. (1982). Infant outcome in relation to second stage labor pushing method. *Birth and the Family Journal, 9*(4)221–229.

Bartnicki, J., & Saling, E. (1994). The influence of maternal oxygen administration on the fetus. *International Journal of Gynaecology and Obstetrics, 45*(2), 87–95.

Blackburn, S. (2005). Free radicals in perinatal and neonatal care, Part 1: The basics. *Journal of Perinatal and Neonatal Nursing, 19*(4), 298–300.

Blackburn, S. (2006). Free radicals in perinatal and neonatal care, Part 2: Oxidative stress during the perinatal and neonatal period. *Journal of Perinatal and Neonatal Nursing, 20*(2), 125–127.

Caldeyro-Barcia, R. (1992). Intrauterine fetal reanimation in acute intrapartum fetal distress. *Early Human Development, 29,* 27–33.

Caldeyro-Barcia, R., Giussi, G., Storch, E., Poseiro, J. J., Lafaurie, N., Kettenhuber, K., et al. (1981). The bearing down efforts and their effects on fetal heart rate, oxygenation and acid base balance. *Journal of Perinatal Medicine, 9*(Suppl. 1), 63–67.

Carbonne, B., Benachi, A., Lévèque, M. L., Cabrol, D., & Papiernik, E. (1996). Maternal position during labor: Effects on fetal oxygen saturation measured by pulse oximetry. *Obstetrics and Gynecology, 88*(5), 797–800.

Carmen, S. (1986). Neonatal hypoglycemia in response to maternal glucose infusion before delivery. *Journal of Obstetric, Gynecologic and Neonatal Nursing, 15*(4), 319–322.

Cerri, V., Tarantini, M., Zuliani, G., Schena, V., Redaelli, C., & Niconlini, U. (2000). Intravenous glucose infusion in labor does not affect maternal and fetal acid base balance. *Journal of Maternal-Fetal Medicine, 9*(4), 204–208.

Clark, S. L., Cotton, D. B., Pivarnik, J. M., Lee, W., Hankins, G. D., Benedetti, T. J., et al. (1991). Position change and central hemodynamic profile during normal third trimester pregnancy and post partum. *American Journal of Obstetrics and Gynecology, 164*(3), 883–887.

Crane, J. M., & Young, D. C. (1998). Meta-analysis of low-dose versus high-dose oxytocin for labour induction. *Journal of the Society of Obstetricians and Gynaecologists of Canada, 20,* 1215–1223.

Crane, J. M., Young, D. C., Butt, K. D., Bennett, K. A., & Hutchens, D. (2001). Excessive uterine activity accompanying induced labor. *American Journal of Obstetrics and Gynecology, 97*(6), 926–931.

Dildy, G. A., Clark, S. L., & Loucks, C. A. (1995). Effects of maternal inhalation of 40% oxygen on fetal oxygen saturation. *American Journal of Obstetrics and Gynecology, 172*(6), 1939–1943.

Eslamian, L., Marsoosi, V., & Pakneeyat, Y. (2006). Increased intravenous fluid intake and the course of labor in nulliparous women. *International Journal of Gynaecology and Obstetrics, 93*(2), 10–15.

Fox, M., Kilpatrick, S., King, T., & Parer, J. T. (2000). Fetal heart rate monitoring: Interpretation and collaborative management. *Journal of Midwifery and Women's Health, 45*(6), 498–507.

Fraser, W. D., Hofmeyr, J., Lede, R., Faron, G., Alexander, S., Goffinet, F., et al. (2005). Amnioinfusion for the prevention of the meconium aspiration syndrome. *New England Journal of Medicine, 353*(9), 909–917.

Fraser, W. D., Marcoux, S., Krauss, I., Douglas, J., Goulet, C., & Boulvain, M. for the PEOPLE (Pushing Early or Pushing Late with Epidurals) Study Group. (2000). Multicenter, randomized, controlled trial of delayed pushing for nulliparous women in the second stage of labor with continuous epidural analgesia. *American Journal of Obstetrics and Gynecology, 182*(5), 1165–1172.

Freeman, R. K., Garite, T. J., & Nageotte, M. P. (2003). *Fetal heart rate monitoring* (3rd ed.). Philadelphia: Lippincott Williams and Wilkins.

Garite, T. J., Weeks, J., Peters-Phair, K., Pattillo, C., & Brewster, W. R. (2000). A randomized controlled trial of the effect of increased intravenous hydration on the course of labor in nulliparous women. *American Journal of Obstetrics and Gynecology, 183*(6), 1544–1548.

Grylack, L. J., Chu, S. S., & Scanlon, J. W. (1984). Use of intravenous fluids before cesarean section: Effects on perinatal glucose, insulin, and sodium homeostasis. *Obstetrics and Gynecology, 63*(5), 654–658.

Gupta, J. K., & Hofmeyr, G. J. (2004). Position for women during second stage labour. *Cochrane Database of Systematic Reviews, 1*, CD002006.

Hansen, S. L., Clark, S. L., & Foster, J. C. (2002). Active pushing versus passive fetal descent in the second stage of labor: A randomized controlled trial. *Obstetrics and Gynecology, 99*(1), 29–34.

Hawkins, J. L. (2003). Anesthesia-related mortality. *Clinical Obstetrics and Gynecology, 46*(3), 679–687.

Haydon, M. L., Gorenberg, D. M., Ghamsary, M., Rumney, P. J., Patillo, C., Nageotte, M., & Garite, T. (2006). The effect of maternal oxygen administration during labor on fetal pulse oximetry. *American Journal of Obstetrics and Gynecology, 195*(3), 735–738.

Hicks, P. (2005). Systematic review of the risk of uterine rupture with the use of amnioinfusion after previous cesarean delivery. *Southern Medical Journal, 98*(4), 458–461.

Higgins, R. D., Bancalari, E., Willinger, M., & Raju, T. N. (2007). Executive summary of the workshop on oxygen in neonatal therapies: Controversies and opportunities. *Pediatrics, 119*(4), 790–796.

Hofmeyr, G. J. (2007). Amnioinfusion for potential or suspected umbilical cord compression in labour. *Cochrane Database of Systematic Reviews,* (2), CD001182.

Johnson, N., van Oudgaarden, E., Montague, I., & McNamara, H. (1994). The effect of oxytocin-induced hyperstimulation on fetal oxygen. *British Journal of Obstetrics and Gynaecology, 101*(9), 805–807.

Kazandi, M., Sendag, F., Akercan, F., Terek, M. C., & Gundem, G. (2003). Different types of variable decelerations and their effects to neonatal outcome. *Singapore Medical Journal, 44*(5), 243–247.

Khaw, K. S., & Ngan Kee, W. D. (2004). Fetal effects of maternal supplementary oxygen during caesarean section. *Current Opinion in Anaesthesiology, 17*(4), 309–313.

Khaw, K. S., Wang, C. C., Ngan Kee, W. D., Pang, C. P., & Rogers, M. S. (2002). Effects of high inspired oxygen fraction during elective caesarean under spinal anaesthesia on maternal and fetal oxygenation and lipid peroxidation. *British Journal of Anaesthesia, 88*(1), 18–23.

Klinger, G., Beyene, J., Shah, P., & Perlman, M. (2005). Do hyperoxaemia and hypocapnia add to the risk of brain damage after intrapartum asphyxia? *Archives of Disease in Childhood: Fetal and Neonatal Edition, 90*(1), F49–F52.

Klingner, M. C., & Kruse, J. (1999). Meconium aspiration syndrome: Pathophysiology and prevention. *Journal of the American Board of Family Practice, 12*(6), 450–466.

Kulier, R., & Hofmeyr, G. J. (2000). Tocolytics for suspected intrapartum fetal distress. *Cochrane Database of Systematic Reviews,* (2): CD000035.

Macones, G. A., Hankins, G. D., Spong, C. Y., Hauth, J. D., & Moore, T. (2008). The 2008 National Institute of Child Health Human Development workshop report on electronic fetal monitoring: Update on definitions, interpretations, and research guidelines. *Obstetrics & Gynecology, 112,* 661–666; and *Journal of Obstetric, Gynecologic and Neonatal Nursing, 37,* 510–515.

Mayberry, L. J., Hammer, R., Kelly, C., True-Driver, B., & De, A. (1999). Use of delayed pushing with epidural anesthesia: Findings from a randomized controlled trial. *Journal of Perinatology, 19*(1), 26–30.

McNamara, H., & Johnson, N. (1995). The effect of uterine contractions on fetal oxygen saturation. *British Journal of Obstetrics and Gynaecology, 102*(8), 644–647.

McNamara, H., Johnson, N., & Lilford, R. (1993). The effect on fetal arteriolar oxygen saturation resulting from giving oxygen to the mother measured by pulse oximetry. *British Journal of Obstetrics and Gynaecology, 100*(5), 446–449.

Mendiola, J., Grylack, L. J., & Scanton, J. W. (1982). Effects of intrapartum maternal glucose infusion on the normal fetus and newborn. *Anesthesia and Analgesia, 61*(1), 32–35.

Miño, M., Puertas, A., Miranda, J. A., & Herruzo, A. J. (1999). Amnioinfusion in term labor with low amniotic fluid due to rupture of the membranes: A new indication. *European Journal of Obstetrics, Gynecology, and Reproductive Biology, 82*(1), 29–34.

Miyazaki, F. S., & Nevarez, F. (1985). Saline amnioinfusion for relief of repetitive variable decelerations: A prospective randomized study. *American Journal of Obstetrics and Gynecology, 153*(3), 301–306.

National Institute of Child Health and Human Development Research Planning Workshop. (1997). Electronic fetal heart rate monitoring: Research guidelines for interpretation. *American Journal of Obstetrics and Gynecology 177*(6), 1385–1390, and *Journal of Obstetric Gynecology and Neonatal Nursing, 26*(6), 635–640.

Nordström, L., Achanna, S., Nuka, K., & Arulkumaran, S. (2001). Fetal and maternal lactate increase during active second stage labour. *British Journal of Obstetrics and Gynaecology, 108*(3), 263–268.

Ouzounian, J. G., Miller, D. A., & Paul, R. H. (1996). Amnioinfusion in women with previous cesarean births: A preliminary report. *American Journal of Obstetrics and Gynecology, 174*(2), 783–786.

Parer, J. T., King, T., Flanders, S., Fox, M., & Kilpatrick, S. J. (2006). Fetal acidemia and electronic fetal heart rate patterns: Is there evidence of an association? *Journal of Maternal-Fetal and Neonatal Medicine, 19*(5), 289–294.

Paternoster, D. M., Micaglio, M., Tambuscio, B., Bracciante, R., & Chiarenza, A. (2001). The effect of epidural analgesia and uterine contractions on fetal oxygen saturation during the first stage of labour. *International Journal of Obstetric Anesthesia, 10*(2), 103–107.

Peebles, D. M., Spencer, J. A., Edwards, A. D., Wyatt, J. S., Reynolds, E. O., Cope, M., et al. (1994). Relation between frequency of uterine contractions and human fetal cerebral oxygen saturation studied during labour by near infrared spectroscopy. *British Journal of Obstetrics and Gynaecology, 101*(1), 44–48.

Philipson, E. H., Kalihan, S. C., Riha, M. M., & Pimental, R. (1987). Effects of maternal glucose infusion on fetal acid-base status in human pregnancy. *American Journal of Obstetrics and Gynecology, 157*(4, Pt. 1), 866–873.

Pierce, J., Gaudier, F. L., & Sanchez-Ramos, L. (2000). Intrapartum amnioinfusion for meconium-stained fluid: Meta-analysis of prospective clinical trials. *Obstetrics and Gynecology, 95*(6, Pt. 2), 1051–1056.

Piquard, F., Hsiung, R., Mettauer, M., Schaefer, A., Haberery, P., & Dellenbach, P. (1988). The validity of fetal heart rate monitoring during second stage of labor. *Obstetrics and Gynecology, 72*(5), 746–751.

Piquard, F., Schaefer, A., Hsiung, R., Dellenbach, P., & Haberey, P. (1989). Are there two biological parts in the second stage of labor? *Acta Obstetricia et Gynecologica Scandinavica, 68*(8), 713–718.

Pullen, K. M., Riley, E. T., Waller, S. A., Taylor, L., Caughey, A. B., Druzin, M. L., et al. (2007). Randomized comparison of intravenous terbutaline vs nitroglycerine for acute intrapartum fetal resuscitation. *American Journal of Obstetrics and Gynecology, 19*, 414e1–414e6.

Roberts, J. E. (2002). The "push" for evidence: Management of the second stage. *Journal of Midwifery and Women's Health, 47*(1), 2–15.

Roberts, J., & Hanson, L. (2007). Best practices in second stage labor care: Maternal bearing down and positioning. *Journal of Midwifery and Women's Health, 52*(3), 238–245.

Rogers, M. S., Mongelli, M., Tsang, K. H., & Wang, C. C. (1999). Fetal and maternal levels of lipid peroxides in term pregnancies. *Acta Obstetricia et Gynecologica Scandinavica, 78*(2), 120–124.

Rogers, M. S., Wang, W., Mongelli, M., Peng, C. P., Duley, J. A., & Chang, A. M. (1997). Lipid peroxidation in cord blood at birth: A marker of fetal hypoxia during labour. *Gynecologic and Obstetric Investigation, 44*(4), 229–233.

Royal College of Obstetricians and Gynaecologists. (2001a). *Induction of labour* (Evidence-Based Clinical Guideline No. 9). London: Author.

Royal College of Obstetricians and Gynaecologists. (2001b). *The use of electronic fetal monitoring* (Evidence-Based Clinical Guideline No. 8). London: Author.

Sameshima, H., & Ikenoue, T. (2005). Predictive value of late decelerations for fetal acidemia in unselective low-risk pregnancies. *American Journal of Perinatology, 22*(1), 19–23.

Seitchik, J., Amico, J., Robinson, A. G., & Castillo, M. (1984). Oxytocin augmentation of dysfunctional labor. IV Oxytocin pharmacokinetics. *American Journal of Obstetrics and Gynecology, 150*(3), 225–228.

Sheiner, E., Hadar, A., Hallak, M., Katz, M., Mazor, M., & Shoham-Vardi, I. (2001). Clinical significance of fetal heart rate tracings during the second stage of labor. *Obstetrics and Gynecology, 97*(5 Pt 1), 747–752.

Shenker, L. (1973). Clinical experience with fetal heart rate monitoring of one thousand patients in labor. *American Journal of Obstetrics and Gynecology, 115*, 1111–1116.

Siira, A. M., Ojala, T. H., Vahlberg, T. J., Jalonen, J. O., Välimäki, B. A., Rosén, K. G., et al. (2005). Marked fetal acidosis and specific changes in power spectrum analysis of fetal heart rate variability recorded during the last hour of labour. *BJOG: International Journal of Obstetrics and Gynaecology, 112*(4), 418–423.

Simpson, K. R. (2006). Critical illness during pregnancy: Considerations for evaluation and treatment of the fetus as the second patient. *Critical Care Nursing Quarterly, 29*(1), 20–31.

Simpson, K. R. (2007). Intrauterine resuscitation during labor: Review of current practice and supportive evidence. *Journal of Midwifery and Women's Health, 52*(3), 229–237.

Simpson, K. R. (2008a). *Cervical ripening, induction and augmentation of labor* (Practice Monograph). Washington, DC: Association of Women's Health, Obstetric, and Neonatal Nurses.

Simpson, K. R. (2008b). Intrauterine resuscitation during labor: Should maternal oxygen administration be a first-line measure? *Seminars in Fetal and Neonatal Medicine,* June 3, epub ahead of print.

Simpson, K. R. (2008c). Labor and birth. In K. R. Simpson & P. A. Creehan (Eds.). *AWHONN's Perinatal Nursing* (3rd ed., pp. 300–375). Philadelphia: Lippincott Williams and Wilkins.

Simpson, K. R., & James, D. C. (2005a). Effects of immediate versus delayed pushing during second stage labor on fetal well-being: A randomized clinical trial. *Nursing Research, 54*(3), 149–157.

Simpson, K. R., & James, D. C. (2005b). Efficacy of intrauterine resuscitation techniques in improving fetal oxygen status during labor. *Obstetrics and Gynecology, 105*(6), 1362–1368.

Simpson, K. R., & James, D. C. (2008). Effects of oxytocin-induced uterine hyperstimulation on fetal oxygen status and fetal heart rate patterns during labor. *American Journal of Obstetrics and Gynecology, 199,* 34.e1-34.e5.

Singhi, S. (1988). Effect of maternal intrapartum glucose therapy on neonatal blood glucose levels and neurobehavioral status of hypoglycemic term infants. *Journal of Perinatal Medicine, 16*(3), 217–224.

Sleutel, M., & Golden, S. S. (1999). Fasting in labor: Relic or requirement. *Journal of Obstetric, Gynecologic and Neonatal Nursing, 28*(5), 507–512.

Smith, J. G., & Merrill, D. C. (2006). Oxytocin for induction of labor. *Clinical Obstetrics and Gynecology, 49*(3), 594–608.

Society of Obstetricians and Gynaecologists of Canada. (2001). *Induction of labour at term* (Clinical Practice Guideline No. 107). *Journal of Obstetrics and Gynaecology in Canada, 111,* 1–12.

Society of Obstetricians and Gynaecologists of Canada. (2007). Fetal health surveillance in labour: Antepartum and intrapartum consensus guideline. *Journal of the Society of Obstetricians and Gynaecologists of Canada, 29*(9 Suppl. 4), S3–S56.

Sommer, P. A., Norr, K., & Roberts, J. (2000). Clinical decision-making regarding intravenous hydration in normal labor in a birth center setting. *Journal of Midwifery and Women's Health, 45*(2), 114–121.

Sprague, A. E., Oppenheimer, L., McCabe, L., Brownlee, J., Graham, I. D., & Davies, B. (2006). The Ottawa Hospital's Clinical Practice Guidelines for the second stage of labour. *Journal of Obstetrics and Gynaecology of Canada, 28*(9), 769–779.

Strong, T. H., Jr. (1997). The effect of amnioinfusion on the duration of labor. *Obstetrics and Gynecology, 89*(6), 1044–1046.

Tucker, S. M., Miller, L. A., & Miller, D. A. (2008). *Fetal monitoring: A multidisciplinary approach* (6th ed.). St. Louis: Mosby.

Ulmsten, U. (1997). Onset and forces of term labor. *Acta Obstetricia et Gynecologica Scandinavica, 76*(6), 499–514.

Vento, M., Asensi, M., Sastre, J., Garcia-Sala, F., Pallardó, F. V., & Viña, J. (2001). Resuscitation with room air instead of 100% oxygen prevents oxidative stress in moderately asphyxiated term neonates. *Pediatrics, 107*(4), 642–647.

Vento, M., Asensi, M., Sastre, J., Lloret, A., García-Sala, F., & Viña, J. (2003). Oxidative stress in asphyxiated term infants resuscitations with 100% oxygen. *Journal of Pediatrics, 142*(3), 240–246.

Wasserstrum, N. (1992). Issues in fluid management during labor: General considerations. *Clinics in Obstetrics and Gynecology, 35,* 505–513.

Williams, K. P., & Galerneau, F. (2002). Fetal heart rate parameters predictive of neonatal outcome in the presence of a prolonged deceleration. *Obstetrics and Gynecology, 100*(5 Pt 1). 951–954.

Williams, K. P., & Galerneau, F. (2003). Intrapartum fetal heart rate patterns in the prediction of neonatal acidemia. *American Journal of Obstetrics and Gynecology, 188*(3), 820–823.

CHAPTER 7

Assessment of Fetal Oxygenation and Acid-Base Status

Rebecca L. Cypher

The primary focus of this chapter is to review techniques that may be used as adjuncts to electronic fetal monitoring (EFM) and intermittent auscultation to provide direct and indirect information concerning the acid-base status of the fetus and newborn. Understanding these concepts requires comprehension of normal glucose metabolism in addition to uteroplacental physiologic factors, as discussed in Chapter 2. General guidelines for the use of selected indirect and direct tools to assess fetal oxygenation are provided. Clinicians should follow their institution's policies and procedures when performing or assisting with indirect and direct tools.

FETAL ACID-BASE BALANCE: KEY CONCEPTS

The placenta is an organ where nutrients for fetal growth and development and exchange of gases between the mother and fetus occurs. The placenta is a low-resistance circuit with oxygenated blood flowing to the fetus via the umbilical vein and deoxygenated blood flowing from the fetus to the placenta via the umbilical arteries. The umbilical arteries branch onto the chorionic plate of the placenta and into the placental villi. Nutrients, oxygen, and waste products are exchanged with maternal blood in the intervillous space. Blood then flows back through the villous blood vessels to the umbilical cord and into the single umbilical vein. Blood flow within the placenta is approximately 500 mL/minute (Blackburn, 2006).

As discussed in Chapter 2, it is at the intervillous space of the placenta that nutrients, oxygen, and waste products are exchanged between the mother and the fetus. Adequate blood flow between the maternal and fetal circulation is necessary to provide for the essential exchange of nutrients, gases, and waste products. Adequate blood flow depends on the structure and function of the uterine arteries, uterine veins, intervillous space, placenta, and umbilical cord (Mescia, 2009; Blackburn, 2007; King & Parer, 2000; Ross, Ervin, & Novak, 2007).

Fetal acid-base balance is determined by a number of factors: adequacy of maternal oxygenation prenatally and in the intrapartum period; blood flow to and across the placenta; and the ability of the fetus to oxygenate the vital organs' tissues (Nageotte & Gilstrap, 2009). Uterine contractions during labor create a temporary interruption in blood flow and exchange of oxygen and carbon dioxide to and from the fetus. The fetus with an adequate oxygen reserve will adapt to this normal decrease in oxygen exchange when there are adequate rest periods between contractions. If the fetus does not have adequate oxygen reserves or there is excessive uterine activity in labor, there may be a progressive accumulation of carbon dioxide (hypercapnia) and a decreased in oxygen content (hypoxemia) that may result in respiratory acidosis, metabolic acidemia, or a combination of metabolic and respiratory acidemia (Bakker & van Geijn, 2008; Greene, 1999; Bakker, Kurver, Kuik, & Van Geijn, 2007). The following sections include terminology used when describing fetal acid-base status or physiology, a description of the means by which the fetus meets its normal metabolic needs, and physiologic and pathophysiologic factors that may affect the fetal acid-base balance.

Terminology

Several terms are used to describe fetal acid-base physiology and blood gas values (Nageotte & Gilstrap, 2009; Blackburn, 2007; King & Parer, 2000):

- Hypoxia: decrease in oxygenation of fetal tissue
- Hypoxemia: decrease in oxygen content in fetal blood
- Hypercapnia: increase in carbon dioxide in fetal blood
- Acidemia: increase in hydrogen ions in fetal blood
- Acidosis: increase in hydrogen ions in fetal tissue
- Metabolic acidosis: low bicarbonate (base excess) in the presence of normal pressure of carbon dioxide (PCO_2) values
- Respiratory acidosis: high PCO_2 with normal bicarbonate levels
- Asphyxia: hypoxia with metabolic acidosis
- Base deficit: HCO_3 concentration lower than normal
- Base excess: HCO_3 concentration higher than normal

The terms "fetal distress" and "birth asphyxia" should not be used in clinical practice because both terms are imprecise and nonspecific. In the past, "fetal distress" has been used in antepartum or intrapartum settings, even though there is little predictive value associated with this term and at birth "the infant may be in good condition as determined by the Apgar score or umbilical cord blood gas analysis or both" (ACOG, 2005a, p.1469). Instead, the interpretation "category II" or "category III" (Macones et al., 2008) followed by a further description of the fetal heart rate (FHR) characteristics is more appropriate than "fetal distress" because it reflects the clinician's assessment of the FHR findings. For example, a clinician may document "category II FHR: BL 175, minimal variability with recurrent late de-

> ### BOX 7-1 Criteria to Define Acute Intrapartum Hypoxic Event
>
> Essential criteria (must meet all four):
> - Evidence of metabolic acidosis in umbilical arterial cord blood sample (pH < 7 and base deficit > 12 mmol/L)
> - Early onset of severe or moderate neonatal encephalopathy in infants born at 34 weeks' gestation or later
> - Cerebral palsy of the spastic quadriplegic or dyskinetic type
> - Exclusion of other etiologies such as trauma, coagulation disorders, infectious conditions, or genetic disorders
>
> Criteria that suggest an intrapartum timing (within close proximity to labor and delivery, e.g., 0-48 hours) but are nonspecific to asphyxial insults:
> - Sentinel hypoxic event occurring immediately before or during labor
> - Sudden and sustained fetal bradycardia or the absence of fetal heart rate variability in the presence of persistent, late, or variable decelerations, usually after a hypoxic sentinel event when the pattern was previously normal
> - Apgar scores of 0 to 3 beyond 5 minutes
> - Onset of multisystem involvement within 72 hours of birth
> - Early imaging study showing evidence of acute nonfocal cerebral abnormality

Source: ACOG/AAP, 2003; ACOG 2005a.

celerations," or "category III FHR: BL 155 with absent variability and recurrent variable decelerations." In the past, the term "birth asphyxia" has been used as a neonatal diagnosis. However, criteria to delineate "an acute intrapartum hypoxic event sufficient enough to lead to cerebral palsy" (ACOG, 2005a, p. 1470) were published in 2003 by American College of Obstetricians and Gynecologists [ACOG] & American Academy of Pediatrics [AAP] (Box 7-1).

Physiologic and Pathophysiologic Factors Affecting Intrapartum Acid-Base Assessment

The energy-consuming process of metabolism is called *anabolism*, whereas *catabolism* refers to the energy-releasing process. There are three phases of catabolism in which proteins, lipids, and polysaccharides are broken down. In phase one, large molecules are broken down into smaller subunits: proteins into amino acids, polysaccharides into simple sugars, and fats into fatty acids and glycerol. In phase two, molecules that enter cells are broken down further in the cytoplasm of the cell. Sugars are broken down into pyruvate, which then enters the mitochondria and is converted to the acetyl groups, which include adenosine triphosphate (ATP). Glycolysis, the breakdown of glucose, can occur both aerobically and anaerobically. In phase three, the acetyl group is degraded to water and carbon dioxide (King & Parer, 2000; McCance & Huether, 2005).

In normal cellular glucose metabolism, ATP is generated from the oxidation of glucose to water and carbon dioxide in the presence of oxygen, and ATP then provides the energy for other cellular processes (Greene, 1999; King & Parer, 2000; McCance & Huether, 2005). For aerobic cellular metabolism to occur, oxygen must be present. Two classes of acids are produced when the fetus exhibits normal metabolism: volatile acids (e.g., carbonic acid) and nonvolatile acids (e.g., lactic acid), also known as fixed acids (Thorp & Rushing, 1999).

The end result of aerobic metabolism in the fetus is carbonic acid, which is formed by the hydration of carbon dioxide during oxidative metabolism. It is found in very low concentrations in the plasma. The fetus can handle the amount of carbonic acid normally produced from aerobic metabolism because carbonic acid dissociates to water and carbon dioxide, which diffuses very rapidly across the placenta as long as there is adequate intervillous and umbilical blood flow (Blackburn, 2007; Garite, 2007).

Under normal circumstances during the labor process, the only variable that alters fetal oxygenation is the brief interruption in blood flow to the placenta that occurs during contractions when the spiral arteries are compressed during the peak of contractions. The duration of spiral artery compression depends on the duration and intensity of the contraction (Figure 7-1). The fetus usually tolerates these transitory interrup-

FIGURE 7-1 Uteroplacental Blood Flow and the Influence of Intramyometrial Pressure

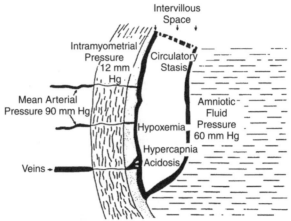

At the acme, or peak of a contraction of greater than 50 mmHg, uteroplacental blood flow ceases temporarily. This causes the fetus to be dependent upon placental reserve. There may be a brief alteration of contraction effectiveness.
Adapted from: Freeman, Garite, & Nageotte, 1991; Poseiro, 1969

tions without a major change in oxygen content (Garite, 2007) because the fetus has several compensatory mechanisms for enduring these transient periods of hypoxia, including a higher hemoglobin concentration and preferential streaming mechanisms (see Chapter 2).

Excessive uterine activity and other factors that affect uterine perfusion can affect fetal oxygenation (Bakker & van Geijn, 2008). When placental transfer of oxygen is restricted over a long period, fetal metabolism proceeds into anaerobic metabolism and lactic acid accumulates (Blechner, 1993). Fetal acid-base status depends on maternal regulation and transplacental transfer of gases. The normoxic fetus has a pH level slightly lower than the maternal pH level and is affected by the acid-base balance of the mother. During labor, uterine arteries are constricted, thereby decreasing blood flow to the fetus and transfer of carbon dioxide away from the fetus. Normally the fetus can adapt to the decrease in oxygen. If fetal oxygen reserves are depleted, there may be a progressive accumulation of carbon dioxide (hypercapnia) that could lead to respiratory acidosis and lack of oxygen (hypoxemia); this may result in metabolic acidemia (Greene, 1999).

Anaerobic metabolism of glucose occurs when oxygen is unavailable for the oxidation of the hydrogen atoms and cellular oxidation of hydrogen cannot take place. When placental transfer of oxygen is restricted over a long period, energy is released through the conversion of pyruvate to lactic acid. Continued hypoxia results in the accumulation of this nonvolatile acid (Blechner, 1993). Buffers in the blood permit the maintenance of the pH at a relatively constant level during short periods of anaerobic metabolism. Plasma bicarbonate and hemoglobin are the two most important buffers in the blood (Nageotte & Gilstrap, 2009).

During the early anaerobic phase of metabolism, when oxygen stores are exhausted, glucose is initially converted to pyruvic acid through a series of chemical reactions, and lactic acid and carbon dioxide build up. As pyruvic and lactic acid accumulate from continued anaerobic metabolism, increasing amounts of hydrogen ion are released. In the absence of oxygen, lactic acid cannot be broken down and it accumulates, resulting in metabolic acidemia. Hydrogen ions are toxic to cells but are buffered by bicarbonate, hemoglobin, and plasma protein. Buffers resist the changes in pH and are a mixture of a weak acid and its salt. Buffers are the first line of defense in counteracting the continuous metabolic production of hydrogen ions by the tissues. They also maintain acid-base homeostasis. Over time, as the ATP supply is exhausted, the fetus will accumulate lactic acid in the bloodstream. When these buffers are saturated, there is marked increase in hydrogen ions and a fall in pH, resulting in acidosis. This starts the chain of events that leads to cell death unless oxygenation is restored (Blackburn, 2007; Blechner, 1993; Green, 1999).

Excretion of nonvolatile acids occurs through the kidneys in the adult. However, fetal excretion of accumulated acids must take place via the placenta because of the immaturity of the fetal renal system. These acids must therefore cross the placenta into the maternal circulation for excretion by the maternal kidneys; however, this diffusion is much slower than carbon dioxide diffusion. It may require hours rather than seconds to completely clear the buildup of nonvolatile acids, even after sufficient oxygen is restored for aerobic metabolism. When these acids accumulate, fetal meta-

bolic acidemia occurs (Thorp & Rushing, 1999). With the addition of oxygen (at the cellular level), lactic acid is converted into carbon dioxide, which enters the umbilical arteries and is transported into the maternal circulation for excretion through the maternal system. The process of reversing metabolic acidosis with adequate oxygenation can take 20 to 30 minutes or longer, depending on the degree of acidosis. Therefore, fetuses with metabolic acidosis in utero may exhibit decreased variability, possible loss of variability, neurologic compromise, and even intrauterine death.

Acidemia, whether respiratory, metabolic, or mixed, is an abnormal increase in the hydrogen ion concentration in the blood resulting from accumulation of an acid or loss of base. Accumulated carbonic acids (weak acids) combine with hydrogen ions and then break down into carbon dioxide and water, which are quickly excreted across the placenta if blood flow is restored in a reasonable time. This principle applies to the adult as well as the fetus.

The fetus can develop respiratory acidemia as a result of several circumstances, including excessive uterine activity (Bakker et al., 2007), an acute onset of decreased umbilical cord perfusion, or decreased uteroplacental perfusion. If these problems are not corrected, respiratory acidemia may occur. For example, repeated umbilical cord compression may occur during a labor complicated by oligohydramnios. When umbilical cord compression or occlusion occurs, carbon dioxide produced by lactic acid conversion cannot be removed from the fetal circulation, resulting in a buildup of carbon dioxide. The excess carbon dioxide is hydrolyzed, and carbonic acid is formed, resulting in respiratory acidosis. However, respiratory acidosis is easily reversed because carbon dioxide is quickly diffused into the maternal circulation for excretion through the maternal system. Depending on the duration of the temporary insult, the fetus will excrete carbon dioxide across the placenta if allowed sufficient time. With adequate cord release, a healthy fetus can be resuscitated in utero.

During labor, a mild maternal metabolic acidemia may develop as a result of muscle activity, catecholamine release, or relative starvation. A mixture of both respiratory and metabolic acidemia also may occur. When the supply of oxygen and the removal of carbon dioxide and fixed acids by the placenta are in balance, the fetus will maintain a normal acid-base balance within a narrow range. If these processes are interrupted, the fetus may develop acidemia (Thorp & Rushing, 1999).

FETAL OXYGENATION AND ACID-BASE ASSESSMENT

Clinicians may need to use additional tools for assessment of fetal acid-base status in order to interpret category II and III FHR findings. These tools may be especially useful in evaluating fetal well-being in the setting of minimal to absent variability with late or variable decelerations (Nageotte & Gilstrap, 2009; Low, Victory, & Derrick, 1999). Fetal well-being can be evaluated when EFM or intermittent auscultation is used with other adjunct methods of evaluation, including indirect and direct approaches (Druzin, Smith, Gabbe, & Reed, 2007; Parer 1997; Society of Obstetricians and Gynaecologists of Canada [SOGC], 2007). Direct methods are those in which actual blood sampling occurs; indirect methods are those in which acid-base levels are implied on the basis of a less direct measure, the fetal response, or both.

Indirect Methods of Acid-Base Assessment during the Intrapartum Period

Indirect methods for evaluation of oxygenation and acid-base values include fetal scalp stimulation and vibroacoustic stimulation (VAS), which are used to elicit an acceleration of 15 beats per minute (bpm) in amplitude for a duration of 15 seconds. This fetal response is typically associated with a nonacidotic fetus, generally with a pH of 7.20 or more and a normoxic central nervous system (Clark, Gimovsky, & Miller, 1982, 1984; Elimian, Figueroa, & Tejani, 1997). The generation of FHR accelerations following scalp stimulation is probably related to a change in the fetal

behavioral state (Porter & Clark, 1999). Although an acceleration response is associated with fetal well-being, the absence of acceleration does not predict fetal compromise. Decisions to use additional assessments of acid-base status are based on various factors, including the maternal-fetal history, labor progress, current maternal status, and individual institutional guidelines.

Fetal Scalp Stimulation

Fetal scalp stimulation is a noninvasive procedure that provides information about the acid-base status of the fetus in the setting of category II or III FHR findings in labor. Historically, scalp stimulation was performed by one of two methods: pinching the fetal scalp with an Allis clamp or applying gentle digital pressure to the scalp through a dilated cervix for 15 seconds. Fetal scalp stimulation is typically used when there is minimal or absent variability and no spontaneous accelerations (ACOG, 2005b) and is performed during segments of baseline, not during decelerations (Clark et al., 1984; Freeman, Garite, & Nagoette, 2003; Garite, 2007). Acceleration of 15 bpm or more in amplitude for a duration of 15 seconds or longer typically reflects a pH of 7.20 or greater (Figure 7-2). The absence of an acceleratory response to stimulation is an indeterminate finding (Macones et al., 2008).

General guidelines for the procedure are as follows:

- Explain the procedure to the patient.
- Place the patient in a lateral position.
- Perform a vaginal examination.
- Apply gentle digital pressure on the fetal scalp.
- Perform stimulation when the FHR is at baseline. It is inappropriate to use fetal scalp stimulation during a deceleration (Clark et al., 1984; Freeman et al., 2003; Garite, 2007).
- Document the procedure and response per institutional policy.

Vibroacoustic Stimulation

FHR accelerations and movement induced by VAS were first reported by Sontag and Wallace in 1936. The acoustic environment of the fetus

FIGURE 7-2 Fetal Scalp Stimulation Elicits FHR Acceleration

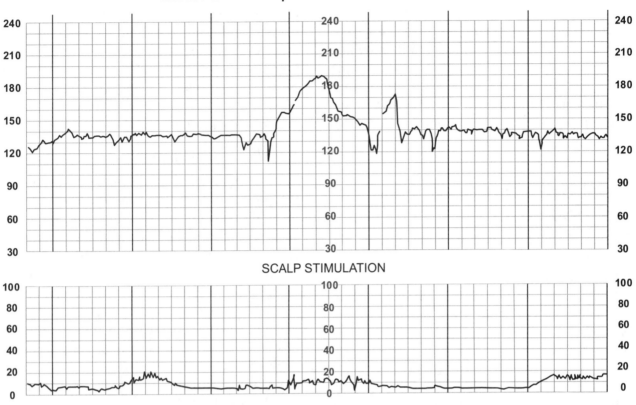

SCALP STIMULATION

is composed of continuous cardiovascular, respiratory, and intestinal sounds of the pregnant woman. Vibrations on the external surface of the mother's abdomen can also induce sounds within the uterus. Sounds penetrate the tissues and fluid surrounding the fetal head and stimulate the inner ear though a bone conduction route. The fetus hears low-frequency sounds below 300 Hz. In fact, the fetus can likely detect vowels and rhythmic patterns of music (Gerhardt & Abrams, 2000). A commercially distributed vibroacoustic stimulator, a battery-powered artificial larynx, or both are used to deliver auditory and vibratory stimulus to the fetus. These devices may be handheld or attached by a connector to the fetal monitor. The vibroacoustic stimulator may be placed over the fetal vertex or fetal breech. Identical FHR responses and increases in fetal movement can be observed after stimulation over either position (Eller, Robinson, & Newman, 1992).

Yao and colleagues (1990) reported that movements occurred more frequently after VAS set at 103 dB and at 109 dB. If the artificial larynx is set at 103 dB, it will usually be sufficient to elicit accelerations (Yao et al.). The static and dynamic forces of the vibrator and the distance from the fetal head are also factors in the transmission of the sound (Gerhardt & Abrams, 2000). The use of VAS in antepartum testing is discussed in Chapter 11.

Intrapartum Use of Vibroacoustic Stimulation

There has been discussion about extending the use of VAS during the intrapartum period for fetal assessment. One of the earliest studies, performed by Smith and colleagues (1986a), found VAS to be as reliable as fetal scalp sampling for determining acidosis during the first stage of labor. Of those fetuses that responded to VAS with an acceleration to 15 bpm above the baseline for a 15-second duration (baseline to baseline), none was found to have an acidotic pH. The predictive value was 100% for a normal scalp pH. Likewise, of the fetuses that did not respond to VAS, 53% had a scalp pH of less than 7.25.

Subsequently, a number of studies considered the use of VAS in the evaluation of fetal well-being in labor. A review by the Cochrane Library of VAS in labor with the presence of a "nonreassuring" tracing showed no randomized controlled trials that addressed the safety and efficacy of VAS in labor. Currently, the evidence on which to base recommendations for use of VAS in the intrapartum period is insufficient (East et al., 2005).

Occasionally, a fetus will respond to VAS with prolonged tachycardia or bradycardia, particularly when oligohydramnios is present (Miller, Rabello, & Paul, 1996). Some medications have been associated with altered responses to VAS. These include beta-adrenergic blocking agents and magnesium sulfate, which have been associated with decreased reactivity and a blunted response (Sherer, 1994; Sherer & Bentolila, 1998). The effect of intrauterine growth restriction on fetal response to VAS has also been studied. It has been noted that FHR accelerations are shorter in duration and body movements are fewer in these fetuses when compared with normal-size fetuses (Porter & Clark, 1999). In fetuses between 26 and 32 weeks gestation that are small for gestational age, researchers reported a limited response, suggesting delayed functional maturation of fetal sensory receptors (Gagnon, Hunse, & Foreman, 1989).

Safety

The benefits of VAS must be weighed against the effect on the predictive reliability of the test and the safety of the procedure. VAS produces significant increases over baseline intrauterine sound pressure levels, which average 72 to 88 decibels (dB) (Smith, Satt, Phelan, & Paul, 1990) to sound levels between 98 and 111 dB. Prolonged exposure to sound levels above 110 dB has been shown to be associated with acoustic injury. Arulkumaran and colleagues (1991) studied the possibility of high-frequency hearing loss in children who had been exposed to VAS in utero and found that none of the children in the study showed evidence of hearing loss.

Randomized controlled trials are lacking in relation to outcomes such as fetal hearing damage, impaired neurologic development, and gestation at birth. These are important safety considerations, particularly those aspects relating to hearing loss, cochlear damage, stress reaction, and perinatal outcome. Therefore, further studies are necessary before routine use can be recommended (Tan & Smyth, 2001).

Fetal Pulse Oximetry

Oximetry was developed in the United States and Great Britain during World War II, when military aircraft did not have pressurized cabins. This technology allowed for the measurement of hemoglobin oxygen saturation in blood or tissue on the basis of the Lambert-Beer relationship (Dildy, Clark, & Loucks, 1996). Pulse oximeters were developed for medical use in the late 1970s, and today, are found in virtually every operating room and critical care unit (Garite & Porreco, 2001). The first reports of continuous fetal arterial oxygen saturation monitoring, also referred to as "fetal pulse oximetry," emerged in the 1980s. These were followed by several observational studies in the 1990s and a large randomized clinical trial published in 2000 (Garite et al., 2000).

The theory behind pulse oximetry is that oxyhemoglobin (hemoglobin carrying oxygen) and deoxyhemoglobin (hemoglobin not carrying oxygen) will absorb light. Oxyhemoglobin weakly absorbs red light and strongly absorbs infrared light. On the other hand, deoxyhemoglobin strongly absorbs red light and weakly absorbs infrared light. During pulse oximetry, red and infrared light are alternately emitted into the tissue through a sensor. The oximeter calculates the ratio of oxygen-saturated and unsaturated hemoglobin by measuring the absorption of each color. The fraction is displayed as a percentage, known as arterial oxygen saturation, via the pulse oximeter (Garite & Porreco, 2001; Mallinckrodt, 2000a; Simpson & Porter, 2001).

The fetal oximetry sensor is a reflectance sensor rather than a transmission sensor. In the traditional transmission sensor, the light-emitting electrodes (LEDs) and photo detector are positioned opposite each other to determine light absorption across the vascular beds. In the reflectance sensor used with fetal pulse oximetry, the LEDs and photodetectors are positioned adjacent to one another on the same skin surface such as the fetal temple, cheek, or forehead (Mallinckrodt, 2000b).

The Critical Threshold

Use of fetal pulse oximetry requires a thorough understanding of the concept of the *critical threshold:* the point below which hypoxia would likely cause metabolic acidosis or above which there would be no risk for acidosis (Garite & Porreco, 2001; Swedlow, 2000). Persistent fetal hypoxia may lead to acidosis, neurologic injury, tissue and organ damage, and ultimately, death (Dildy, Clark, & Loucks, 1996). However, because the fetus often becomes hypoxemic for short periods of time and may revert to a normal acid-base balance without becoming acidotic, it was necessary to establish a critical threshold. The goal of intrapartum monitoring is to intervene early enough to avoid these complications whenever possible.

Based on the research, normal oxygen saturation for the fetus in labor is 30% to 65% saturation (Dildy, Thorp, Yeast, & Clark, 1996; Nijland, Jongsma, Nijhuis, van den Berg, & Oeseburg, 1995; Richardson, Carmichael, Homan, & Patrick, 1992; Swedlow, 2000). The fetus is presumed to be adequately oxygenated in this range of values. Metabolic acidosis does not develop until the saturation level falls below 30% for at least 10 to 15 minutes (Seelbach-Gobel, Heupel, Kuhnert, & Butterwegge, 1999). Thus, the critical threshold was established at 30%. This value was also validated in a randomized controlled trial

conducted concurrently in nine medical centers across the United States (Garite et al., 2000).

Current Status of Fetal Pulse Oximetry Technology

In May 2000, the U.S. Food and Drug Administration approved fetal pulse oximetry as a method of assessing fetal oxygen status during labor. However, the adoption of fetal pulse oximetry as a standard clinical practice was not endorsed by the ACOG (2001, 2005b) or the SOGC (2007) because of concerns that it would increase obstetric care costs without improving outcomes. Although one randomized controlled trial reported a decrease in the cesarean operative birth rates for "nonreassuring" FHR findings, there was no difference in the overall cesarean or operative birth rates because more cesarean births were performed for dystocia (Kuhnert & Schmidt, 2004). In 2006, Bloom and colleagues concluded that there were no significant differences in the overall rates of cesarean birth associated with a "nonreassuring" FHR and dystocia. The manufacturer removed the product from the market in January 2006. The use of fetal pulse oximetry in research has contributed significantly to our understanding of the effects of common interventions on fetal oxygenation (Haydon et al., 2006; Simpson & James, 2005, 2008).

DIRECT METHODS OF ACID-BASE ASSESSMENT

Direct methods of acid-base assessment, such as fetal scalp sampling and umbilical cord blood sampling, are those in which actual blood sampling occurs. Other examples of direct assessment include sampling obtained via in utero methods (e.g., cordocentesis or percutaneous umbilical blood sampling), but these methods are rarely used and are not discussed in this chapter. Fetal scalp sampling can provide additional information about acid-base status during labor. Umbilical cord sampling can provide fetal acid-base information at the moment of birth as well as data for newborn stabilization if needed (ACOG, 2006b; Nageotte & Gilstrap, 2009; Sonek & Nicolaides, 1994).

Fetal Scalp Sampling

Fetal scalp sampling is a reliable ancillary test of fetal well-being in labor (ACOG, 2005b). However, today in the United States fetal scalp sampling is rarely used outside of residency training facilities (Dildy, 2005; Goodwin, Milner-Masterson, & Paul, 1994) because of the inconvenience to the patient and clinicians as well as its invasiveness to the fetus (Dildy; Greene, 1999) and does not provide information on a continuous basis. The need for fetal scalp sampling has been dramatically reduced by the use of other, less invasive, tests such as fetal stimulation which indicates a normal pH when an acceleration is elicited (Ecker & Parer, 1999; Freeman et al., 2003; Sarno, Ahn, Phelan, & Paul, 1990; Skupski, Rosenberg, & Eglinton, 2002).

Fetal scalp sampling should be performed in institutions that have 24-hour access to blood gas analysis with a 10- to 15-minute turnaround. A protocol should be developed in facilities where fetal scalp sampling is performed.

Contraindications

Contraindications to fetal scalp sampling may include (ACOG, 1999a, 2007; SOGC, 2007)

- Suspected or identified fetal coagulopathy (hemophilia).
- Maternal infections with risk of maternal-fetal transmission (e.g., human immunodeficiency virus, hepatitis, herpes simplex)
- Prematurity

Factors and Limitations That Affect Fetal Scalp Sampling

Factors and limitations that may affect fetal scalp sampling include (Clark & Paul, 1985; Dildy, 2005; Freeman et al., 2003; SOGC, 2007; Whitworth & Bricker, 2006):

- Availability of equipment and insufficient initial training or continuing opportunity to maintain individual proficiency

- Ruptured membranes and accessible presenting part
- Fetal presentation, position, station, and presence of fetal caput; maternal cervical dilation and effacement (which may limit feasibility of obtaining sample)
- Maternal positioning
- Cooperation of the patient
- Time lapse for filling the capillary tube
- Machine calibration
- Misinterpretation of pH data or lack of reporting of base deficit or base excess
- Contamination of the sample with hair, caput, air from slow blood flow, and meconium (which may affect accuracy of results)
- Blood clotting in capillary tube before sample reaches the laboratory

A study performed by Bowen, Kochenour, Rehm, and Wooley (1986) showed that 10% of samples obtained at the time of birth were found to be below the values found in the umbilical artery; this suggests that there may be factors in the fetal scalp that are responsible for the falsely low fetal scalp pH value.

Interpretation of Results from Fetal Scalp Sampling

Results obtained from fetal scalp sampling reflect fetal acid-base status only at the time of the sampling (Freeman et al., 2003); thus, repeat testing is often necessary. The information should be evaluated in the context of the total clinical situation at the time of sampling, including FHR characteristics and patterns, uterine contraction pattern, and any maternal factors that could affect the fetal acid-base status. Repeat testing is typically performed to assess trends in values, for example, whether the pH is rising or falling. Furthermore, pH as a sole value reported is a less satisfactory measure of acidemia than a combination of pH and base deficit because of variations of acidemia that may be present at the time of blood sampling (SOGC, 2007).

Mothers with complications such as asthma, dehydration and hyperventilation may need a simultaneous arterial blood gas sample for comparative evaluation with the fetal scalp sample. Typically, fetal scalp blood pH is approximately 0.1 unit below the maternal pH, which will guide the clinician when significant maternal acidosis or alkalosis is suspected.

Umbilical Cord Blood Sampling

Umbilical cord blood acid-base analysis can be used as an objective method of quantifying fetal acid-base balance and oxygenation at birth (Table 7-1). The pH, PCO_2, and PO_2 of the blood can be measured; the bicarbonate concentration and percentage oxygen saturation are determined from these measurements. From the measured values and the hemoglobin level, the base excess and base deficit can be calculated. The pH and the base excess or base deficit are the most useful values in assessing the fetal condition at the time of collection (Yeomans & Ramin, 2007). Box 7-2 describes the process of neonatal cord blood sampling. A finding of normal umbilical blood gas measurements precludes the presence of acidemia at or immediately before birth (Gregg & Weiner, 1993) and is a more objective measure than the Apgar score, especially in the preterm fetus (ACOG, 2006a; Dickinson, Erikson, Meyer, & Parisi, 1992).

When indicated, a double-clamped segment of the umbilical cord is obtained immediately after birth and before or as near to the first neonatal breath as possible. Umbilical cord blood acid-base values can change quickly, within 5 to 10 seconds of neonatal breathing after birth. This includes a decrease in the pH as well as an increase in PCO_2 and base deficit (Lievaart & de Jong, 1984; Yeomans & Ramin, 2007).

Indications and Contraindications

Umbilical cord blood sampling may be helpful in clarifying fetal acid-base status at or near birth and may also assist planning the clinical management of selected newborns (Thorp & Rushing, 1999).

Indications for umbilical cord blood sampling may include but may not be limited to the following (ACOG, 2006a; Johnson & Riley, 1993):

- Category II or III FHR patterns
- Severe intrauterine growth restriction
- Low 5-minute Apgar score
- Cesarean birth for fetal compromise
- Delivery of high-risk patients (e.g., maternal thyroid disease, multifetal gestations)
- Intrapartum fever
- Newborn depression
- Premature and postterm pregnancies
- Thick meconium
- Breech birth
- Abnormal labor
- Abnormal biophysical profile

There are no known contraindications for the use of umbilical cord blood sampling, but it may preclude other uses of the cord, such as harvesting blood for stem cells.

Analysis of the cord blood can be delayed while Apgar scores are being assigned. A double-clamped segment of the umbilical cord is stable for blood gas assessment for at least

Table 7-1	Normal Ranges of Umbilical Cord Arterial Blood Gas Values	
ARTERIAL MEASURE[a]	**NORMAL MEAN VALUE RANGE**[b]	**RANGE (±2 STANDARD DEVIATIONS)**
pH	7.20–7.29	7.02–7.43
PCO_2 (mm Hg)	49.2–56.3	21.5–78.3
Bicarbonate (mEq/L)	22.0–24.1	14.8–29.2
Base deficit (mEq/L)	2.7–8.3	−2.0–16.3
PO_2 (mm Hg)	15.1–23.7	2.0–37.8

[a]Venous values reflect maternal acid-base status and are generally higher than arterial values that reflect fetal acid-base status. Venous values may be normal despite arterial values reflecting fetal acidemia.
[b]These figures represent the range of normal mean values reported in a review of studies of umbilical arterial cord blood gases.
Source: Thorp & Rushing, 1999.

When indicated, blood gas analysis of the umbilical cord blood collected at delivery provides an objective means of assessing fetal oxygenation and acid-base status at birth (Thorp & Rushing, 1999). Obtaining cord blood samples will document the presence and type of acidemia, as well as provide information for resuscitation efforts and neonatal care.

General Guidelines
- Obtain two or three 1-mL heparinized syringes with a short, small-gauge needle for optimal control with minimal injury to the vessels.
- Heparin is the only acceptable anticoagulant for umbilical cord blood gases.
- Prepare labels with patient's name, medical record number, and sample site.
- Obtain a double-clamped cord segment immediately after birth.
- Obtain a blood sample from the umbilical artery first, because it is often more difficult to get, and the umbilical vein may help support the umbilical artery. Obtain samples from both an artery and the vein whenever possible.
- Avoid air bubbles or carefully expel excess air from each syringe.
- Cap each syringe.
- Label the specimen(s) and send specimen(s) to the laboratory for analysis.
- Document that the cord blood samples were collected and sent to the laboratory for analysis; document the results when available.

Sources: ACOG, 2006a; Thorp & Rushing, 1999; Wallman, 1997.

1 hour (ACOG, 2006a; Duerbeck, Chaffin, & Seeds, 1992). The cord blood sample in a heparinized syringe is stable for up to 1 hour (ACOG), but not longer. Residual heparin and air should be expelled because it has been reported that the addition of heparin or air can decrease the pH, PCO_2, and bicarbonate (Kirshon & Moise, 1989). Umbilical cord segments and cord blood samples do not need to be placed on ice because they will remain relatively stable at room temperature for up to 1 hour with no significant changes in the pH value (Yeomans & Ramin, 2007). Many facilities no longer transport samples on ice because of the short amount of time

required between obtaining the specimen and performing the test.

The cord blood should be analyzed if "a serious abnormality that arose during the birth process or a problem with the neonate's condition, or if both persist at or beyond the first 5 minutes" (ACOG, 2006a, p.1321) or according to facility protocol. "If the 5-minute Apgar score is satisfactory and the infant appears stable, the umbilical cord segment may be discarded" (ACOG, p. 1321) or depending on facility protocol.

Samples from the umbilical artery demonstrate the presence and severity of fetal acidosis at or near birth, whereas samples obtained from the umbilical vein reflect placental tissue acid-base status at or near birth. Analysis of both the umbilical vein and artery samples should prevent debate over whether a true arterial specimen was obtained (ACOG, 2006a; Riley & Johnson, 1993; Thorp & Rushing, 1999).

Umbilical arterial and venous samples should be collected separately. The sample values can then be reviewed to verify that the samples come from two separate vessels and are accurate (Westgate, Garibaldi, & Greene, 1994). This will also assist in identifying the general cause of fetal acidosis, if present (Riley & Johnson, 1993). For example, in an umbilical cord prolapse, the values in the umbilical arterial blood may be more acidotic compared with the normal values in the venous sample (Riley & Johnson). The umbilical arterial values are also the most accurate assessment of fetal metabolic status and appear to correlate best with the Apgar score (Thorp, Dildy, Yeomans, Meyer, & Parisi, 1996; Thorp, Sampson, Parisi, & Creasy, 1989). The umbilical venous values are an important addition to umbilical cord sampling (Riley & Johnson).

Obtaining cord blood samples from the umbilical cord can be difficult at times. The umbilical arteries, which carry deoxygenated blood away from the fetus, have smaller lumens, have thicker walls, and contain less blood than the umbilical vein. Therefore, the distended umbilical vein that carries oxygenated blood to the fetus may provide some support to the artery, making sampling easier when the arterial sample is obtained first (ACOG,

2006a; Benirschke & Kaufmann, 2000). If the umbilical cord vessels are poorly filled, blood can be milked with the thumb and forefinger from the placenta toward the clamp. After the umbilical vessels become distended, the cord can be clamped again to isolate a segment that can be used for sampling (Riley & Johnson, 1993).

In the event that the umbilical cord samples are inadequate, such as when the cord is thin, a sample can be obtained from the umbilical vessels that traverse the chorionic surface of the placenta. These vessels are easy to distinguish because the smaller, thick-walled arteries cross over the larger, thin-walled veins. These vessels become very obvious when they are traced back to the umbilical cord (ACOG, 2006a; Riley & Johnson, 1993; Thorp & Rushing, 1999). When compared with each other, samples from the umbilical cord and the placental vessels of non-smoking patients show little difference in acid-base characteristics (Riley & Johnson). Some reports have indicated that there is greater deterioration of acid-base values in smokers when umbilical cord gases are obtained from the placental vessels (Nageotte & Gilstrap, 2009).

Factors Affecting Sampling and Interpretation of Results

Factors that may affect umbilical cord blood sampling and interpretation include the following:

- Differences in methodology, such as duration of procedure or air bubbles in sample
- Differences in heparin concentration
  - Spurious metabolic acidosis resulting from use of too much heparin or too concentrated a solution (Thorp & Rushing, 1999)

  - Bicarbonate and partial PCO_2 values show an inverse relationship with the volume of heparin (Duerbeck et al., 1992)
- Sampling of venous and not arterial blood

Interpretation of Umbilical Cord Blood Acid-Base Values

Interpretation of the results of cord blood gas analysis requires basic understanding of both respiratory and metabolic acidosis and the clinical implications of each. As previously discussed, respiratory acidosis occurs when an elevated PCO_2 level is present (i.e., the value is more than 2 standard deviations above the mean). Normally, carbon dioxide diffuses rapidly across the pla-

Table 7-3	Single-Digit Value Guideline for Initial Assessment of Normal and Abnormal Umbilical Cord Blood Acid-Base Values		
	NORMAL VALUES	METABOLIC ACIDEMIA	RESPIRATORY ACIDEMIA
pH	≥7.10	<7.10	<7.10
PO_2 (mm Hg)	≥>20	<20	Variable
PCO_2 (mm Hg)	<60	<60	>60
Bicarbonate (mEq/L)	>22	<22	≥22
Base deficit (mEq/L)	≤12	>12	<12
Base excess (mEq/L)	≥−12	<−12	>−12

The values presented are suggested as a guide for evaluating acid-base status. All umbilical cord blood values should be evaluated in relation to the specific clinical findings and situation for a given patient. Note that greater absolute values of base deficit or excess are associated with acidemia.
Sources: Andres et al., 1999; Nageotte & Gilstrap, 2009; Low, Lindsey, & Derrick, 1997.

Table 7-2	Significance of Deviation from Normal Values				
TYPE OF ACIDOSIS	pH	PO_2	PCO_2	HCO_3	BASE DEFICIT
Respiratory	Decreased	Variable	Increased	Normal	Normal
Metabolic	Decreased	Decreased	Normal	Decreased	Increased
Mixed	Decreased	Decreased	Increased	Decreased	Increased

Sources: Freeman et al., 2003; King & Parer, 2000.

centa. The rate of carbon dioxide diffusion is related to the rate of blood flow on both sides of the placenta. Respiratory acidosis can develop rapidly but also can be corrected rapidly.

Metabolic acidosis takes longer to develop and longer to resolve; it is present when levels of lactic acid and other acids become elevated. These acids are the end product of anaerobic metabolism. Elevation of the acids consumes fetal base buffers, exhausting the fetal capacity to regulate pH. Metabolic acidosis is more serious than respiratory acidosis because it reflects a more prolonged hypoxic insult (Wallman, 1997).

A fetus may experience respiratory and metabolic acidosis simultaneously. When this occurs it is referred to as mixed acidosis (Table 7-2).

For umbilical cord blood, the normal mean arterial blood pH values ranged from 7.20 to 7.29 in a review of studies that monitored umbilical cord arterial blood gas values, with a full range of normal pH values (±2 standard deviations) from 7.02 to 7.43 (Thorp & Rushing, 1999). Traditionally, cord blood pH values below 7.20, defined as acidemia, have been considered pathologic or clinically significant. However, published data suggest that the lower range of normal for umbilical artery pH is between 7.10 and 7.19 and that the original threshold of 7.2 may not be reasonable (Blackstone & Young, 1993; Dildy, 2005; Gilstrap, Leveno, Burris, Williams, & Little, 1989; Goldaber & Gilstrap, 1993; Low, 1988; Riley & Johnson, 1993; Sykes et al., 1982; Thorp et al., 1989; Yeomans, Hauth, Gilstrap, & Strickland, 1985). Blood pH values below 7.00 have been associated with adverse neonatal outcomes and more clearly represent a threshold for significant fetal acidemia (Andres et al., 1999; Gilstrap et al.; Goldaber, Gilstrap, Leveno, Dax, & McIntire, 1991). Mean values for arterial and venous blood gas results in the preterm infant are similar to those of the term infant (Dickinson, Erikson, Meyer, & Parisi, 1992).

Although normal blood values are often described in ranges, it may be helpful to identify a specific number to use a frame of reference when evaluating cord blood values (see Table 7-3). All umbilical cord blood values should be evaluated in relationship to the specific clinical findings and situation for any given infant. In addition to pH levels, the PO_2, PCO_2, bicarbonate, and base deficit or excess values are also considered.

Plasma bicarbonate is one base buffer used to raise (or normalize) pH levels. In metabolic acidosis, an excess of hydrogen ions is released. As a result, bicarbonate is depleted, so the values are decreased in metabolic acidosis (Cohen & Schifrin, 1989; Gimovsky & Caritis, 1982). Thus, a base deficit exists when fetal base buffers are below normal values. The base deficit or excess is not measured directly but is calculated from the pH, PCO_2, and bicarbonate blood values. The terms "base deficit" and "base excess" are often confusing, but they basically measure the same thing: base buffers in the blood specimen. When the base buffers are depleted, a base deficit exists and metabolic acidosis is present. Although this is expressed as a negative base excess by some laboratories, the principle is the same. Numbers further from zero, whether expressed as base deficit or negative base excess, indicate inadequate base buffer reserves and increasing metabolic acidosis (the larger the absolute value, the more severe the acidosis). Conversely, the closer to "0" either the base deficit or negative base excess is, the more buffers remain in the specimen.

SUMMARY

Assessment of fetal well-being is an important component of antepartum and intrapartum care. A variety of methods for direct and indirect fetal acid-base monitoring have been developed, each with potential challenges to successful clinical implementation (Dildy, 2005). Research to identify additional effective assessment strategies is needed. Health care providers are challenged to understand the circumstances that affect fetal oxygenation, select the appropriate method of acid-base assessment, and intervene in a timely manner to maximize fetal oxygenation.

REFERENCES

American College of Obstetricians & Gynecologists. (1999a). *Thrombocytopenia in pregnancy* (Practice Bulletin No. 6). Washington, DC: Author.

American College of Obstetricians and Gynecologists. (1999b). *Antepartum fetal surveillance* (Practice Bulletin No. 9). Washington, DC: Author.

American College of Obstetricians and Gynecologists. (2001). *Fetal pulse oximetry* (ACOG Committee Opinion No. 258). Washington, DC: Author.

American College of Obstetricians and Gynecologists. (2005a). *Inappropriate use of the terms fetal distress and birth asphyxia* (ACOG Committee Opinion No. 326). Washington, DC: Author.

American College of Obstetricians and Gynecologists. (2005b). *Intrapartum fetal heart rate monitoring* (ACOG Practice Bulletin No. 70). Washington, DC: Author.

American College of Obstetricians and Gynecologists. (2006a). *Umbilical cord blood gas and acid-base analysis* (ACOG Committee Opinion No. 348). Washington, DC: Author.

American College of Obstetricians and Gynecologists. (2006b). *The Apgar score* (ACOG Committee Opinion. No. 333). Washington, DC: Author.

American College of Obstetricians and Gynecologists, & American Academy of Pediatrics. (2003). *Neonatal encephalopathy and cerebral palsy: Defining the pathogenesis & pathophysiology*. Washington, DC: Author.

Andres, R. L., Saade, G., Gilstrap, L. C., Wilkins, I., Witlin, A., Zlatnik, F., et al. (1999). Association between umbilical blood gas parameters and neonatal morbidity and death in neonates with pathologic fetal acidemia. *American Journal of Obstetrics and Gynecology, 181,* 867–871.

Arulkumaran, S., Skurr, B., Tong, H., Kek, L. P., Yeoh, K. H., & Ratnam, S. S. (1991). No evidence of hearing loss due to fetal acoustic stimulation test. *Obstetrics & Gynecology, 78,* 283–285.

Bakker, P., & van Geijn, H. P. (2008). Uterine activity: Implications for the condition of the fetus. *Journal of Perinatal Medicine, 36,* 30-37.

Bakker, P. C., Kurver, P. H., Kuik, D. J., & Van Geijn, H. P. (2007). Elevated uterine activity increases the risk of fetal acidosis at birth. *American Journal of Obstetrics and Gynecology, 196,* 311–316.

Benirschke, K., & Kaufmann, P. (2000). *Pathology of the human placenta* (4th ed.). New York: Springer Verlag.

Blackburn, S. (2006). Placental, fetal, and transitional circulation revisited. *Journal of Perinatal and Neonatal Nursing, 20*(4), 290–294.

Blackburn, S. T. (2007). *Maternal, fetal, and neonatal physiology: A clinical perspective* (3rd ed.). St. Louis: Saunders.

Blackstone, J., & Young, B. K. (1993). Umbilical cord blood acid-base values and other descriptors of fetal condition. *Clinical Obstetrics and Gynecology, 36,* 33–46.

Blechner, J. N. (1993). Maternal-fetal acid-base physiology. *Clinical Obstetrics and Gynecology, 36, 3*–12.

Bloom, S. L., Spong, C. Y., Thom, E., Varner, M. W., Rouse, D. J., Weininger, S., et al. (2006). Fetal pulse oximetry and cesarean delivery. *New England Journal of Medicine, 355,* 2195–2202.

Bowen, L. W., Kochenour, N. K., Rehm, N. E., & Woolley, F. R. (1986). Maternal-fetal pH difference and fetal scalp pH as predictors of neonatal outcome. *Obstetrics & Gynecology, 67,* 487–495.

Clark, S. L., Gimovsky, M. L., & Miller, F. C. (1982). Fetal heart rate response to scalp blood sampling. *American Journal of Obstetrics and Gynecology, 144,* 706–708.

Clark, S. L., Gimovsky, M. L., & Miller, F. C. (1984). The scalp stimulation test: A clinical alternative to fetal scalp blood sampling. *American Journal of Obstetrics and Gynecology, 148,* 274–277.

Clark, S. L., & Paul, R. H. (1985). Intrapartum fetal surveillance: The role of fetal scalp blood sampling. *American Journal of Obstetrics and Gynecology, 153,* 717–720.

Cohen, W. R., & Schifrin, B. S. (1989). Clinical management of fetal hypoxemia. In W. R. Cohen, W. R. Aker, & E. A. Friedman (Eds.), *Management of labor* (pp. 283-316). Baltimore, MD: University Park Press.

Dickinson, J. E., Eriksen, N. L., Meyer, B. A., & Parisi, V. M. (1992). The effect of preterm birth on umbilical cord blood gases. *Obstetrics and Gynecology, 79,* 575–578.

Dildy, G. A., 3rd. (2005). Intrapartum assessment of the fetus: Historical and evidence-based practice. *Obstetrics and Gynecology Clinics of North America, 32,* 255–271, ix.

Dildy, G. A., Clark, S. L., & Loucks, C. A. (1996). Intrapartum fetal pulse oximetry: Past, present, and future. *American Journal of Obstetrics and Gynecology, 175,* 1–9.

Dildy, G. A., Thorp, J. A., Yeast, J. D., & Clark, S. L. (1996). The relationship between oxygen saturation and pH in umbilical blood: Implications for intrapartum fetal oxygen saturation monitoring. *American Journal of Obstetrics and Gynecology, 175*(3 Pt. 1), 682–687.

Druzin, M. L., Smith, F., Gabbe, S. G., & Reed, K. L. (2007). Antepartum fetal evaluation. In S. G. Gabbe, J. R. Niebyl, & J. L. Simpson (Eds.), *Obstetrics: Normal and problem pregnancies* (5th ed., pp. 267–300). Philadelphia: Elsevier.

Duerbeck, N. B., Chaffin, D. G., & Seeds, J. W. (1992). A practical approach to umbilical artery pH and blood gas determinations. *Obstetrics and Gynecology, 79,* 959–962.

East, C. E., Smyth, R., Leader, L. R., Henshall, N. E., Colditz, P. B., & Tan, K. H. (2005). *Vibroacoustic stimulation for fetal assessment in labour in the presence of a nonreassuring fetal heart rate trace.* Cochrane Database Systematic Reviews (2), CD004664.

Ecker, J. L., & Parer, J. T. (1999). Obstetric evaluation of fetal acid-base balance. *Critical Reviews in Clinical Laboratory Sciences, 36,* 407–451.

Elimian, A., Figueroa, R., & Tejani, N. (1997). Intrapartum assessment of fetal well-being: A comparison of scalp stimulation with scalp blood pH sampling. *Obstetrics and Gynecology, 89,* 373–376.

Eller, D. P., Robinson, L. J., & Newman, R. B. (1992). Position of the vibroacoustic stimulator does not affect fetal response. *American Journal of Obstetrics and Gynecology, 167*(4 Pt. 1), 1137–1139.

Freeman, R. K., Garite, T. J., & Nageotte, M. P. (2003). *Fetal heart rate monitoring* (3rd ed.). Philadelphia: Lippincott Williams & Wilkins.

Gagnon, R., Benzaquen, S., & Hunse, C. (1992). The fetal sound environment during vibroacoustic stimulation in labor: Effect on fetal heart rate response. *Obstetrics and Gynecology, 79,* 950–955.

Gagnon, R., Hunse, C., & Foreman, J. (1989). Human fetal behavioral states after vibratory stimulation. *American Journal of Obstetrics and Gynecology, 161*(6 Pt. 1), 1470–1476.

Garite, T. J. (2007). Intrapartum evaluation. In S. G. Gabbe, J. R. Neibyl, & J. L. Simpson (Eds.), *Obstetrics: Normal and problem pregnancies* (5th ed., pp. 364–395). Philadelphia: Elsevier.

Garite, T. J., Dildy, G. A., McNamara, H., Nageotte, M. P., Boehm, F. H., Dellinger, E. H., et al. (2000). A multicenter controlled trial of fetal pulse oximetry in the intrapartum management of nonreassuring fetal heart rate patterns. *American Journal of Obstetrics and Gynecology, 183,* 1049–1058.

Garite, T. J., & Porreco, R. P. (2001). Evaluating fetal hypoxia with pulse oximetry. *Contemporary OB/GYN, 46*(7), 12–26.

Gegor, C. L., Paine, L. L., & Johnson, T. R. (1991). Antepartum fetal assessment. A nurse-midwifery perspective. *Journal of Nurse Midwifery, 36,* 153–167.

Gerhardt, K. J., & Abrams, R. M. (2000). Fetal exposures to sound and vibroacoustic stimulation. *Journal of Perinatology, 20*(8 Pt. 2), S21–S30.

Gilstrap, L. C., Leveno, K. J., Burris, J., Williams, M. L., & Little, B. B. (1989). Diagnosis of birth asphyxia on the basis of fetal pH, Apgar score, and newborn cerebral dysfunction. *American Journal of Obstetrics and Gynecology, 161,* 825–830.

Gimovsky, M. L., & Caritis, S. N. (1982). Diagnosis and management of hypoxic fetal heart rate patterns. *Clinical Perinatology, 9,* 313–324.

Goldaber, K. G., & Gilstrap, L. C., 3rd. (1993). Correlations between obstetric clinical events and umbilical cord blood acid-base and blood gas values. *Clinical Obstetrics and Gynecology, 36,* 47–59.

Goldaber, K. G., Gilstrap, L. C., Leveno, K. J., Dax, J. S., & McIntire, D. D. (1991). Pathologic fetal academia. *Obstetrics and Gynecology, 78,* 1103-1107.

Goodwin, T. M., Milner-Masterson, L., & Paul, R. H. (1994). Elimination of fetal scalp blood sampling on a large clinical service. *Obstetrics and Gynecology, 83,* 971–974.

Greene, K. R. (1999). Scalp blood gas analysis. *Obstetrics and Gynecology Clinics of North America, 26,* 641–656, vii.

Gregg, A. R., & Weiner, C. P. (1993). "Normal" umbilical arterial and venous acid-base and blood gas values. *Clinical Obstetrics and Gynecology, 36,* 24–32.

Haydon, M. L., Gorenberg, D. M., Nageotte, M. P., Ghamsary, M., Rumney, P. J., Patillo, C., et al. (2006). The effect of maternal oxygen administration on fetal pulse oximetry during labor in fetuses with nonreassuring fetal heart rate patterns. *American Journal of Obstetrics and Gynecology, 195,* 735–738.

Johnson, J. W., & Riley, W. (1993). Cord blood gas studies: A survey. *Clinical Obstetrics and Gynecology, 36,* 99–101.

King, T., & Parer, J. (2000). The physiology of fetal heart rate patterns and perinatal asphyxia. *Journal of Perinatal and Neonatal Nursing, 14*(3), 19–39; quiz 102–103.

Kirshon, B., & Moise, K. J., Jr. (1989). Effect of heparin on umbilical arterial blood gases. *Journal of Reproductive Medicine, 34,* 267–269.

Kuhnert, M., & Schmidt, S. (2004). Intrapartum management of nonreassuring fetal heart rate patterns: A randomized controlled trial of fetal pulse oximetry. *American Journal of Obstetrics and Gynecology, 191,* 1989–1995.

Lievaart, M., & de Jong, P. A. (1984). Acid-base equilibrium in umbilical cord blood and time of cord clamping. *Obstetrics and Gynecology, 63,* 44–47.

Lindsay, M. K. (1999). Intrauterine resuscitation of the compromised fetus. *Clinical Perinatology, 26,* 569–584

Low, J. A. (1988). The role of blood gas and acid-base assessment in the diagnosis of intrapartum fetal asphyxia. *American Journal of Obstetrics and Gynecology, 159,* 1235–1240.

Low, J. A., Lindsay, B. G., & Derrick, E. J. (1997). Threshold of metabolic acidosis associated with newborn complications. *American Journal of Obstetrics and Gynecology, 177,* 1391–1394.

Low, J. A., Victory, R., & Derrick, E. J. (1999). Predictive value of electronic fetal monitoring for intrapartum fetal asphyxia with metabolic acidosis. *Obstetrics and Gynecology, 93,* 285–291.

Macones, G. A., Hankins, G. D., Spong, C. Y., Hauth, J. D., & Moore, T. (2008). The 2008 National Institute of Child Health Human Development workshop report on electronic fetal monitoring: Update on definitions, interpretations, and research guidelines. *Obstetrics & Gynecology, 112,* 661–666; and *Journal of Obstetric, Gynecologic and Neonatal Nursing, 37,* 510–515.

Mallinckrodt, Inc. Healthy Mother and Baby Division. (2000a). *Oxifirst fetal oxygen saturation monitoring system: The technology.* Pleasanton, CA: Author.

Mallinckrodt, Inc. Healthy Mother and Baby Division (2000b). *Questions and answers for medical professionals.* Pleasanton, CA: Author.

McCance, K., & Huether, S. E. (2005). *Pathophysiology: The biologic basis for disease in adults and children* (3th ed.). St. Louis: Mosby.

Mendez-Bauer, C., Arnt, I. C., Gulin, L., Escarcena, L., & Caldeyro-Barcia, R. (1967). Relationship between blood pH and heart rate in the human fetus during labor. *American Journal of Obstetrics and Gynecology, 97,* 530–545.

Mescia, G. (2009). Placental respiratory gas exchange and fetal oxygenation. In R. K. Creasy, R. Resnik, J. D. Iams, C. Lockwood, & T. R. Moore (Eds.), *Maternal-fetal medicine: Principles and practice* (6th ed., pp. 181-191). Philadelphia: W. B. Saunders.

Miller, D. A., Rabello, Y. A., & Paul, R. H. (1996). The modified biophysical profile: Antepartum testing in the 1990s. *American Journal of Obstetrics and Gynecology, 174,* 812–817.

Nageotte, M. & Gilstrap, L. (2009). Intrapartum fetal surveillance. In R. K. Creasy, R. Resnik, J. D. Iams, C. Lockwood, & T. R. Moore (Eds.), *Maternal-fetal medicine: Principles and practice* (6th ed., pp. 397-417). Philadelphia: W. B. Saunders.

Nijland, R., Jongsma, H. W., Nijhuis, J. G., van den Berg, P. P., & Oeseburg, B. (1995). Arterial oxygen saturation in relation to metabolic acidosis in fetal lambs. *American Journal of Obstetrics and Gynecology, 172,* 810–819.

Parer, J. T. (1997). *Handbook of fetal heart monitoring* (2nd ed.). Philadelphia: W. B. Saunders.

Pearson, J. F., & Weaver, J. B. (1976). Fetal activity and fetal wellbeing: An evaluation. *British Medicine Journal, 1*(6021), 1305–1307.

Porter, T. F., & Clark, S. L. (1999). Vibroacoustic and scalp stimulation. *Obstetrics and Gynecology Clinics of North America, 26,* 657–669.

Richardson, B. S., Carmichael, L., Homan, J., & Patrick, J. E. (1992). Electrocortical activity, electroocular activity, and breathing movements in fetal sheep with prolonged and graded hypoxemia. *American Journal of Obstetrics and Gynecology, 167,* 553–558.

Riley, R. J., & Johnson, J. W. (1993). Collecting and analyzing cord blood gases. *Clinical Obstetrics and Gynecology, 36,* 13–23.

Ross, M. G., Ervin, M. G., & Novak, D. (2007). Placental and fetal physiology. In S. G. Gabbe, J. R. Niebyl, & J. L. Simpson (Eds.), *Obstetrics normal and problem pregnancies* (pp. 26–34). Philadelphia: Churchill Livingstone.

Sarno, A. P., Ahn, M. O., Phelan, J. P., & Paul, R. H. (1990). Fetal acoustic stimulation in the early intrapartum period as a predictor of subsequent fetal condition. *American Journal of Obstetrics and Gynecology, 162,* 762–767.

Seelbach-Gobel, B., Heupel, M., Kuhnert, M., & Butterwegge, M. (1999). The prediction of fetal acidosis by means of intrapartum fetal pulse oximetry. *American Journal of Obstetrics and Gynecology, 180*(1 Pt. 1), 73–81.

Sherer, D. M. (1994). Blunted fetal response to vibroacoustic stimulation associated with maternal intravenous magnesium sulfate therapy. *American Journal of Perinatology, 11,* 401–403.

Sherer, D. M., & Bentolila, E. (1998). Blunted fetal response to vibroacoustic stimulation following chronic exposure to propranolol. *American Journal of Perinatology, 15,* 495–498.

Simpson, K. R., & James, D. C. (2005). Efficacy of intrauterine resuscitation techniques in improving fetal oxygen status during labor. *Obstetrics and Gynecology, 105,* 1362–1368.

Simpson, K. R., & James, D. (2008). Effects of oxytocin-induced uterine hyperstimulation on fetal oxygen status and fetal heart rate patterns during labor. *American Journal of Obstetrics and Gynecology, 199,* 34 e1-34e5.

Simpson, K. R., & Porter, M. L. (2001). Fetal oxygen saturation monitoring. Using this new technology for fetal assessment during labor. *Association of Women's Health, Obstetric and Neonatal Nurses (AWHONN) Lifelines, 5*(2), 26–33.

Skupski, D. W., Rosenberg, C. R., & Eglinton, G. S. (2002). Intrapartum fetal stimulation tests: A meta-analysis. *Obstetrics and Gynecology, 99,* 129–134.

Smith, C. V., Nguyen, H. N., Phelan, J. P., & Paul, R. H. (1986a). Intrapartum assessment of fetal well-being: A comparison of fetal acoustic stimulation with acid-base determinations. *American Journal of Obstetrics and Gynecology, 155,* 726–728.

Smith, C. V., Phelan, J. P., Platt, L. D., Broussard, P., & Paul, R. H. (1986b). Fetal acoustic stimulation testing.

II. A randomized clinical comparison with the non-stress test. *American Journal of Obstetrics and Gynecology, 155,* 131–134.

Smith, C. V., Satt, B., Phelan, J. P., & Paul, R. H. (1990). Intrauterine sound levels: Intrapartum assessment with an intrauterine microphone. *American Journal of Perinatology, 7,* 312–315.

Society of Obstetricians and Gynaecologists of Canada. (2007). Fetal health surveillance: Antepartum and intrapartum consensus guideline. *Journal of Obstetrics and Gynaecology Canada, 29,* 1–59.

Sonek, J., & Nicolaides, K. (1994). The role of cordocentesis in the diagnosis of fetal well-being. *Clinical Perinatology, 21,* 743–764.

Swedlow, D.B. (2000). *Review of evidence for a fetal SPO₂ critical threshold of 30 percent* (Reference Note No. 2). Pleasanton, CA: Mallinckrodt, Inc.

Sykes, G. S., Molloy, P. M., Johnson, P., Gu, W., Ashworth, F., Stirrat, G. M., et al. (1982). Do Apgar scores indicate asphyxia? *Lancet, 1*(8270), 494–496.

Tan, K. H., & Smyth, R. (2001). *Fetal vibroacoustic stimulation for facilitation of tests of fetal wellbeing.* Cochrane Database Systematic Reviews (1), CD002963.

Thorp, J. A., Dildy, G. A., Yeomans, E. R., Meyer, B. A., & Parisi, V. M. (1996). Umbilical cord blood gas analysis at delivery. *American Journal of Obstetrics and Gynecology, 175*(3 Pt. 1), 517–522.

Thorp, J. A., & Rushing, R. S. (1999). Umbilical cord blood gas analysis. *Obstetrics and Gynecology Clinics of North America, 26,* 695–709.

Thorp, J. A., Sampson, J. E., Parisi, V. M., & Creasy, R. K. (1989). Routine umbilical cord blood gas determinations? *American Journal of Obstetrics and Gynecology, 161,* 600–605.

Wallman, C. M. (1997). Interpretation of fetal cord blood gases. *Neonatal Network, 16*(1), 72–75.

Westgate, J., Garibaldi, J. M., & Greene, K. R. (1994). Umbilical cord blood gas analysis at delivery: A time for quality data. *British Journal of Obstetrics and Gynaecology, 101,* 1054–1063.

Whitworth, M. K., & Bricker, L. (2006). How to perform intrapartum fetal blood sampling. *British Journal of Hospital Medicine, 67*(9), 162–164.

Yao, Q. W., Jakobsson, J., Nyman, M., Rabaeus, H., Till, O., & Westgren, M. (1990). Fetal responses to different intensity levels of vibroacoustic stimulation. *Obstetrics and Gynecology, 75,* 206–209.

Yeomans, E. R., Hauth, J. C., Gilstrap, L. C., 3rd, & Strickland, D. M. (1985). Umbilical cord pH, PCO₂, and bicarbonate following uncomplicated term vaginal deliveries. *American Journal of Obstetrics and Gynecology, 151,* 798–800.

Yeomans, E. R., & Ramin, S. M. (2007). *Umbilical cord blood acid-base analysis.* UpToDate®. Accessed October 12, 2007. http://utdol.com/utd/contenttopic.do?toppicKey+labordel/11115&view=text.

Application of Fetal Heart Monitoring Data

1. Read This Book
2. Take the On-Line Test
3. Earn Continuing Nursing Education Credit

www.awhonn.org/fhm

AWHONN is accredited as a provider of continuing nursing education by the American Nurses Credentialing Center's Commission on Accreditation.

CHAPTER 8

Communication of Fetal Heart Monitoring Information

Kathleen Rice Simpson
G. Eric Knox

PURPOSE AND SIGNIFICANCE

Communication is an integral component of clinical care. The quality of communication can significantly influence patient safety, quality of care, and outcomes for mothers and babies. Communication that is open, direct, accurate, and concise will increase the likelihood that information regarding patient status is known and appropriately acted on by all professionals in a timely manner. Common communication channels include those between the clinician and the laboring woman (and her family or support persons), among nurses and primary health care providers, among primary health care providers, and among nurses. Although most of the communication between a clinician and patient is verbal, it is important to consider that a nonverbal cue from the clinician may influence how the woman interprets the message. Communication among clinicians is both verbal and written. Verbal communication among providers may not always be face to face. For example, communication about ongoing maternal-fetal status during labor can occur while the nurse is at the bedside and the physician or midwife is in the office or at home. Medical record documentation serves to communicate the previous and ongoing patient condition and care to the nurse, midwife, physician, and other members of the health care team.

This chapter covers communications regarding fetal status, including discussions among professional colleagues and discussions with the woman and her family and support person(s). Strategies to promote respectful, collaborative communication among colleagues are included. Trends and issues related to medical record documentation are discussed with examples that can be used or adapted according to individual institutional protocols. Perspectives on risk management, conflict management, and the chain of command (also known as chain of authority) as they relate to fetal assessment are presented as suggestions to promote safe care for mothers and babies and to decrease professional liability exposure.

COMMUNICATION AMONG PROFESSIONAL COLLEAGUES

Perinatal services in each institution are provided by teams of professional colleagues. Teamwork is a key factor in achieving excellence in clinical practice. In any situation requiring a real-time combination of multiple skills, experiences, and judgment, teams—not individuals—create superior performance (Merry & Brown, 2002; Risser et al., 1999). Ideally, a perinatal team consists of health care professionals working collectively and in nonhierarchical fashion toward a mutually agreed on and common goal: the best possible outcomes for mothers and babies (Simpson, James, & Knox, 2006). Each member contributes and is valued for his or her talents, education, experience, background, and perspective. Individual member contributions are evaluated by merit without re-

177

gard for the member's status in a traditional health care hierarchy. For example, the input of a staff nurse has as much value as that of an attending physician, and the input from a resident physician is considered just as important as that of an advanced-practice nurse. The value of individual contributions is defined by existing data or merit rather than presumed organizational position (Sherwood, Thomas, Bennett, & Lewis, 2002). The hallmark of successful teamwork is effective communication.

Achieving an environment in which perinatal teamwork is a reality can be a challenge because universal and institution-specific barriers may exist. Those barriers are complex and involve many interrelated factors (Box 8-1). Although some factors can be changed or overcome, others represent challenges embedded in the structure of our current health care system (Simpson & Knox, 2001). Each factor influences how well nurses, midwives, and physicians communicate.

Although teamwork is a key component of safe and effective perinatal care, nurses, midwives, and physicians are accountable for their individual actions and contributions to the team.

BOX 8-1 Factors That Impede Teamwork in Perinatal Care

Historical roles of women in society
Traditional roles of physicians and nurses
Institutional territory and politics
Licensure and professional accountability
Type and quantity of education
Different styles of learning and information
    exchange
Socialization of each group
Methods and amounts of compensation
Power of social and professional position
Collaboration—an impediment because it assumes separation of groups
Unresolved conflict, setting the stage for the
    expectation of future discord
Inability to establish common incentives

From: Simpson, K. R., & Knox, G. E. (2001). Perinatal teamwork: Turning rhetoric into reality. In K. R. Simpson & P. A. Creehan (Eds.), *AWHONN's Perinatal Nursing* (pp. 53–67). Philadelphia: Lippincott.

Professionals are responsible members of the health care team who have a body of knowledge and skills that contain an ethos of good practice. That ethos includes practice based on valid, current science; appropriate use of technology; a fiduciary relationship to the patient and family; and responsible behavior in relation to other health care providers to uphold patient safety standards (Benner et al., 2002). Health care professionals are responsible for accurate and timely assessments, clinical interventions, follow-up, and documentation of all critical events in the medical record. The nursing process (Figure 8-1) is a scientific problem solving model. Effective communication with women and between professional colleagues is an essential component embedded in all stages of the process.

Nurse to Primary Health Care Provider Communication

Nurse to primary health care provider (e.g., physician or midwife) communication includes information about maternal-fetal assessments and needs, and in relation to FHM, interpretation of fetal heart rate (FHR) and uterine activity data; changes in maternal or fetal status; interventions already taken with maternal-fetal responses; and specific requests for primary care provider orders or actions, as well as expectations as to when requested actions will occur. Data concerning the FHR pattern should ideally be conveyed using the definitions provided in the proceedings of the National Institute of Child Health and Human Development 2008 guidelines for EFM definitions, interpretation, and research (Macones, Hankins, Spong, Hauth, & Moore, 2008). If the nurse is concerned about indeterminate (category II) or abnormal (category III) patterns, the data that should be communicated includes but is not limited to the following:

- Baseline FHR
- Variability (absent, minimal, moderate, or marked)
- Presence or absence of accelerations (appropriate for gestational age)

FIGURE 8-1   The Nursing Process and Fetal Heart Monitoring: Communication

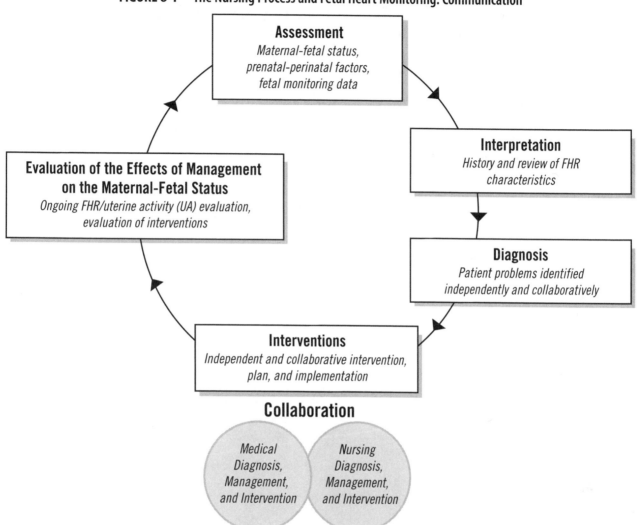

- Presence or absence of decelerations:
  - o If decelerations are noted, type of decelerations (early, late, variable, prolonged), and whether the decelerations are recurrent
  - o Clinical context (e.g., tachysystole, vaginal bleeding, recent epidural dose, rupture of membranes)
- Timeframe of indeterminate or abnormal FHR changes (e.g., how long has this pattern been evolving?)
- Specific intrauterine resuscitation techniques initiated and the maternal-fetal response
- Specific, clearly stated requests for additional orders and/or direct bedside evaluation by the primary health care provider (Fox, Kilpatrick, King, & Parer, 2000)

A structured format for communicating clinical information works well. One example of a structured communication format is **S**ituation, **B**ackground, **A**ssessment and **R**ecommendation, also known as SBAR. (An example of this type of format for indeterminate or abnormal FHR patterns is provided in Box 8-2.) CHAT (**C**ontext, **H**istory, **A**ssessment, **T**entative plan) is a similar framework. The format of communication can be whatever the perinatal team agrees it should be as long as it is direct, clear, concise, timely, and respectful. No specific method has been demonstrated to produce better outcomes than another method.

Interaction and communication among physicians and nurses commonly occurs in a hierarchical model (based on tradition and education)

BOX 8-2   SBAR Communication: Indeterminate or Abnormal Fetal Heart Rate Pattern

Call to Dr/CNM_____@_____
Patient_____
Nurse_____

Perinatal SBAR: Indeterminate or Abnormal FHR Pattern

Situation	I'm calling about _____(patient name) I'm concerned about the FHR pattern. The FHR is _____ with (absent, minimal, moderate, or marked) variability. Accelerations are (absent, present). There are (late, variable, or prolonged) decelerations. They are/are not recurrent. Contractions are every ___ minutes of (mild, moderate, strong; or ____ mg Hg) intensity, lasting _____ seconds. G_____, P_____ Cervical dilation_____ Labor progress_____ (Progressing 1 cm per hour/slow progression/nonprogression since _____)
Background	She's here for _____ (e.g., rule out labor/labor/induction of labor/VBAC labor, etc.). I've (repositioned her, given an IV fluid bolus, discontinued oxytocin, given oxygen); however, the pattern has not resolved. She was receiving _____ mU of oxytocin before I discontinued it.
Assessment	The FHR is (indeterminate, abnormal) and this has been going on for about 30 minutes despite my interventions. Her vital signs are (normal; hypotensive/hypertensive; elevated temperature). Provide clinical impression (should include context, e.g., bleeding, elevated temperature and pattern evolution, e.g., how long has this been going on?). Examples of a clinical impression: She hasn't progressed in labor for 2 hours despite adequate contractions. Her temperature is 100.1 F. There is caput and cervical swelling. She's had a lot of bloody show that has progressed to frank bleeding.
Response	Please come to the hospital to review the tracing (now, as soon as possible, within the hour, after you're done in the office). When can I expect to see you? Because it will be _____ before you can get here, I'd like to have the in-house physician evaluate the patient in the interim. Read back orders and expected response.

FHR, Fetal heart rate; G, gravidity; IV, intravenous; P, parity; VBAC, vaginal birth after cesarean birth.

---

even though hierarchy can be hazardous and create conditions that decrease patient safety (Knox & Simpson, 2003). Physician-nurse interaction and communication patterns and the effects of those patterns have been examined; however, little is known about interactions and communication among nurses and other care providers (e.g., midwives). Therefore, the following discussion refers to nurse-physician communication. In a hierarchical model, physicians give orders and nurses may be expected to follow those orders without question (Clancy & Tornberg, 2007; Keenan, Cooke, & Hillis, 1998; Simpson et al., 2006; Sleutel, 2000). Communication of this nature regarding fetal status does not always create optimal patient care and has the potential to increase the risk of preventable adverse outcomes. Examples of situations in which a traditional hierarchical model creates barriers to clear communication include (1) situations of rapidly changing fetal status, where the nurse at the bedside has more information than the physician or CNM at home or in the office; (2) teaching situations in which the nurse has more experience than the student or resident physician in training; and (3) situations in which the nurse has learned important information from the woman or family that the family has chosen not to communicate with the physician. In circumstances such as these, experienced nurses may initiate strategies designed to overcome provider discomfort with nurses' critical thinking skills or clinical suggestions concerning how their patients should be cared for, thus circumventing the expected hierarchal model of communication (Simpson & Knox, 2001; Simpson et al., 2006).

Nurses and physicians often develop a "negotiated order" (Corser, 2000) to structure their communication and behavioral patterns to facilitate work interactions. This negotiated order has been described as "a coordinated management of meanings" among professionals accustomed to working together under long-standing perpetual differences (Pearce & Cronen, 1980). Nurses and physicians have repeatedly been shown to engage in numerous strategies designed to evade the fundamental contradictions that exist between nursing and medical paradigms (Corser). "Interpretive communication events" consisting of scripted messages and response patterns are often modified by nurses and physicians for each clinical context as they attempt to make patient care decisions under challenging or conflicted conditions (McMahan, Hoffman, & McGee, 1994).

Instead of direct communication leading to a plan of care developed through the wisdom and experience of two knowledgeable professionals, nurses at times feel forced by conditions imposed in a hierarchical system to revert to the "doctor-nurse game" to achieve what they believe is in the patient's best interest (Stein, Watts, & Howell, 1990). Although this technique was described more than 40 years ago (Stein, 1967), it appears to be still operational today. Tips on how to interact effectively with members of the health care team are often given by experienced

nurses to new graduates as part of socialization to the role of the professional registered nurse (Willis & Parish, 1997). One technique often taught is how to encourage the physician to think a plan of action was his or her idea rather than that of the nurse. Using this communication technique may avoid open disagreement and/or conflict and allow the nurse to give recommendations and the physician to request recommendations without appearing to do so (Peter, 2000). However, indirect ("hinting and hoping"), inefficient, and inaccurate communication can occur and may lead to adverse outcomes in multiple ways such as (1) when nurses have difficulty finding the right "story" to convey the emergent nature of an evolving clinical situation (Knaus, Draper, & Wagner, 1986); (2) when the assessment is not complete because of a clinical fact known to the physician but not the nurse; or (3) when the assessment is correct but the description is misunderstood by the physician. Dysfunctional communication using less direct and respectful techniques can have a negative impact on safe patient care (Knox & Simpson, 2003).

Trust, open communication, and effective interdisciplinary teamwork are integral to promoting safe patient care. Communication implies a transfer of information. Ideally that information is accurate, timely, and conveyed with mutual respect. Teamwork is a complementary relationship of interdependence (Sherwood et al., 2002). Nurses and physicians must rely on each other, each contributing a unique aspect of care needed for optimal outcomes. Effective teamwork requires ongoing, consistent communication, full participation, working in synchrony, effective conflict management, ongoing feedback, knowledge of team goals, and acknowledgment of each other's roles and responsibilities to achieve those goals (Firth-Cozens, 2001; Katzenbach & Smith, 1993).

One hallmark of team behavior is clear language, agreed on and understood by all members (Knox & Simpson, 2003). Terminology related to FHM should be defined in each facility's policies and procedures so that all members of the perinatal team communicate using an agreed upon common terminology. AWHONN and ACOG support the use of the 2008 NICHD guidelines (Macones et al., 2008) for EFM definitions, interpretation, and research.

Clear language is particularly important when communication does not occur face to face. Telephone communication with the physician or midwife should be direct and to the point. For example:

- "Based on my initial assessment, this patient is having recurrent variable decelerations. May I have an order for an amnioinfusion, and can you please come in to see this patient as soon as possible?"
- "I am having difficulty obtaining a continuous tracing of the fetal heart rate. May I have an order to place a fetal spiral electrode? I'll call you back and let you know how the baby is doing after I have a period of fetal heart rate tracing with the spiral electrode."
- "I am uncomfortable with your order to start oxytocin because of the fetal heart rate pattern. I am going to wait until you are able to come in and see this patient and we can review the tracing together. When can I expect to see you?"
- "I wanted to let you know that I discontinued the oxytocin infusion because of tachysystole. I also gave an IV fluid bolus of 500 mL of lactated Ringer's solution and assisted the patient to a lateral position to decrease uterine activity. The FHR tracing is normal. As soon as the uterine activity has returned to normal, I'll restart the oxytocin. Do you want me to call you in an hour with a status report?"
- "You ordered intermittent auscultation of the fetal heart rate, but what I am hearing during auscultation suggests decelerations. I'm calling to let you know that I am going to use continuous monitoring at least for a while until I have a normal fetal heart rate tracing. I'll call you back after I assess the patient and review the tracing to let you know what is happening with the baby."

- "Your patient is fully dilated, but she doesn't feel the urge to push. I'm going to delay pushing until she feels pressure, but if she doesn't have an urge to push in an hour, I'll see what I can do to help her push effectively. I'll let you know when I need you to come."
- "I'm calling for ____. She just checked your patient during a prolonged deceleration and noted a prolapsed cord. We are transferring your patient to the OR and need you to come now. We'll let the anesthesiologist and the neonatal team know that they need to come too. We'll be ready to proceed when you get here."
- "Fetal status is deteriorating quickly, and I need you here now."

In a classic study of how the quality of interactions between nurses and physicians in an intensive care setting affects patient outcomes, Knaus et al. (1986) demonstrated that the most powerful determinant of severity-adjusted patient death rates was how well nurses and physicians worked together in planning and subsequently delivering patient care. They concluded that a high degree of involvement and interaction among nurses and physicians directly influences patient outcomes. Other researchers found that for each severity level of medical condition studied, patients were at greater risk of dying or being readmitted when nurses and resident physicians failed to communicate and effectively work together (Baggs, Ryan, Phelps, Richeson, & Johnson, 1992). These findings were supported by a later study (Baggs et al., 1999). In summary, knowledgeable, clear, direct, and respectful communication is an important key to promoting patient safety.

Handoff Communications

The "handoff" or transfer of patient care from one care provider to another occurs multiple times each day in the health care setting, yet it is prone to errors and omissions that have the potential to negatively affect outcomes (Patterson, Roth, Woods, Chow, & Gomes, 2004). During labor, nursing care is often transferred from one nurse to another. These transfers can be temporary or permanent and may be the result of change of shift, covering for nursing breaks, a change in patient acuity, or a move to the surgical suite for cesarean birth. Although the handoff process is meant to promote continuity and efficiency, there are inherent vulnerabilities because of the human factors involved in the relay of critical information (Simpson, 2005). Other industries such as aviation, nuclear power, and emergency dispatch have developed strategies to increase the likelihood that accurate and comprehensive information is transferred and that information is received and fully understood (Patterson et al., 2004). Some of these strategies are listed in Box 8-3 and others have been added and adapted to perinatal care (Simpson, 2005). To ensure the robustness of patient safety system during handoffs, the perinatal team should develop and continually reevaluate effective communication and coordination strategies (Patterson et al., 2004). This is particularly impor-

tant in emergent situations such as a sudden, profound fetal bradycardia when the stress is high (Simpson, 2005). The fresh perspective of the oncoming team should be valued and open interaction regarding prior, ongoing, and anticipated maternal-fetal status should be routinely expected.

One communication strategy is the confirmation summary.

- "Just to confirm…Mrs. Smith has been having recurrent variable decelerations for the last 30 minutes that are unresolved by position changes. You have orders for an amnioinfusion from Dr. Jones, but you haven't started the infusion yet. Yes?"
- "I understand that Dr. Black has requested a change from intermittent auscultation to continuous fetal monitoring for Ms. Clancy. Am I correct?"
- "Before you leave, I want to make sure I understand you correctly. Mrs. Miller has been push-

---

BOX 8-3 Strategies for Promoting Safe Handoffs

These strategies for handing off patient care to another clinician can be used both individually and collectively. They are useful for all team members and across all disciplines.

- Use face-to-face communication whenever possible with interactive questioning encouraged.
- Use confirmation summaries for verifying communication content.
- Limit interruptions during updates and handoffs.
- Develop protocols for what type and amount of information must be included in a handoff for each clinical situation (i.e., admission, labor, birth, discharge).
- Solicit outgoing team's opinions about ongoing patient status and contingency plans for various potential variations in clinical condition.
- Assess patient status together (incoming and outgoing clinicians at the bedside).
- Provide a written summary of critical information.
- Ensure incoming clinicians have knowledge of and access to the most up-to-date information.
- Ensure an unambiguous transfer of responsibility for key tasks that are left undone.
- Delay transfer of care responsibility when there is concern about status of the process or the ability of the incoming clinician to safely handle the situation.
- During emergencies, remain involved until there is assurance and evidence that each piece of critical information has been accurately transferred and received by all members of the accepting team.
- Use role playing to teach new team members how to effectively communicate during handoffs.
- Regularly observe handoffs in progress to evaluate the process and develop ideas for improvement.
- Use handoffs that are ideal and less than ideal as learning opportunities.

Adapted from: Simpson, K. R. (2005). Handling handoffs safely. *MCN American Journal of Maternal Child Nursing, 30*, 76.

ing for the last 2 hours and the baby is still at +1 station. The fetal heart rate pattern is normal. Dr. Ross is aware and wants her to continue pushing. He wants me to call him with an update in 45 minutes. Is this accurate?"

Communication of fetal assessment data among clinicians varies with institutional practice models and staffing patterns. In some situations, nursing handoffs may be limited to change-of-shift reporting. In other situations, handoffs may be required when a woman's condition changes so that she temporarily needs one-to-one care, for example, during epidural placement, an indeterminate or abnormal FHR pattern, second-stage labor pushing, or birth. A significant amount of data regarding maternal-fetal status must be communicated accurately and concisely to the relief nurse who will be covering the other nurse's patient. Verbal reports should be accompanied by complete and timely medical record documentation. Some practice models involve team nursing, in which several nurses care for a team of patients. It is important in this model to identify which nurse has primary responsibility for the patient and to keep all members of the team informed about ongoing maternal-fetal status. At times an acute event necessitates that one clinician cover another clinician's patient without the benefit of a comprehensive verbal report. If the medical record documentation is up-to-date, a review of the electronic fetal monitoring (EFM) tracing and labor flow record should be adequate for the clinician to assume care and ensure patient safety.

Communication among clinicians during change of shift or change of responsibility for patient care should be comprehensive. For example, a handoff report from one clinician to another about a woman in labor should include the following:

- Important maternal-fetal admission data, including pertinent laboratory tests and results
- Current assessment, including how well the mother and fetus are tolerating labor
- Characteristics of the FHR pattern and uterine activity

- Any intrauterine resuscitation measures that have been initiated, indications for the measures, and the maternal-fetal response
- Other interventions or procedures planned or completed
- Progress of labor
- Maternal vital signs
- Current and previous dosages of pharmacologic agents that were used to ripen the cervix or induce or augment labor, if applicable, including the maternal-fetal response
- Pain status, including current and previous pain relief and comfort measures that have been used
- The woman's desires for labor and birth
- Pertinent psychosocial issues

When possible, clinicians should review the medical record and fetal monitor tracing together before the clinician who is giving the report leaves the unit. Doing so will ensure that all data are covered and give the clinician who is leaving an opportunity to answer questions and address concerns that the relief or oncoming clinician may have. Ideally, a report between nurses is followed by a visit to the patient's room, where the reporting nurse introduces the relief nurse to the patient and support persons in attendance.

STRATEGIES FOR SUCCESSFUL COMMUNICATION AMONG PROFESSIONAL COLLEAGUES

Common Expectations and Standardized Definitions of Fetal Heart Rate Patterns

Each institution should have policies related to FHR pattern interpretation, expected interventions if there is concern for maternal or fetal status (Fox et al., 2000), and medical record documentation, ideally developed by an interdisciplinary perinatal team (Simpson & Knox, 2005). These mutually agreed-on practices can then be routinely used by all providers to enhance both interdisciplinary communication and patient safety. The potential for miscommunication among care providers, especially during telephone conversations regarding fetal status, are decreased when everyone is using the same terminology to describe EFM data. Thus, appropriate and timely intervention for indeterminate or abnormal FHR patterns is more likely. The Association of Women's Health, Obstetric and Neonatal Nurses' (AWHONN, 2005) and the American College of Obstetricians and Gynecologists' (ACOG, 2005) endorsement of the NICHD (1997) definitions and co-publication of the 2008 updates to these definitions for FHR patterns are a positive step in promoting effective, concise communication regarding FHR patterns.

Joint Nurse–Midwife–Physician Education Regarding Fetal Assessment

Nurses, midwives, and physicians jointly assess and manage maternal-fetal status during labor. Therefore, interdisciplinary continuing education programs provide one way to promote effective communication among providers (Simpson & Knox, 2001). These interdisciplinary educational programs concerning electronic fetal monitoring can potentially accomplish the following:

- Decrease the frequency of clinical disagreement among physicians, midwives, and nurses regarding the description and interpretation of FHR patterns
- Increase the opportunity for interaction and role modeling professional communication techniques
- Promote collaborative problem solving in the clinical setting

EFM tracing reviews work well as a form of interdisciplinary education because the presentation and discussion are associated with specific clinical cases and graphic display of FHR patterns. A group process can be used to review expected responses, appropriate interpretations, and related interventions. Team discussions can lead to an increased knowledge of EFM principles for everyone involved. Developing case

studies containing clinical ambiguity can be an ideal way to clarify ongoing clinical issues and expose differing levels of individual clinician tolerance of risk when interpretation and expectations of provider groups may not always be the same (Simpson, 2008a). An interdisciplinary team in each institution can identify clinical situations for which there are varying opinions regarding management or that can result in varying opinions. For example, physicians may expect a series of nursing interventions for a specific FHR pattern that are not the routine of nurses on the unit. In another example, there may be clinical disagreement about what to do when tachysystole is the result of oxytocin administration but the FHR pattern remains normal. Opinions may vary among nurses and primary care providers concerning when and under what circumstances oxytocin dosages should be increased or decreased, and thus may be a source of frustration (Simpson et al., 2006; Sleutel, Schultz, & Wyble, 2007). An open and proactive discussion of physiologic principles related to oxytocin administration and rationale for a course of action can result in standardization of policies and enhanced communication among providers (Simpson et al.).

One way to explicitly demonstrate that knowledge of fetal monitoring is not discipline-specific is to engage all disciplines in ongoing collaborative FHR monitoring education through interdisciplinary case reviews and joint FHM continuing education or certification activities. Educational collaboration among nurses, midwives, and physicians who are jointly responsible for FHR pattern interpretation and clinical interventions can enhance collaboration in everyday clinical interactions and thus promote patient safety. Funai et al. (2007) reported reduced rates of adverse perinatal events, improved staff perception of the overall perinatal patient safety climate, and decreased costs of malpractice claims related to obstetric care following the implementation of a multidimensional patient safety project. Adoption of the 1997 NICHD definitions for FHR patterns, team training, and interdisciplinary fetal monitoring education culminating in a national certification examination in EFM by all members of the perinatal team were included among the components of their comprehensive obstetric patient safety program.

COMMUNICATION WITH PREGNANT WOMEN AND THEIR FAMILIES OR SUPPORT PERSONS

Preparation for any method of fetal monitoring should ideally include an explanation of how data will be obtained (i.e., explain the use of auscultation or EFM) and time for answering the woman's questions and those of her support person(s). The clinician should describe how monitoring equipment will be used, and for EFM, the clinician should also explain the heart rate sounds and, in lay terms, the meaning of the data on the tracing. In addition, clinicians should discuss the fluidity of FHR characteristics and what might happen if the FHR pattern is not normal so that the woman and her family can be prepared if intrauterine resuscitation techniques are initiated quickly. In one study, the higher women rated the amount and quality of information about EFM provided by the nurse during initial monitor application, the more positively they viewed their overall EFM experience during labor (Simpson, 1991). In addition, women who felt that they were adequately informed about routine interventions during "nonreassuring" FHR patterns were less likely to be overly concerned when such patterns occurred.

Ideally, the most low-tech and least-invasive methods of fetal assessment are used for women in labor (AWHONN, 2009). Intermittent auscultation of the FHR at prescribed frequencies during labor has been shown to be as efficacious as continuous EFM (AAP & ACOG, 2007) and is recommended as the preferred method for low-risk women by some professional associations (Society of Obstetricians and Gynaecologists of Canada [SOGC], 2007). Women may know prior to labor that some form of EFM or auscultation may be used. Ideally, the primary health care provider discusses common methods of fetal assessment during labor with the woman during the prenatal period so that potential concerns or objections may be reviewed prior to admission for childbirth.

MEDICAL RECORD DOCUMENTATION
Overview

Documentation has become one of the most time-consuming of nursing activities and, therefore, one that is prone to omissions. Nurses often are concerned that medical record documentation forces them to focus on "paperwork" rather than patient care. Cumbersome documentation systems that require duplicate and triplicate entries of the same data contribute to this real problem. The ongoing challenge is to create a streamlined system for documentation that is cost-effective, easy to use, time efficient for clinicians, and sufficiently comprehensive for current or subsequent review. There can be ramifications for inaccuracies and omissions in medical record documentation. Documentation deficiencies may result in decreased communication among team members; denial of reimbursement by insurance carriers for care rendered; loss of information for statistical or outcome data for quality purposes; and, in the case of litigation, increased liability exposure for institutions and health care providers (Simpson, 2008c).

The medical record should provide a factual and objective account of care provided, including direct and indirect communication with other members of the health care team. There should be guidelines in each institution regarding how to document initiation and steps of notification in the chain of command or authority. See Figure 8-2 for an example of a chain of command or authority. Facility guidelines may include chain-of-command documentation in the medical record or on quality improvement or incident reports. It is important to be knowledgeable about and adhere to individual institutional policies about chain-of-command or -authority documentation.

FIGURE 8-2 Example of Problem Resolution Relying on Chain-of-Command or Chain-of-Authority

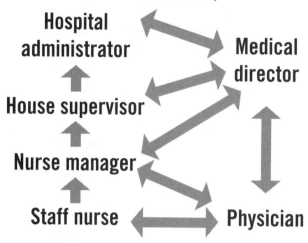

Decreasing Liability Exposure Related to Documentation

The medical record is often the single most important document available in the defense of an allegation of negligent care. The time from event to formal legal inquiry may involve several years, and clinicians may have limited independent recall without the documentation in the medical record. In issues of litigation, clinicians frequently rely on written notes or data entered into an electronic medical record at the time of patient contact. A complete, legible medical record is an asset when defending against allegations of improper care. Because lack of documentation can result in a presumed lack of care, omissions are challenging to defend. According to risk-claims data from a professional liability insurance carrier, documentation ranks second only to patient monitoring and assessment in the area of nursing-related risk exposure, accounting for 20.7% of all exposures (Berry, 1999).

Litigation can follow clinical events that result in adverse outcomes, regardless of whether or not the outcome was preventable. Documentation of events preceding, during, and following an emergent clinical situation should reflect all care provided. During emergent situations, medical record documentation may occur retrospectively. The first priority during an emergency is to provide immediate patient care. Post-event documentation should focus on reconstructing a summary of all of the assessments, actions, and communication that transpired as accurately and in as timely a manner as possible. For example, in the case of an acute onset of an FHR pattern resulting in an emergent cesarean birth, summary documentation should include but may not be limited to the following:

- Time the FHR pattern leading to the cesarean birth was recognized
- Clinical actions initiated for maternal and/or fetal resuscitation
- Continued assessment to evaluate the maternal-fetal responses to interventions
- Communication with team members and their responses
- Time the woman was taken to the surgical suite, time of arrival of other members of the surgical team, time of anesthesia, time of the incision, and time of birth
- Newborn status at birth, Apgar scores, and chronologies of interventions performed (including by which personnel) for newborn resuscitation, if necessary
- A narrative note reflecting discussion among health care providers and the woman and her family

Most medical record documentation systems (paper or electronic) have cues for data entry of these and other critical aspects of emergent birth care. During emergent intrapartum situations, some nurses believe that documentation directly on the paper version of the fetal monitoring tracing can assist them in constructing notes after patient stabilization. If this approach is used, it is important to ensure that the content and times included in the narrative notes written later coincide with the fetal monitoring tracing annotations (including the time, if present on the fetal monitoring tracing). Retrospective charting is better than no documentation. However, late entries can be areas of focus in litigation if they are written days after the event. Give careful attention to ensuring that charting occurs as soon after the event as possible and that the data entered are accurate and objective. Do not alter the medical record to include data that are not accurate even if asked to do so.

Although notations directly on the paper version of an FHR tracing can be useful during emergent situations, the practice of duplicate documentation of routine care on both the FHR tracing and the medical record is no longer recommended (Chez, 1997). Previously, perinatal nurses believed that there should be enough documentation on the FHR tracing so that the tracing could "stand alone" for subsequent review. However, not only does handwriting on the tracing about routine care increase the amount of nursing time spent on nonpatient care activities, but this practice can also lead to errors in documentation and can contribute to delays in transcription to the medical record. If the FHR tracings are electronically archived, handwritten notes on the paper tracing do not become part of the permanent medical record. As more institutions adopt electronic information systems with the ability to enter data that can be noted electronically on both the FHR tracing and labor record, this issue may be minimized or eliminated.

It is appropriate for nurses and health care providers to document FHR patterns by name in the medical record. In 1986, ACOG and AWHONN (then known as NAACOG, the Nurses Association of the American College of Obstetricians and Gynecologists) issued a joint publication on electronic fetal monitoring that included recommendations for identification, documentation, and communication of FHR patterns (ACOG & NAACOG, 1986). According to this joint statement, fetal monitoring patterns were given descriptive names (e.g., accelerations and early, late, variable, and prolonged decelerations) and the statement recommended that clinicians, including nurses, use these terms in written medical record documentation and in verbal communication regarding fetal status among providers. Since at least 1986, perinatal nurses have been encouraged to identify FHR patterns by the appropriate name in the medical

record, and it remains appropriate to do so (AAP & ACOG, 2007).

In the past, nurses were often taught to provide extensive detail about all FHR decelerations (e.g., deceleration down to the 60s lasting for 70 seconds with a slow return to baseline *or* decelerations occurring after each contraction down to the 100s lasting for 40 seconds) in the medical record so that they would be able to reconstruct the FHR pattern from their notes. Describing FHR patterns in the narrative notes was previously taught for two reasons: (1) fear that the paper EFM tracing could be lost and these descriptions would be crucial if the case involved a future lawsuit, and (2) "diagnosing" was not considered to be within the scope of nursing practice, thus descriptions of the patterns rather than identifying the FHR pattern by name was preferable.

Routine detailed description of deceleration patterns is time-consuming, may be unnecessary, and in some situations may increase liability exposure. For example, if the nurse has documented descriptive details of decelerations in the narrative notes and a subsequent adverse outcome occurs followed by litigation, experts may disagree about the details of each FHR deceleration. Repeated expert testimony that decelerations lasted 60 seconds rather than 55 seconds and/or reached a low point of 100 beats per minute (bpm) rather than 105 bpm may be challenging to defend when presented to a jury. There is typically little clinical significance between 100 bpm and 105 bpm and/or a 5-second difference in the duration of the FHR deceleration; however, these perceived differences in documentation can create the impression that the clinician was inaccurate in his or her interpretation of the clinical situation, when in reality there was no relationship between the FHR *documentation* and the condition of the infant (Simpson & Knox, 2000). Detailed narrative descriptions of FHR patterns may be necessary only when there is uncertainty about how to name a pattern with unusual characteristics.

In addition to the previous considerations, facilities may need backup systems for EFM data storage to ensure later retrieval if necessary.

The ink on the paper monitor tracings has the potential to fade over time. Microfilming the tracings prior to storing or discarding them can prevent loss of data. If paper tracings are routinely discarded after electronic or microfilm archiving, consider saving for education and peer review paper tracings associated with a selected set of clinical indicators that reflect complex or challenging case scenarios. Facilities should have a mechanism in place to ensure safe storage of EFM data. Electronic archiving systems are at risk for data corruption and software obsolescence like any other computerized storage system, and facilities should have appropriate backup systems for reading archived data. Because many states have statutes of limitations for litigation related to labor and birth that extend to 21 years after the event, it is important to consider whether current data and storage systems can be accessed by information systems 21 years in the future.

Flow Sheets and Narrative Notes

A written or electronic flow sheet at the point of care as the primary source of comprehensive data regarding maternal-fetal status, clinical interventions, and the events of labor and birth can facilitate timely and accurate medical record data entry. Well-designed flow sheets are useful to prompt notations and practice consistent with unit guidelines, especially in the labor and birth setting (see Figure 8-3 for a sample labor flow sheet). Routine assessments and interventions can easily be documented in the flow sheet format (see Figures 8-4 through and 8-9 for examples of documentation based on common clinical situations with EFM tracings). Figure 8-10 is an example of documentation based on intermittent auscultation and palpation. Abbreviations can be useful for speeding the documentation process. If abbreviations are used, there should be a "key to abbreviations" on the labor flow record, and the abbreviations should be consistent with the documentation policy of the institution. (See Table 8-1 for a list of common abbreviations used for documentation of maternal-fetal assessment data.)

Narrative notes should be used to document care or events that are other than routine and not included on the flow sheet. Narrative notes may also be used to document the following:

- Nurse-physician and/or midwife communication
- Ongoing interventions for indeterminate or abnormal FHR patterns that do not resolve with the usual intrauterine resuscitation techniques
- Changes in maternal status
- Patient concerns or requests
- Details and outcome of emergent situations

Text continued on p. 194

Table 8-1	Common Abbreviations Used in Medical Record Documentation during Labor
Abbreviation	**Term**
AFI	Amniotic fluid index
AFV	Amniotic fluid volume
bpm	Beats per minute
ED	Early deceleration
EFM	Electronic fetal monitoring
FHR	Fetal heart rate
FSE	Fetal spiral electrode
IA	Intermittent auscultation
IUPC	Intrauterine pressure catheter
LD	Late deceleration
MVU	Montevideo units
PD	Prolonged deceleration
TOCO	Tocodynamometer
UC	Uterine contractions
US	Ultrasound
VAS	Vibroacoustic stimulation
VD	Variable deceleration
VE	Vaginal examination

FIGURE 8-3   Sample Labor Flow Record

Patient Name:		Physician/CNM:			
	DATE:				**KEY**
	TIME:				**Variability** Ab = Absent (undetectable) Min = Minimal (>0 but ≤5 bpm)
Cervix — **Dilation**					Mod = Moderate (6-25 bpm) Mar = Marked (>25 bpm)
Cervix — **Effacement**					**Accelerations** + = Present and appropriate
Cervix — **Station**					for gestational age Ø = Absent
Fetal Heart — **Baseline Rate**					**Decelerations** E = Early
Fetal Heart — **Variability**					L = Late V = Variable
Fetal Heart — **Accelerations**					P = Prolonged **Stim/pH**
Fetal Heart — **Decelerations**					+ = Acceleration in response to stimulation
Fetal Heart — **STIM/pH**					Ø = No response to stimulation
Fetal Heart — **Monitor Mode**					Record number for scalp pH **Monitor mode**
Uterine Activity — **Frequency**					A = Auscultation/Palpation E = External u/s or toco
Uterine Activity — **Duration**					FSE = Fetal spiral electrode IUPC = Intrauterine pressure
Uterine Activity — **Intensity**					catheter **Frequency of uterine activity**
Uterine Activity — **Resting Tone**					Ø = None
Uterine Activity — **Monitor Mode**					Irreg = Irregular **Intensity of uterine activity**
Uterine Activity — **Oxytocin milliunits/min**					M = Mild Mod = Moderate
Pain					Str = Strong By IUPC = mm Hg
Coping					**Resting tone** R = Relaxed
Maternal Position					By IUPC = mm Hg **Coping**
O2/LPM/Mask					W = Well S = Support provided
IV					For pain use 0-10 scale **Maternal position**
Nurse Initials					A = Ambulatory U = Upright SF = Semi-Fowlers
Narrative notes:					RL = Right lateral LL = Left lateral MS = Modified Sims'

FIGURE 8-4 Sample EFM Documentation: Normal Tracing

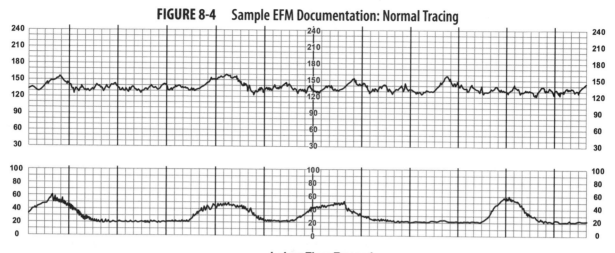

Labor Flow Record

					KEY
	DATE:	12/22/06			**KEY**
	TIME:	12:15			**Variability**
Cervix	Dilation	4			Ab = Absent (undetectable)
	Effacement	80			Min = Minimal (>0 but ≤5 bpm)
	Station	-2			Mod = Moderate (6-25 bpm)
					Mar = Marked (>25 bpm)
Fetal Heart	Baseline Rate	135			**Accelerations**
	Variability	Mod			+ = Present and appropriate for gestational age
	Accelerations	+			Ø = Absent
	Decelerations	Ø			**Decelerations**
	STIM/pH				E = Early
					L = Late
	Monitor Mode	E			V = Variable
					P = Prolonged
					Stim/pH
Uterine Activity	Frequency	2-4			+ = Acceleration in response to stimulation
	Duration	80-90			Ø = No response to stimulation
	Intensity	mod			Record number for scalp pH
	Resting Tone	R			**Monitor mode**
					A = Auscultation/Palpation
	Monitor Mode	E			E = External u/s or toco
	Oxytocin milliunits/min				FSE = Fetal spiral electrode
					IUPC = Intrauterine pressure catheter
	Pain	5			**Frequency of uterine activity**
	Coping	W/S			Ø = None
					Irreg = Irregular
	Maternal Position	U			**Intensity of uterine activity**
	O2/LPM/Mask				M = Mild
					Mod = Moderate
	IV				Str = Strong
					By IUPC = mm Hg
	Nurse Initials	KLW			**Resting tone**
					R = Relaxed
					By IUPC = mm Hg

Narrative notes: 12:15 FHR Normal. Tolerating contractions well with support. In rocking chair.

Patient Name: Physician/CNM:

Coping
W = Well
S = Support provided
For pain use 0-10 scale
Maternal position
A = Ambulatory
U = Upright
SF = Semi-Fowlers
RL = Right lateral
LL = Left lateral
MS = Modified Sims'

FIGURE 8-5   Sample EFM Documentation with Early Decelerations

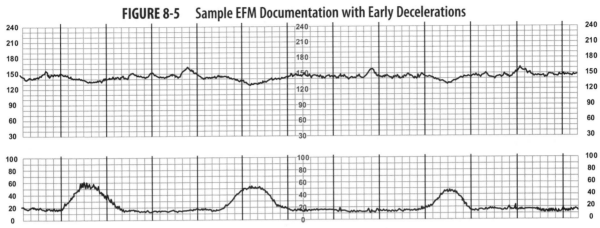

	LABOR FLOW RECORD				
Patient Name:		Physician/CNM:			
	DATE:	7/31/06			**KEY**
	TIME:	14:15			**Variability** Ab = Absent (undetectable) Min = Minimal (>0 but ≤5 bpm)
Cervix	Dilation	7			Mod = Moderate (6-25 bpm) Mar = Marked (>25 bpm) **Accelerations**
	Effacement	100			+ = Present and appropriate for gestational age
	Station	0			Ø = Absent **Decelerations**
Fetal Heart	Baseline Rate	145			E = Early
	Variability	Mod			L = Late V = Variable
	Accelerations	+			P = Prolonged **Stim/pH**
	Decelerations	E			+ = Acceleration in response to stimulation
	STIM/pH				Ø = No response to stimulation
	Monitor Mode	E			Record number for scalp pH **Monitor mode** A = Auscultation/Palpation
Uterine Activity	Frequency	3-4			E = External u/s or toco
	Duration	60-80			FSE = Fetal spiral electrode IUPC = Intrauterine pressure
	Intensity	mod			catheter **Frequency of uterine activity**
	Resting Tone	R			Ø = None Irreg = Irregular
	Monitor Mode	E			**Intensity of uterine activity** M = Mild
	Oxytocin milliunits/min	8			Mod = Moderate Str = Strong
	Pain	2			By IUPC = mm Hg **Resting tone**
	Coping	W/S			R = Relaxed By IUPC = mm Hg
	Maternal Position	RL			**Coping** W = Well
	O2/LPM/Mask				S = Support provided For pain use 0-10 scale
	IV				**Maternal position** A = Ambulatory
	Nurse Initials	JCW			U = Upright SF = Semi-Fowlers RL = Right lateral LL = Left lateral MS = Modified Sims'
Narrative notes:					

FIGURE 8-6 Sample EFM Documentation with Late Decelerations

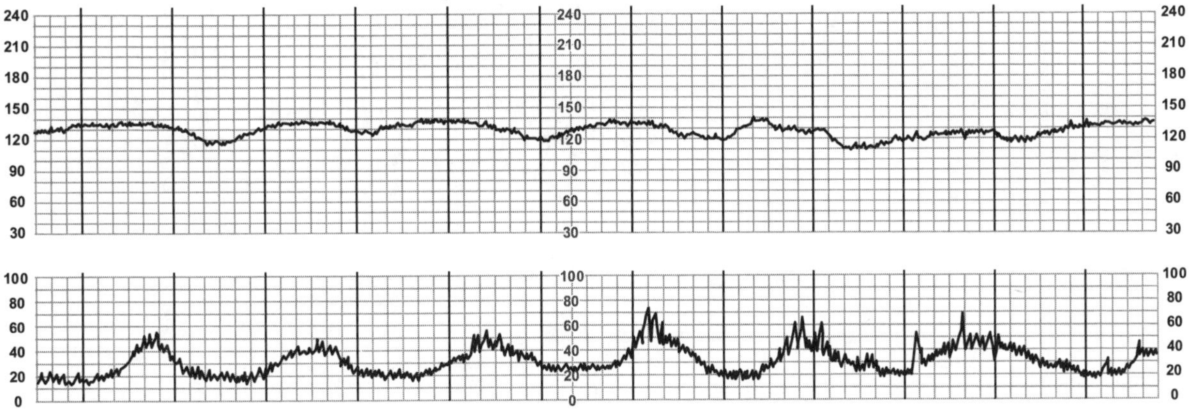

LABOR FLOW RECORD

Patient Name: **Physician/CNM:**

	DATE:	8/28/07		
	TIME:	18:30	18:40	
Cervix	**Dilation**	3		
	Effacement	50		
	Station	-2		
Fetal Heart	**Baseline Rate**	135	135	
	Variability	Min	Min	
	Accelerations	Ø	Ø	
	Decelerations	L	L	
	STIM/pH			
	Monitor Mode	E	E	
Uterine Activity	**Frequency**	1½-2	1½-2	
	Duration	60-80		
	Intensity	M		
	Resting Tone	R	R	
	Monitor Mode	E		
	Oxytocin milliunits/min	Off	Off	
	Pain	3		
	Coping	W/S		
	Maternal Position	RL		
	O2/LPM/Mask		10	
	IV	bolus		
	Nurse Initials	NLW	NLW	

Narrative notes: 18:30 Tachysystole & late decelerations noted. Uterine resting tone soft. Oxytocin discontinued; turned to RL; 500 ml IV fluid bolus. Dr Smith notified of all of above; will be here in 20 min to see pt.18:40 Ø change in FHR. O2 applied.

KEY

Variability
Ab = Absent (undetectable)
Min = Minimal (>0 but ≤5 bpm)
Mod = Moderate (6-25 bpm)
Mar = Marked (>25 bpm)
Accelerations
+ = Present and appropriate for gestational age
Ø = Absent
Decelerations
E = Early
L = Late
V = Variable
P = Prolonged
Stim/pH
+ = Acceleration in response to stimulation
Ø = No response to stimulation
Record number for scalp pH
Monitor mode
A = Auscultation/Palpation
E = External u/s or toco
FSE = Fetal spiral electrode
IUPC = Intrauterine pressure catheter
Frequency of uterine activity
Ø = None
Irreg = Irregular
Intensity of uterine activity
M = Mild
Mod = Moderate
Str = Strong
By IUPC = mm Hg
Resting tone
R = Relaxed
By IUPC = mm Hg
Coping
W = Well
S = Support provided
For pain use 0-10 scale
Maternal position
A = Ambulatory
U = Upright
SF = Semi-Fowlers
RL = Right lateral
LL = Left lateral
MS = Modified Sims'

FIGURE 8-7 Sample EFM Documentation with Variable Decelerations

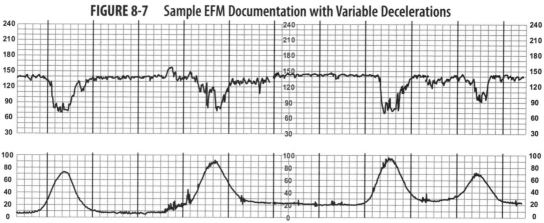

LABOR FLOW RECORD

Patient Name: **Physician/CNM:**

		DATE:	9/24/07		
		TIME:	05:30		
Cervix	Dilation		9		
	Effacement		100		
	Station		+2		
Fetal Heart	Baseline Rate		140		
	Variability		Mod		
	Accelerations		+		
	Decelerations		V		
	STIM/pH				
	Monitor Mode		FSE		
Uterine Activity	Frequency		2-4		
	Duration		60-90		
	Intensity		70-95		
	Resting Tone		8-28		
	Monitor Mode		IUPC		
	Oxytocin milliunits/min				
	Pain		1		
	Coping		W/S		
	Maternal Position		RL		
	O2/LPM/Mask				
	IV				
	Nurse Initials		RS		

KEY

Variability
Ab = Absent (undetectable)
Min = Minimal (>0 but ≤5 bpm)
Mod = Moderate (6-25 bpm)
Mar = Marked (>25 bpm)
Accelerations
+ = Present and appropriate for gestational age
Ø = Absent
Decelerations
E = Early
L = Late
V = Variable
P = Prolonged
Stim/pH
+ = Acceleration in response to stimulation
Ø = No response to stimulation
Record number for scalp pH
Monitor mode
A = Auscultation/Palpation
E = External u/s or toco
FSE = Fetal spiral electrode
IUPC = Intrauterine pressure catheter
Frequency of uterine activity
Ø = None
Irreg = Irregular
Intensity of uterine activity
M = Mild
Mod = Moderate
Str = Strong
By IUPC = mm Hg
Resting tone
R = Relaxed
By IUPC = mm Hg
Coping
W = Well
S = Support provided
For pain use 0-10 scale
Maternal position
A = Ambulatory
U = Upright
SF = Semi-Fowlers
RL = Right lateral
LL = Left lateral
MS = Modified Sims'

Narrative notes: 16:40. Position change for variable decelerations. Dr. Jones notified of FHR findings as above, and rapid labor progress. On his way to hospital.

FIGURE 8-8   Sample EFM Documentation with Prolonged Decelerations

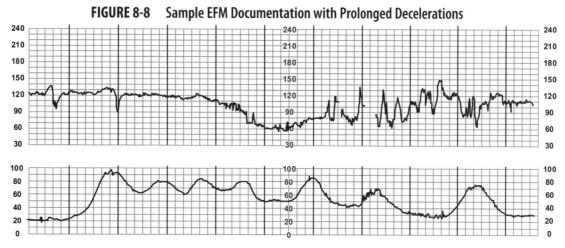

LABOR FLOW RECORD				
Patient Name:		**Physician/CNM:**		

		DATE:	5/1/07			KEY
		TIME:	16:40			**Variability**
Cervix	Dilation	3-4				Ab = Absent (undetectable) Min = Minimal (>0 but ≤5 bpm)
	Effacement	100				Mod = Moderate (6-25 bpm) Mar = Marked (>25 bpm)
	Station	-2				**Accelerations** + = Present and appropriate
Fetal Heart	Baseline Rate	125				for gestational age Ø = Absent
	Variability	Mod				**Decelerations**
	Accelerations	Ø				E = Early L = Late
	Decelerations	P				V = Variable P = Prolonged
	STIM/pH					**Stim/pH** + = Acceleration in response
	Monitor Mode	FSE				to stimulation Ø = No response to stimulation
Uterine Activity	Frequency	Tachysystole				Record number for scalp pH **Monitor mode** A = Auscultation/Palpation
	Duration					E = External u/s or toco
	Intensity					FSE = Fetal spiral electrode IUPC = Intrauterine pressure
	Resting Tone					catheter **Frequency of uterine activity**
	Monitor Mode	IUPC				Ø = None Irreg = Irregular
	Oxytocin milliunits/min	Off				**Intensity of uterine activity** M = Mild
	Pain	1				Mod = Moderate Str = Strong
	Coping	W/S				By IUPC = mm Hg **Resting tone**
	Maternal Position	RL				R = Relaxed By IUPC = mm Hg
	O2/LPM/Mask					**Coping** W = Well
	IV	bolus				S = Support provided For pain use 0-10 scale
	Nurse Initials	MM				**Maternal position** A = Ambulatory

Narrative notes: Tachysystole and hypertonus noted. Oxytocin discontinued; position change; 500ml IV fluid bolus; VE. Dr. Brown notified of above, coming over from office to evaluate pt. 16:45 FHR & UA recovering.

U = Upright
SF = Semi-Fowlers
RL = Right lateral
LL = Left lateral
MS = Modified Sims'

FIGURE 8-9   Sample EFM Documentation with Twins

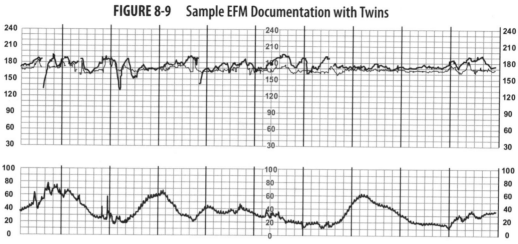

LABOR FLOW RECORD							
Patient Name:			**Physician/CNM:**				

		DATE	1/12/07				**KEY**
		TIME	04:15				**Variability**
Cervix	Dilation		9				Ab = Absent (undetectable) Min = Minimal (>0 but ≤5 bpm)
	Effacement		100				Mod = Moderate (6-25 bpm)
	Station		+2				Mar = Marked (>25 bpm) **Accelerations**
		TWIN	A	B	A	B	A	B	+ = Present and appropriate for gestational age
Fetal Heart	Baseline Rate		175	165						Ø = Absent **Decelerations**
	Variability		Mod	Mod						E = Early
	Accelerations		+	+						L = Late V = Variable
	Decelerations									P = Prolonged **Stim/pH**
	STIM/pH									+ = Acceleration in response to stimulation
	Monitor Mode		FSE	E						Ø = No response to stimulation
Uterine Activity	Frequency		2-3							Record number for scalp pH **Monitor mode**
	Duration		80-120							A = Auscultation/Palpation E = External u/s or toco
	Intensity		Mod							FSE = Fetal spiral electrode IUPC = Intrauterine pressure
	Resting Tone		R							catheter **Frequency of uterine activity**
	Monitor Mode		E							Ø = None
	Oxytocin milliunits/min									Irreg = Irregular **Intensity of uterine activity**
	Pain		2							M = Mild Mod = Moderate
	Coping		W/S							Str = Strong By IUPC = mm Hg
	Maternal Position		SF							**Resting tone** R = Relaxed
	O2/LPM/Mask									By IUPC = mm Hg **Coping**
	IV									W = Well S = Support provided
	Nurse Initials		MDF							For pain use 0-10 scale **Maternal position**

Narrative notes: Comfortable with epidural. Dr. Jackson here to see pt.

A = Ambulatory
U = Upright
SF = Semi-Fowlers
RL = Right lateral
LL = Left lateral
MS = Modified Sims'

FIGURE 8-10   Sample Documentation of Intermittent Auscultation

					KEY
	**LABOR FLOW RECORD**				

Patient Name:		**Physician/CNM:**			

		DATE	2/28/07			**KEY**
		TIME	08:00			**Variability**
Cervix	Dilation		3			Ab = Absent (undetectable)
	Effacement		80			Min = Minimal (>0 but ≤5 bpm)
	Station		-1			Mod = Moderate (6-25 bpm)
Fetal Heart	Baseline Rate		140s/Reg			Mar = Marked (>25 bpm)
	Variability					**Accelerations**
	Accelerations		↑ to 160			+ = Present and appropriate for gestational age
	Decelerations		Ø			Ø = Absent
	STIM/pH					**Decelerations**
	Monitor Mode		A			E = Early
Uterine Activity	Frequency		3-4			L = Late
	Duration		60-70			V = Variable
	Intensity		mod			P = Prolonged
	Resting Tone		R			**Stim/pH**
	Monitor Mode		A			+ = Acceleration in response to stimulation
	Oxytocin milliunits/min					Ø = No response to stimulation
	Pain		3			Record number for scalp pH
	Coping		W/S			**Monitor mode**
	Maternal Position		U			A = Auscultation/Palpation
	O2/LPM/Mask					E = External u/s or toco
	IV					FSE = Fetal spiral electrode
	Nurse Initials		KP			IUPC = Intrauterine pressure catheter

KEY

Variability
Ab = Absent (undetectable)
Min = Minimal (>0 but ≤5 bpm)
Mod = Moderate (6-25 bpm)
Mar = Marked (>25 bpm)
Accelerations
+ = Present and appropriate for gestational age
Ø = Absent
Decelerations
E = Early
L = Late
V = Variable
P = Prolonged
Stim/pH
+ = Acceleration in response to stimulation
Ø = No response to stimulation
Record number for scalp pH
Monitor mode
A = Auscultation/Palpation
E = External u/s or toco
FSE = Fetal spiral electrode
IUPC = Intrauterine pressure catheter
Frequency of uterine activity
Ø = None
Irreg = Irregular
Intensity of uterine activity
M = Mild
Mod = Moderate
Str = Strong
By IUPC = mm Hg
Resting tone
R = Relaxed
By IUPC = mm Hg
Coping
W = Well
S = Support provided
For pain use 0-10 scale
Maternal position
A = Ambulatory
U = Upright
SF = Semi-Fowlers
RL = Right lateral
LL = Left lateral
MS = Modified Sims'

Narrative note: 08:00 FHR Normal. Tolerating contractions well with coaching. On birthing ball.

Avoid forms with preprinted times and limited space for notations. These types of forms may contribute to inaccurate or inadequate documentation. Vital signs and other maternal and fetal assessments and/or emergencies do not always occur at predetermined 15-minute intervals. Care should be documented at the time it is provided, not at some artificially pre-determined time.

Fetal Heart Rate and Uterine Activity Assessment and Documentation

The frequency of FHR and uterine activity assessment and documentation are guided by professional organizations and institutional guidelines and take into consideration the particular clinical circumstances (ACOG, 2005; AWHONN, 2009; SOGC, 2007). Guidelines for ongoing labor assessments are described in the Position Statement *Fetal Heart Monitoring* (AWHONN, 2009), *Guidelines for Perinatal Care* (AAP & ACOG, 2007), the Practice Bulletin *Intrapartum Fetal Heart Rate Monitoring* (ACOG, 2005) and the *Fetal Health Surveillance: Antepartum and Intrapartum Consensus Guideline* (SOGC, 2007). The *Comprehensive Accreditation Manual for Hospitals* (Joint Commission, 2007), perinatal nursing textbooks, and some state board of health publications are other resources that provide guidelines for initial and ongoing nursing assessments of women in labor. Based on these guidelines, each perinatal center develops policies and procedures related to maternal and fetal assessment. See Box 8-4 for suggested guidelines for maternal and fetal assessment and documentation during a normal, uncomplicated labor and

---

BOX 8-4 Maternal-Fetal Assessments during Labor and Birth

Maternal Vital Signs

Maternal vital signs should be assessed and recorded at regular intervals, at least every 4 hours. This frequency may be increased, particularly as active labor progresses, according to clinical signs and symptoms (AAP & ACOG, 2007).

Fetal Heart Rate

In the absence of risk factors:

Determine and evaluate the FHR every 30 minutes during the active phase of the first stage of labor and every 15 minutes during the [active pushing phase of the] second stage of labor (AWHONN, 2009, AAP & ACOG, 2007). In Canada the FHR is evaluated every 5 minutes in the active pushing phase of the second stage of labor (SOGC, 2007).

When risk factors are present, continuous EFM is recommended:

During the active phase of the first stage of labor, the FHR should be determined and evaluated every 15 minutes (AWHONN, 2009, AAP & ACOG, 2007).

During the active pushing phase of the second stage of labor, the FHR should be determined and evaluated at least every 5 minutes (AWHONN 2008, 2009).

During oxytocin induction or augmentation, the FHR should be determined and evaluated every 15 minutes during the active phase of the first stage of labor and every 5 minutes during [the active pushing phase of] the second stage of labor (AAP & ACOG, 2007; AWHONN, 2008, 2009).

When EFM is used to record FHR data permanently, periodic documentation can be used to summarize evaluation of fetal status at the recommended frequencies, as outlined by institutional protocols. Thus, while evaluation of the FHR may be occurring every 15 minutes, a summary note including findings of fetal status may be documented in the medical record less frequently. During oxytocin induction or augmentation, the FHR should be evaluated and documented before each dose increase. During the active pushing phase of the second stage of labor, summary documentation of fetal status approximately every 30 minutes indicating that there was continuous nursing bedside attendance and evaluation seems reasonable (AWHONN, 2009; Simpson, 2008b).

BOX 8-4 Maternal-Fetal Assessments during Labor and Birth—cont'd

Fetal Heart Rate—cont'd

Misoprostol should be administered at or near the labor and birth suite, where the FHR can be monitored continuously (ACOG, 1999).

Dinoprostone vaginal insert [prostaglandin E_2 (PGE_2)] should be administered at or near the labor and birth suite, where the FHR can be monitored continuously while in place and for at least 15 minutes after removal (ACOG, 1999).

Dinoprostone gel [prostaglandin E_2 (PGE_2)] should be administered at or near the labor and birth suite, where the FHR can be monitored continuously for 30 minutes to 2 hours after administration (ACOG, 1999).

Uterine Activity/Labor Progress

For women who are at no increased risk for complications, evaluation of the quality of uterine contractions should be sufficient to detect abnormalities in the progress of labor (AAP & ACOG, 2007).

Generally, uterine activity should be assessed each time the FHR is assessed because uterine activity has implications for fetal status.

When EFM is used to record uterine activity data permanently, periodic documentation can be used to summarize evaluation of uterine activity as outlined by institutional protocols. Thus, while evaluation of uterine activity may be occurring every 15 minutes, a summary note including findings of uterine activity may be documented less frequently in the medical record. During oxytocin induction or augmentation, uterine activity should be evaluated and documented before each dose increase. During the active pushing phase of the second stage of labor, summary documentation of uterine activity approximately every 30 minutes indicating that there was continuous nursing bedside attendance and evaluation seems reasonable (AWHONN, 2009; Simpson, 2008b).

Misoprostol should be administered at or near the labor and birth suite, where uterine activity can be monitored continuously (ACOG, 1999)

Dinoprostone vaginal insert [prostaglandin E_2 (PGE_2)] should be administered at or near the labor and birth suite, where uterine activity can be monitored continuously while in place and for at least 15 minutes after removal (ACOG, 1999).

Dinoprostone gel [prostaglandin E_2 (PGE_2)] should be administered at or near the labor and birth suite, where uterine activity can be monitored continuously for at least 30 minutes to 2 hours after placement (ACOG, 1999).

Vaginal examinations and evaluation of the quality of uterine contractions should be sufficient to detect abnormalities in the progress of labor (AAP & ACOG, 2007). Vaginal examinations include assessment of dilation and effacement of the cervix and station of the fetal presenting part.

Monitoring and Assessment during Regional Analgesia/Anesthesia

Women who receive epidural analgesia should be monitored in a manner similar to that used for any patient in labor.

For women in labor receiving regional anesthesia, vital signs and FHR should be monitored and documented at regular intervals by a qualified individual (AAP & ACOG, 2007; ASA, 2000).

Before epidural anesthesia/analgesia is initiated, the nurse should assess and document maternal vital signs. The FHR should be assessed before and after the procedure, either intermittently or continuously, and as possible during the procedure. Additional monitoring of the patient should be provided during epidural anesthesia/analgesia as the patient's condition warrants (AWHONN, 2001). A suggested protocol includes assessing "…the FHR after the initiation or re-bolus of a regional block, including PCEA. FHR may be assessed every 5 minutes for the first 15 minutes. More or less frequent monitoring may be indicated based on consideration of factors such as the type of analgesia/anesthesia, route and dose of medication used, the maternal-fetal response to medication, maternal-fetal consideration, the stage of labor, or facility protocol" (AWHONN, 2001, p. 13).

Continued

BOX 8-4 Maternal-Fetal Assessments during Labor and Birth—cont'd

Documentation of Additional Assessment Parameters Should Include:
Character and amount of amniotic fluid (e.g., clear, bloody, meconium stained, odorous)
Character and amount of bloody show/vaginal bleeding
Maternal and fetal response to labor
Level of maternal discomfort, coping, and effectiveness of pain management/pain relief measures
Labor support person(s)' interactions with the woman and contributions to labor support as indicated

---

PCEA, Patient-controlled epidural analgesia.
Adapted from: Simpson, K. R. (2008b). Labor and birth. In K. R. Simpson & P. A. Creehan (Eds.), *AWHONN's Perinatal Nursing* (3rd ed., pp. 300–398). Philadelphia: Lippincott Williams and Wilkins.

Figure 8-3 for a sample medical record form for documentation during labor.

Documentation reflects the systematic assessment the FHR and uterine activity. Systematic assessment and documentation of the FHR via auscultation includes FHR baseline rate, rhythm, increases (accelerations) and decreases (decelerations) from the baseline rate. Systematic assessment and documentation of the FHR via EFM includes determination of the baseline rate, variability, and presence or absence of accelerations and decelerations (Table 8-2). If decelerations are noted with EFM, assessments include the type and duration. Systematic assessments of uterine activity, including frequency, duration, intensity, and resting tonus, are documented according to the method of uterine activity monitoring being used (Table 8-3).

When auscultation is used, FHR and uterine activity findings are documented in the patient's record according to facility established intervals because no other record (e. g., EFM tracing) of the findings is available. A reasonable approach would be to document auscultation findings each time they are determined, except when assessing the FHR at q 5 minute intervals. When this level of assessment is occurring, it may be reasonable to summarize findings at approximately 15 minute intervals, due to the clinical difficulty of documenting every 5 minutes while also conducting maternal-fetal and labor assessments and providing labor support.

Table 8-2	Documentation of the Fetal Heart Rate with Different Assessment Methods	
AUSCULTATION	**ULTRASOUND**	**SPIRAL ELECTRODE**
Rate Rhythm	Rate	Rate
	Variability	Variability
Increases and decreases	Periodic patterns Episodic patterns	Periodic patterns Episodic patterns

Table 8-3	Documentation of Uterine Activity with Different Assessment Methods	
PALPATION	**TOCODYNAMOMETER**	**INTRAUTERINE PRESSURE CATHETER**
Frequency	Frequency	Frequency
Duration	Duration	Duration
Tone	Tone (assessed by palpation)	Tone (verified by palpation)
Intensity	Intensity (assessed by palpation)	Intensity (verified by palpation)

When EFM is used, the FHR findings are recorded electronically. Therefore documentation of the clinician's interpretation of EFM findings may occur at intervals that are different from the assessment interval, as indicated by institutional policy and procedure. For example, it may be appropriate for a nurse who is at the bedside continuously assessing the FHR during the active pushing phase of the second stage of labor to document FHR interpretation in a summary note at intervals of 15 to 30 minutes or more.

During the active phase of the first stage of labor, the FHR should be determined, and evaluated at 30-minute intervals, preferably just after a contraction. During the active pushing phase of the second stage of labor, the FHR should be determined and evaluated at 15-minute intervals unless fetal risk status or response to labor indicates the need for more frequent assessment (AAP & ACOG, 2007; AWHONN, 2008, 2009). If risk factors are present on admission or develop during the course of labor, the FHR should be determined and evaluated every 15 minutes (preferably just after a contraction), during the active phase of the first stage of labor, and every 5 minutes during the [active pushing phase of the] second stage of labor (AAP & ACOG, 2007; AWHONN, 2008, 2009). SOGC (2007) recommends assessment every 15 to 30 minutes during the active phase of labor regardless of risk status, every 5 minutes for 30 minutes after initiation of epidural analgesia, and every 5 minutes after pushing is initiated. These assessments can occur via intermittent auscultation of the FHR in low-risk women or via continuous electronic fetal monitoring (ACOG, 2005; AWHONN, 2009; SOGC, 2007). ACOG (2005) and SOGC (2007) recommend continuous fetal monitoring for women with complications presenting a risk for adverse perinatal outcome, such as suspected fetal growth restriction, preeclampsia, and type 1 diabetes. The use of regional analgesia, oxytocin dosage rate, and intervals between increases in oxytocin dosage rate are additional considerations when determining how often to assess and document maternal-fetal well-being during labor.

Also documented are clinical interventions based on assessment of all characteristics of the electronic FHR tracing or noted during auscultation; and the individual clinical situation of the mother and fetus, including, but not limited to, gestational age and medications administered to the mother.

Additional assessments of fetal oxygenation using indirect and direct methods (see Chapter 7) also are documented in the medical record. For example, with scalp stimulation, the fetal response to the stimulation is documented.

If there are difficulties in obtaining an interpretable FHR tracing, documentation in the medical record concerning ongoing efforts to improve the tracing should be noted. A tracing of uterine activity is just as important as the FHR tracing. Identification of characteristics of FHR patterns depends on their relationship to uterine activity. In order to be able to make clinically appropriate decisions, both must be determined as accurately as possible. This attention to accuracy is often not noted when a retrospective review occurs as part of the quality monitoring process (Simpson & Knox, 2000) (see Chapter 4 for troubleshooting strategies to improve the FHM data). Prolonged periods of uninterpretable FHR and uterine activity tracing may erroneously imply that there was no one attending the mother and fetus. Sometimes a simple maternal position change or adjustment of the monitoring equipment will facilitate obtaining a continuous tracing. Documentation of troubleshooting efforts and results should be included in the medical record. If there is a need for more accurate assessment data, consideration should be given to placing an internal fetal spiral electrode (FSE) and/or intrauterine pressure catheter (IUPC) if clinically appropriate. The discussion among providers regarding the need for an FSE and/or IUPC, orders received, interventions initiated, data obtained as a result about maternal-fetal status, and follow-up communication with the physician or midwife should be documented in the medical record.

Evaluating the Quality of Medical Record Documentation

Periodic continuing education and institutional protocols, policies, and procedures provide the foundation for expectations of medical record documentation. One way that institutions can create a learning environment to decrease omissions and inaccuracies in medical record documentation is to conduct periodic medical record audits. See Box 8-5 - for an example of a medical record audit tool (Simpson, 2008c).

Medical record audits provide data concerning the perinatal nurse's requisite knowledge base and clinical skills during the intrapartum period and can provide insight into the level of teamwork and coordination of care among clinicians (Simpson, 2008c). A well-documented medical record should be comparable with the electronic monitor tracing and include appropriate ongoing assessment, intervention, and evaluation. This objective information can be used to verify clinical skills and plan ongoing continuing education to improve skills, clinical integration, and documentation.

Risk Management and Communication of Fetal Heart Monitoring Information

Along with emergency departments and perioperative services, perinatal units account for most of the claims of patient injuries and death (Knox, Simpson, & Garite, 1999). Some of these patient injuries are related to human error and are preventable. Fetal and neonatal injuries are more common than maternal injuries. Several common recurring clinical situations account for the majority of fetal and neonatal injuries (Knox, Simpson, & Townsend, 2003; Simpson & Knox, 2005):

• Inability to recognize and/or appropriately respond to both antepartum and intrapartum fetal compromise

• Inappropriate use of oxytocin or misoprostol leading to tachysystole, uterine rupture, and fetal compromise and/or death
• Inappropriate continued coached second-stage pushing despite an indeterminate FHR pattern with decelerations or an abnormal FHR pattern
• Inability to effect a timely cesarean birth (30 minutes from decision to incision) when indicated by fetal or maternal condition
• Inability to appropriately resuscitate a depressed baby
• Inappropriate use of forceps/vacuum/fundal pressure leading to fetal trauma and/or preventable shoulder dystocia
• Inability to resolve clinical conflicts related to interpretation of and interventions for deteriorating maternal or fetal status

It is important to note that these same clinical situations have been the source of the majority of legal claims related to fetal/neonatal injuries for more than 20 years, when these data first began to be collected (Knox et al., 2003). Communication inadequacies and omissions can be associated with these recurring clinical situations. Failure to resolve a clinical conflict in a timely manner may contribute to patient injuries.

When cerebral palsy or other brain injury is diagnosed and the medical record indicates that there have been periods of abnormal or some types of indeterminate FHR patterns during labor without evidence of identification and timely intervention, there is a risk of liability exposure to the health care providers and the institution despite the fact that not all adverse or unexpected outcomes are preventable (Simpson & Knox, 2001). Under these circumstances, an argument can be made that the FHR was not normal and that the lack of timely intervention is directly associated with the condition of the infant. In some cases, experts who testify in medical malpractice cases for the defense and for the plaintiff offer differing opinions. Sometimes these opinions may appear to be completely dichotomous. The differences in opinion may include description and characterization

BOX 8-5 Suggested Components of a Medical Record Audit

- Is medical record documentation regarding FHR patterns consistent with the NICHD definitions?
- Are hand-written clinicians' notes legible?
- Are the times noted on the Admission Assessment, Labor Flow Chart, and the initial EFM tracing consistent with each other within a reasonable time frame?
- If elective labor induction, is gestational age of at least 39 completed weeks confirmed?
- Is there documentation of notification of the physician or midwife of admission within the time frame outlined in the policies and procedures?
- Is fetal well-being established on admission?
- Is fetal well-being established prior to ambulation?
- Is fetal well-being established prior to medication administration?
- Does the EFM FHR baseline rate match the FHR baseline documented?
- Does the EFM FHR baseline variability match the FHR baseline variability documented?
- If there is evidence of absent or minimal FHR variability, is it documented?
- If there is evidence of absent or minimal FHR variability, are appropriate interventions documented?
- If there are FHR decelerations on the EFM tracing, are they correctly documented?
- Are appropriate interventions documented during indeterminate or abnormal FHR patterns?
- Is there documentation of physician or midwife notification of indeterminate or abnormal FHR patterns?
- If FHR accelerations are documented, are they present on the EFM tracing?
- Are maternal assessments documented according to policy?
- If there is evidence of an indeterminate FHR pattern with decelerations or an abnormal FHR pattern, is oxytocin dosage increased?
- If there is evidence of a deteriorating or abnormal FHR pattern, is oxytocin dosage discontinued?
- If there is evidence of tachysystole, are appropriate interventions documented?
- If there is evidence of adequate labor, is oxytocin dosage increased?
- If there is evidence of tachysystole, is oxytocin dosage increased or decreased?
- Does the frequency of uterine contractions on the EFM tracing match what is documented?
- Is the uterine activity monitor (external tocodynamometer or IUPC) adjusted to maintain an accurate uterine activity baseline?
- Are oxytocin dosage increases charted when there is an inaccurate uterine baseline tracing or an uninterpretable FHR tracing?
- Is the physicians' or midwife's documentation of fetal status consistent with the nurses' documentation?
- Are automatically generated data from BP and SpO$_2$ devices accurate (i.e., do data correlate with maternal condition)?
- Does documentation continue during the second stage of labor?
- Is there evidence of the woman's urge to push in the record at the time pushing is initiated?
- When the FHR is indeterminate or abnormal during the second stage of labor, is pushing discontinued or encouraged with every other or every third contraction to help maintain a stable baseline rate and minimize decelerations?
- If the FHR is indeterminate or abnormal during the second stage of labor, is oxytocin discontinued?
- If continuous EFM is being used for fetal assessment during second stage labor, are uterine contractions likewise continuously monitored via external tocodynamometer or IUPC?
- Does the time of birth on the medical record match the time of birth at end of the EFM tracing?
- If the woman received regional analgesia/anesthesia, is a qualified anesthesia provider involved in the decision to discharge from PACU care?
- If the woman had regional analgesia/anesthesia, is the discharge from PACU care scoring evaluation documented?
- Are maternal assessments documented during the immediate postpartum period every 15 minutes for the first two hours?
- Are newborn assessments documented during the transition to extrauterine life at least every 30 minutes until the newborn's condition has been stable for 2 hours?

BP, Blood pressure; CNM, certified nurse midwife; EFM, electronic fetal monitor(ing); FHR, fetal heart rate; IUPC, intrauterine pressure catheter; NICHD, National Institute of Child Health and Human Development; PACU, postanesthesia care unit; SpO$_2$, oxygen saturation.
Adapted from Simpson, K. R. (2008c). Perinatal patient safety and professional liability issues. In K. R. Simpson & P. A. Creehan (Eds.), *AWHONN's Perinatal Nursing*. Philadelphia: Lippincott Williams and Wilkins. ©AWHONN.

and interpretation of the FHR patterns displayed, clinical implications, need for intervention, and probable impact on the present condition of the plaintiff. It is sometimes challenging for lay juries to sort out the technical language and determine which expert's opinion is closer to solid scientific principles and professional standards. Under these circumstances it may be difficult, if not impossible, for a jury to come to a reasonable decision about whether the health care providers met professional standards.

There are two key components to a successful risk management program: avoiding preventable adverse outcomes and decreasing risk of liability exposure (Simpson & Knox, 2000). Although somewhat similar, these are two distinct concepts. Avoiding preventable adverse outcomes to the fetus during labor requires competent care providers who use consistent FHR monitoring language and who are in a practice environment with systems in place that permit timely clinical intervention. Decreasing risk of liability exposure includes methods to demonstrate evidence that appropriate, timely care was provided and that accurately reflect maternal-fetal status before, during, and after interventions occurred (Knox & Simpson, 2003). Risk management strategies that meet both components of a successful program are included in Box 8-6.

EFFECTIVE CONFLICT MANAGEMENT

There are many challenges to achieving teamwork in the perinatal setting. Interpretation of maternal-fetal data and subsequent communication regarding those data among professional colleagues may sometimes result in conflict. It is helpful to acknowledge that no group of individuals can work together in an organization and always have the same expectations, goals, and perspectives. Conflict is an inevitable result when situations do not meet with individual expectations. Although individual expectations may differ, usually there exists among caregivers a basic commitment to quality and to the best possible outcomes for mothers and babies. Mutual trust and respect and the capacity to engage in agreeable disagreement are the hallmarks of a professional unit. When involved in a clinical or administrative situation that may potentially cause conflict, consider that both parties probably have the best interests of the patient in mind, although there may be very different approaches proposed to achieve that goal (Simpson, 2008c). At times, clinical practice issues arise when the "way we've always done it" conflicts with a new or an alternate approach.

Classic principles of conflict resolution (Mayer, 2000) can be used to successfully resolve the inevitable differences of opinion that occur in everyday clinical practice. If the conflict is not related to an emergent patient situation (e.g., there is at least some time for discussion), effective communication techniques can facilitate conflict resolution to the satisfaction of both parties, or at least help them reach a workable compromise (Simpson, 2008c). Taking time to really listen and understand the intent of the other person is a helpful starting point. While the other person is expressing himself or herself, give visual and verbal feedback to ensure that the other person's concern is important and being taken seriously. For example, nodding your head or saying "I see, please go on..." or summarizing what the other person is concerned about by indicating, "let me see if I am understanding you correctly...." Phrases such as, "I have a different perspective" usually work better in conflict resolution than, "You are wrong." Other successful strategies include a calm, collected attitude and careful consideration of the goal to be accomplished.

Communication in situations of conflict may not always be rational. This is especially true when dealing with difficult people, particularly those who exhibit hostile or aggressive behavior that is abusive, abrupt, intimidating, or overwhelming (Mayer, 2000). Being confronted by this behavior often catches one by surprise and can generate feelings of helplessness. Under these circumstances, it is important to stand up

> **BOX 8-6 Key Components of Risk Management Related to Use of Electronic Fetal Monitoring**
>
> 1. Common definitions of FHR patterns in all professional communication and medical record documentation
> 2. Collaborative, interdisciplinary nurse, midwife, and physician education about EFM
> 3. Competent care providers
> 4. Collaboration and mutual respect among care providers; zero tolerance for disruptive clinician behavior
> 5. Clear definition for fetal well-being and assessment of fetal well-being on admission
> 6. Ongoing assessment and determination of fetal well-being during labor
> 7. Appropriate use of intrauterine resuscitation techniques
> 8. Accurate monitoring of the FHR and uterine activity via EFM
> 9. Accurate interpretation of EFM data
> 10. Appreciation for the potential physiologic stress involved with tachysystole and second-stage pushing; efforts to minimize this stress by avoiding tachysystole and treating it in a timely manner when identified rather than waiting until the FHR is indeterminate or abnormal; using fetal status to guide coaching of maternal pushing efforts during the active pushing phase of the second stage of labor
> 11. Organizational resources and systems to support clinically timely and physiologically appropriate interventions when the FHR pattern is indeterminate or abnormal.
> 12. Continuation of fetal and uterine activity assessment until birth
> 13. Neonatal resuscitation team in attendance at birth if there is any question of fetal compromise
> 14. Interdisciplinary case reviews for near misses and adverse outcomes

CNM, Certified nurse midwife; EFM, electronic fetal monitor(ing); FHR, fetal heart rate.
Adapted from Simpson, K. R., & Knox, G. E. (2000). Risk management and EFM: Decreasing risk of adverse outcomes and liability exposure. *Journal of Perinatal and Neonatal Nursing, 14*(3), 40–52. © Lippincott Williams and Wilkins. Reprinted with permission.

for yourself and command respect. Try to be calm, and then diffuse the situation in an assertive manner. For example, saying, "I am willing to discuss this with you when you are ready to speak to me with respect," may help stop the behavior and allow time for more respectful and rational discussion (Henrikson, 1999).

Selecting the best time and place for interaction is also essential (Mayer, 2000). Ideally, the setting should be private and away from patients, family members, or other colleagues. The focus of the discussion should remain on the issue, preferably on the potential impact on patient care. If the conversation deteriorates beyond personal capacity to handle it or the colleague becomes verbally abusive, it is helpful to end the discussion until a later time and inform a third party who has the ability to help or the responsibility to know about the interaction (Simpson, 2008c).

An important strategy for promoting positive long-term professional collaboration is the devel-opment of interdisciplinary specialty practice opportunities when colleagues can come together to work toward a common goal (Simpson & Knox, 1999). This can include the development of unit guidelines, learning from a case review or grand rounds, examining quality or research findings, designing unit projects, or discussing conflict resolution. When colleagues come together to identify problems, define objectives, address alternatives, integrate changes, remain patient focused, disagree agreeably, negotiate, demonstrate mutual respect, and recognize and praise positive attributes and actions, they can facilitate a professional culture for positive conflict management and promote mutual respect.

Chain of Command or Authority

Some issues of conflict in the clinical setting cannot be resolved between the caregivers immediately involved and yet need to be resolved quickly. Clinicians must initiate an appropriate course of action when, after careful deliberation, the issue is determined to be a matter of maternal/fetal well-being or there is potential for the clinical situation to deteriorate rapidly (e.g., when a primary health care provider does not respond to a deteriorating maternal or fetal condition). Decisive, timely nursing intervention may be necessary to avoid a potentially adverse outcome. Clinical knowledge and the use of the chain of command or authority are ways to attempt to resolve differences of opinion in clinical practice settings. An example of chain of command or authority is presented in Figure 8-2. Steps or levels in the chain are determined by the positions and availability of personnel in each individual institution. Generally, larger institutions and academic medical centers have more steps in the chain of command or authority than community and rural hospitals. If discussions with the physician or midwife do not result in appropriate care for the clinical situation, the nurse has the responsibility to use the perinatal unit institutional chain of command or authority to ensure appropriate and timely intervention (Simpson, 2008c).

At the first level, the staff nurse notifies the appropriately available immediate supervisory nurse as outlined in their institution's chain of command or authority (i.e., charge nurse, nurse manager, or nursing supervisor) to provide assistance and to review the conflict situation and possible actions and then documents in the medical record or variance report that this action has been taken as outlined in the institutional policies and protocols. In selected instances, it may be necessary to go further up the chain if the situation cannot be resolved. It is important to realize that this process may require more time than the situation can accommodate. Thus, invoking the complete use of the chain of command or authority is generally more successful when there is an urgent situation (e.g., progressively deteriorating FHR tracing) rather than an overt emergency (e.g., shoulder dystocia).

Institutions should support nurses who use the chain of command or authority. Nurses may be reluctant to initiate this process because of intimidation, a perceived sense of personal or professional jeopardy, fear of retribution, and/or lack of confidence in the institutional lines of authority and responsibility. Nurses and physicians need to know the institution's policy for chain of command or authority. Data concerning use of the chain of command or authority can be collected and analyzed so that the process can be optimized and personnel can receive positive feedback for its appropriate use (Simpson, 2008c). Chain of command or authority should not be used as a routine method of conflict resolution. Clinical disagreements that result in initiation of the chain of command or authority can be detrimental to nurse-physician relationships. Soon after a clinical disagreement resulting in the use of the chain of command or authority, all those involved should meet and calmly discuss what happened and why. Having an objective third party, such as the risk manager, present during this discussion may facilitate the interaction. Prospective plans should then be developed to avoid this situation in the future. A positive corporate culture supports use of the chain of command or authority. When personnel are given the resources, support, and guidance that are necessary to carry out the responsibilities of their positions, everyone generally benefits: the institution, their employees, the medical staff, and the patients (Simpson, 2008c).

SUMMARY

Communication regarding fetal status is a critical aspect of perinatal care. Verbal and written communication should be accurate, timely, and concise. Common communication avenues include nurse to primary care provider, primary provider to primary provider, nurse to nurse, and clinician to patient and her family members/support person(s). A collaborative attitude and mutual respect are the foundations of a healthy interpersonal interaction. Over time, with patience and a joint commitment to the best possible outcomes for mothers and babies, respectful nonhierarchical communication styles among professional colleagues can be promoted and enhanced.

Perinatal care providers should develop common strategies as a team for intervening when the FHR pattern is suggestive of fetal compromise. Patient safety related to FHR assessment is dependent on competent care providers, adequate and accurate monitoring of maternal-fetal status, and timely implementation of appropriate clinical interventions. Nurses, midwives, and physicians benefit from learning about FHM in joint continuing education classes. Such classes enhance consistent communication of FHM data among professionals and provide opportunities to discuss clinical controversies and propose potential resolutions. Consistent and timely medical record documentation is important for effective communication and successful risk management. A single source of data entry at the point of care generally works best, rather than charting events on multiple forms. One way to validate requisite knowledge and clinical skills is by use of medical record audits. Effective communication involves management of conflict that is often part of work among professionals with differing views and perspectives. Policies for use of the chain of command or authority are helpful when conflict resolution efforts are not successful.

REFERENCES

American Academy of Pediatrics & American College of Obstetricians and Gynecologists. (2007). *Guidelines for perinatal care* (6th ed.). Elk Grove Village, IL: Authors.

American College of Obstetricians and Gynecologists. (1999). *Induction of labor* (ACOG Practice Bulletin No. 10). Washington, DC: Author.

American College of Obstetricians and Gynecologists. (2005). *Intrapartum fetal heart rate monitoring* (ACOG Practice Bulletin No. 70). Washington, DC: Author.

American College of Obstetricians and Gynecologist & Nurses' Association of the American College of Obstetricians and Gynecologists. (1986). *Joint ACOG/NAACOG statement on electronic fetal monitoring.* Washington, DC: Authors. (withdrawn).

American Society of Anesthesiologists. (2000). *Guidelines for regional anesthesia in obstetrics.* Park Ridge, IL: Author.

Association of Women's Health, Obstetric and Neonatal Nurses. (2001). *Nursing care of the woman receiving regional analgesia/anesthesia in labor* (Evidence-Based Clinical Practice Guideline). Washington, DC: Author.

Association of Women's Health, Obstetric and Neonatal Nurses. (2005). *Fetal heart monitoring program.* Washington, DC: Author.

Association of Women's Health, Obstetric and Neonatal Nurses. (2008). *Nursing management of the second stage of labor.* (Evidence-Based Clinical Practice Guideline). Washington, DC: Author.

Association of Women's Health, Obstetric and Neonatal Nurses. (2009). *Fetal heart monitoring* (Position Statement). Washington, DC: Author.

Baggs, J. G., Ryan, S. A., Phelps, C. E., Richeson, J. F., & Johnson, J. E. (1992). The association between interdisciplinary collaboration and patient outcomes in a medical intensive care unit. *Heart and Lung, 21*(1), 18–24.

Baggs, J. G., Schmitt, M. H., Mushlin, A. I., Mitchell, P. H., Eldredge, D. H., & Hutson, A. D. (1999). Association between nurse–physician collaboration and patient outcomes in three intensive care units. *Critical Care Medicine, 27*(9), 1991–1998.

Benner, P., Sheets, V., Uris, P., Malloch, K., Schwed, K., & Jamison, D. (2002). Individual practice and system causes of errors in nursing: A taxonomy. *Journal of Nursing Administration, 32*(10), 509–523.

Berry, M. C. (1999). Changes in the nursing environment create new liability exposures. *MMI Advisory, 15*(3), 1–4.

Chez, B. F. (1997). Electronic fetal monitoring: Then and now. *Journal of Perinatal and Neonatal Nursing, 10*(4), 1–4.

Chez. B. F., Harvey, C. J., & Murray, M. L. (1990). *Critical concepts in fetal heart rate monitoring.* Baltimore: Williams & Wilkins.

Clancy, C. M., & Tornberg, D. N. (2007). TeamSTEPPS: Assuring optimal teamwork in clinical settings. *American Journal of Medical Quality, 22*(3), 214–217.

Corser, W. D. (2000). The contemporary nurse-physician relationship: Insights from scholars outside the two professions. *Nursing Outlook, 48*(6), 263–268.

Firth-Cozens, J. (2001). Teams, culture and managing risk. In C. Vincent (Ed.), *Clinical risk management: Enhancing patient safety* (2nd ed., pp. 335–368). London: BMJ Books.

Fox, M., Kilpatrick, S., King, T., & Parer, J. T. (2000). Fetal heart rate monitoring: Interpretation and collaborative management. *Journal of Midwifery and Women's Health. 45*(6), 498-507.

Funai, E., Pettker, C., Thung, S., Raab, C., Norwitz, E., Buhimschi, C. et al., (2007). Impact of a comprehensive strategy to reduce obstetric adverse events. *American Journal of Obstetrics and Gynecology, 197*(6, Suppl), S36.

Henrikson, M. L. (1999). Dealing with difficult people: Tips and techniques for enhancing communication. *AWHONN Lifelines, 3*(3), 51–52.

Joint Commission. (2007). *Comprehensive accreditation manual for hospitals.* Oak Brook, IL: Author.

Katzenbach, J. R., & Smith, D. K. (1993). *The wisdom of teams: Creating the high-performance organization.* Boston: Harvard Business School Press.

Keenan, G. M., Cooke, R., & Hillis, S. L. (1998). Norms and nurse management of conflicts: Keys to understanding nurse–physician collaboration. *Research in Nursing and Health, 21*(1), 59–72.

Knaus, W. A., Draper, E. A., Wagner, D. P., & Zimmerman, J. E. (1986). An evaluation of outcome from intensive care units in major medical centers. *Annals of Internal Medicine, 104*(3), 410–418.

Knox, G. E., & Simpson, K. R. (2003). Teamwork: The fundamental building block of high reliability organizations and patient safety. In B. Youngberg & M. J. Hatlie (Eds.), *The patient safety handbook* (pp. 379–414). Chicago: American Hospital Association.

Knox, G. E., & Simpson, K. R. (2006). Perinatal patient safety. *Risk Management Handbook for Health Care Organizations* (5th ed., pp. 391–404*).* Chicago: American Society for Healthcare Risk Management (ASHRM).

Knox, G. E., Simpson, K. R., & Garite, T. J. (1999). High reliability perinatal units: An approach to the prevention of patient injury and medical malpractice claims. *Journal of Healthcare Risk Management, 19*(2), 24–32.

Knox, G. E., Simpson, K. R., & Townsend, K. E. (2003). High reliability perinatal units: Further observations and a suggested plan for action. *Journal of Healthcare Risk Management, 23*(4), 17–21.

Macones, G. A., Hankins, G. D., Spong, C. Y., Hauth, J. D., & Moore, T. (2008). The 2008 National Institute of Child Health Human Development workshop report on electronic fetal monitoring: Update on definitions, interpretations, and research guidelines. *Obstetrics & Gynecology, 112,* 661-666, and *Journal of Obstetric, Gynecologic, and Neonatal Nursing, 37,* 510-515.

Mayer, B. S. (2000). *The dynamics of conflict resolution: A practitioner's guide.* San Francisco: Jossey-Bass.

McMahan, E. M., Hoffman, K., & McGee, G. W. (1994). Physician-nurse relationships in clinical settings: A review and critique of the literature. *Medical Care Review, 51*(1), 83–112.

Merry, M. D., & Brown, J. P. (2002). From a culture of safety to a culture of excellence: Quality science, human factors, and the future of healthcare quality. *Journal of Innovative Management, 7*(2), 29–46.

National Institute of Child Health and Human Development (NICHD) Research Planning Workshop. (1997). Electronic fetal heart rate monitoring: Research guidelines for interpretation. *American Journal of Obstetrics and Gynecology, 177*(6), 1385–1390, and *Journal of Obstetric Gynecology and Neonatal Nursing, 26*(6), 635–640.

Patterson, E. S., Roth, E. M., Woods, D. D., Chow, R. & Gomes, J. O. (2004). Handoff strategies in settings with high consequences for failure: Lessons for health care operations. *International Journal for Quality in Health Care, 16*(2), 125–132.

Pearce, W. B., & Cronen, V. E. (1980). *Communication, action and meaning: The creation of social realities.* New York: Praeger.

Peter, E. (2000). Commentary: Ethical conflicts or political problems in intrapartum nursing care. *Birth: Issues in Perinatal Care, 27*(1), 46–48.

Risser, D. T., Rice, M. M., Salisbury, M. L., Simon, R., Jay, G. D., & Berns, S. D. (1999). The potential for improved teamwork to reduce medical errors in the emergency department: The MedTeams Research Consortium. *Annals of Emergency Medicine, 34*(3), 370–383.

Sherwood, G., Thomas, E., Bennett, D. S., & Lewis, P. (2002). A teamwork model to promote safety in critical care. *Critical Care Nursing Clinics of North America, 14*(4), 333–340.

Simpson, K. R. (1991). *Attitudes of laboring women towards continuous electronic fetal monitoring.* Unpublished masters thesis, University of Missouri–St. Louis, School of Nursing.

Simpson, K. R. (2005). Handling handoffs safely. *MCN The American Journal of Maternal Child Nursing, 30*(2), 152.

Simpson, K. R. (2008a). EFM competence validation. In C. A. Menihan & E. K. Zottoli (Eds.), *Electronic fetal monitoring: Concepts and applications* (2nd ed., pp. 243–252). Philadelphia: Lippincott Williams and Wilkins.

Simpson, K. R. (2008b). Labor and birth. In K. R. Simpson & P. A. Creehan (Eds.), *AWHONN's perinatal nursing* (3rd ed., pp 300–398). Philadelphia: Lippincott Williams and Wilkins.

Simpson, K. R. (2008c). Perinatal patient safety and professional liability issues. In K. R. Simpson & P. A. Creehan (Eds.), *AWHONN's perinatal nursing* (3rd ed., pp. 21–52). Philadelphia: Lippincott Williams and Wilkins.

Simpson, K. R., James, D. C., & Knox, G. E. (2006). Nurse-physician communication during labor and birth: Implications for patient safety. *Journal of Obstetric, Gynecologic, and Neonatal Nursing, 35*(4), 547–556.

Simpson, K. R., & Knox, G. E. (1999). Strategies for developing an evidence-based approach to perinatal care. *MCN: The American Journal of Maternal Child Nursing, 24*(3), 122–132.

Simpson, K. R., & Knox, G. E. (2000). Risk management and electronic fetal monitoring: Decreasing risk of adverse outcomes and liability exposure. *Journal of Perinatal and Neonatal Nursing, 14*(3), 40–52.

Simpson, K. R., & Knox, G. E. (2001). Perinatal teamwork: Turning rhetoric into reality. In K. R. Simpson & P. A. Creehan (Eds.), *AWHONN's perinatal nursing* (2nd ed., pp. 53–67). Philadelphia: Lippincott Williams and Wilkins.

Simpson, K. R., & Knox, G. E. (2005). Perinatal patient safety: Essential criteria for safe care for mothers and babies during labor and birth. *AWHONN Lifelines, 9*(6), 478–483.

Sleutel, M. R. (2000). Intrapartum nursing care: A case study of supportive interventions and ethical conflicts. *Birth: Issues in Perinatal Care, 27*(1), 38–45.

Sleutel, M., Schultz, S., & Wyble, K. (2007). Nurses' views of factors that help and hinder their intrapartum care. *Journal of Obstetric, Gynecologic and Neonatal Nursing, 36*(3), 203–211.

Society of Obstetricians and Gynaecologists of Canada (SOGC). (2007). Fetal health surveillance: Antepartum and intrapartum consensus guideline. *Journal of Obstetrics and Gynaecology Canada, 29*(9 Suppl. 4), S1-S56.

Stein, L. I. (1967). The doctor–nurse game. *Archives in General Psychiatry, 16*(6), 699–703.

Stein, L. I., Watts, D. T., & Howell, T. (1990). The doctor–nurse game revisited. *New England Journal of Medicine, 322*(8), 546–549.

Willis, E., & Parish, K. (1997). Managing the doctor–nurse game: A nursing and social science analysis. *Contemporary Nurse, 6*(3), 136–144.

CHAPTER 9

Intermediate Fetal Heart Monitoring Course Skills Station

Linda Usher Ali

OVERVIEW

This chapter focuses specifically on the skills stations for the Intermediate Course of the Fetal Heart Monitoring Program (FHMP). It is *essential* reading for all FHMP Course participants and may also be a useful guide or refresher for others. FHMP Course participants must complete the following skills stations:

- Leopold's maneuvers
- Auscultation of the fetal heart
- Fetal spiral electrode (FSE) and intrauterine pressure catheter (IUPC) placement
- Integration of fetal heart monitoring knowledge and practice
- Communication of fetal monitoring data

For each skill station, the objectives, principles, steps in skill performance, and requirements to successfully pass are identified. The participant is encouraged to refer to the relevant chapters of the text for further detail as needed.

Intermediate Course participants review DVDs, listen to audio, and use anatomic models to achieve learning objectives for each skill station. Each skill station includes a practice session that contains elements similar to those that course participants will be required to address in the evaluation portion of the skill station. The instructor will notify participants of the amount of time allocated for completion of practice and evaluation portions for each skill station. Participants will be required to complete the skill station within the allotted timeframe. *To successfully complete the Intermediate Course, the participant must pass each skill station.*

To prepare for the skills stations, course participants should read this chapter and familiarize themselves with the objectives. If auscultation is not a regular part of their current clinical practice, participants are encouraged to practice counting fetal heart rates (FHRs) using a watch with a second hand and a fetoscope, Doppler device, or the electronic fetal monitor (EFM) prior to the course. This may assist in becoming more comfortable counting the FHR in the auscultation skill station. A watch with a second hand is required for both the didactic course and the auscultation skill station.

LEOPOLD'S MANEUVERS

This skill station focuses on performing Leopold's maneuvers to determine fetal lie, presentation and position, and the optimal site for FHR auscultation. Patient education related to the procedure and comfort measures are also included.

Objectives

In this skill station, the participant will complete the following:

1. Explain the purpose of Leopold's maneuvers.
2. Describe measures for patient comfort.
3. Perform the four steps of Leopold's maneuvers.
4. Identify the optimal site for FHR auscultation based on Leopold's maneuvers assessment.

Principles of Leopold's Maneuvers

1. Evaluation of uterine tone, irritability, tenderness, consistency, and the presence or absence of contractions can be assessed by palpation.
2. Estimated fetal weight and fetal movement can be assessed during abdominal examination.
3. Fetal lie (longitudinal, transverse, oblique), presentation (cephalic, breech, shoulder), and position (anterior, posterior, transverse, right, left) may be evaluated with Leopold's maneuvers and confirmed by vaginal examination.
4. Correct placement of the instrument used for auscultating the FHR can be determined by completing Leopold's maneuvers.
5. Performing Leopold's maneuvers expedites location of the FHR.

Steps in Skill Performance

1. Use measures to make the woman comfortable.
   a. Wash hands and warm them.
   b. Encourage the woman to empty her bladder.
   c. Expose the woman's abdomen from the symphysis pubis to the xiphoid process.
   d. Drape the woman appropriately.
   e. Position the woman with a pillow under her head, flex her knees, and rest her arms at her sides.
   f. Place a small wedge under the woman's hip.
   g. Explain the purpose of the procedure (to determine fetal lie, presentation, position, and the site for auscultation of the FHR) and the steps of the Leopold's maneuvers.
   h. Place warmed hands on the woman's abdomen while explaining the procedure to assist her in relaxing her abdominal muscles.
2. Prepare to perform Leopold's maneuvers.
   a. Inspect the woman's abdomen for bulges (small parts), fetal movement, and the long axis of the fetus.
   b. Use the palmar surface of the hands with fingers together for a gentle but firm examination.
   c. Stand at the woman's right or left side (e.g., a right-handed examiner should stand at the woman's right side; a left-handed examiner should stand at the woman's left side).
3. Perform Leopold's maneuvers (Figure 9-1).
   a. Begin with the first maneuver. Face the woman and place your hands at the top and side of the fundus. Be attentive to the size, shape, and consistency of the fetal part that is in the fundus (note where the longitudinal axis of the fetus is located).
   b. For the second maneuver, remain standing at the woman's side, facing her, with hands placed on either side at the middle of the abdomen. One hand will push the contents of the abdomen toward the other hand to stabilize the fetus for palpation. The hand that is palpating begins at the middle of the abdomen near the fundus and moves posterior toward the woman's back. Continue this process, progressing downward to the symphysis pubis. Determine which part of the fetus lies at the side of the abdomen. If firm, smooth, and consistent, it is likely to be the back. If smaller, protruding, and irregular, it is likely to be the small parts. Note the location of the small parts and the back. Reverse the hands and repeat the maneuver.
   c. For the third maneuver, remain facing the woman. With the middle finger and thumb grasp the part of the fetus situated over the pelvic brim. With firm, gentle pressure, determine whether the head is the presenting part. This maneuver should confirm what was felt during the first two maneuvers. If the presenting part is moveable, it is not engaged in the pelvis. If the presenting part is fixed and difficult to move, it is likely to be engaged. The third maneuver also is known as "Pallach's maneuver" or "Pallach's grip."

FIGURE 9-1   The Four Steps in Performing Leopold's Maneuvers

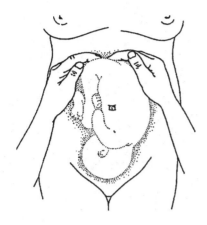

1st Maneuver
Assess part of fetus
in the upper uterus

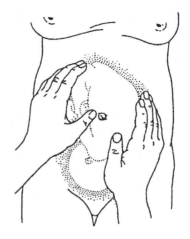

2nd Maneuver
Assess location
of the fetal back

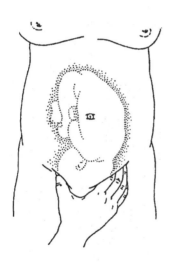

3rd Maneuver
Identify presenting part

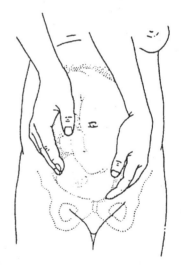

4th Maneuver
Determine the descent
of the presenting part

d. For the fourth maneuver, turn and face the woman's feet. Place your hands at the sides of the uterus, below the umbilicus, pointing toward the symphysis pubis. Press deeply, with fingertips toward the pelvic inlet, feeling for the cephalic prominence. If the cephalic prominence is felt on the same side as the fetus's back, it will be the oc- ciput (crown), and the head will be slightly extended. If the cephalic prominence is felt on the same side as the small parts, it is likely to be the sinciput (forehead), and the fetus will be in a vertex or well-tucked position. If the cephalic prominence is felt equally on each side, the fetus's head may be in a military position, which is common when the fetus is in a posterior position. Finally, move the hands toward the pelvic brim. If the hands come together around the presenting part, the presenting part is floating. If the hands stay apart, the presenting part is either dipping or engaged in the pelvis.

4. Share the information obtained with the woman, and ask if she would like to feel her fetus through palpation, if appropriate.
5. Locate and verify the FHR, which generally can be heard over the curved part of the fetus closest to the anterior wall of the uterus.
6. Document the findings of Leopold's maneuvers, the FHR and rhythm, and appropriate nursing interventions.

Criteria for Passing

Participants are required to meet all of the following criteria:

1. Explain the purpose of Leopold's maneuvers and describe patient comfort measures that should be provided before the procedure.
2. Perform *all four steps* of the Leopold's maneuvers:
   a. Assess and identify the part of fetus in the upper uterus.
   b. Assess the location of the fetal back.
   c. Identify the presenting part.
   d. Determine the descent of the presenting part.
3. Accurately indicate the optimal area for auscultation based on Leopold's maneuvers.

⌐AUSCULTATION OF THE FETAL HEART

This skill station focuses on auscultation skills to identify the FHR baseline rate, rhythm, increases and decreases, and nursing responses or interventions appropriate to the auscultated FHR.

Objectives

The participant will complete the following:

1. Choose the appropriate timing of auscultation in relation to uterine contractions.

2. Identify accurate baseline FHR and rhythm.
3. Recognize changes from the baseline FHR as increases (accelerations) or decreases (decelerations) as appropriate.
4. Select appropriate clinical responses and interventions corresponding to auscultated FHR and rhythm, including timing, method, and frequency of assessment of the FHR.

Principles of Auscultation

1. Auscultation is a means of assessment that provides data for interpretation of rate, rhythm, presence of increases and decreases in the FHR, and data for determining appropriate and timely interventions.
2. Use of auscultation requires the ability to integrate underlying physiology, elements of the maternal and fetal histories, and physical assessment data with information gathered by auscultation.
3. Auscultation requires the development of auditory skills to establish baseline rates and identify changes in rate and rhythm.
4. Use of auscultation presumes knowledge and understanding of the indications, benefits, and limitations of this method of fetal assessment.

Steps in Skill Performance

1. Perform Leopold's maneuver to locate the site for auscultation over the fetal back. (Verbalize only for this skill station.)
2. Check maternal pulse and compare with auscultated FHR. (Verbalize only for this skill station.)
3. Palpate contractions to clarify relationship between FHR and uterine contractions. (Verbalize only for this skill station.)
4. Count the FHR between uterine contractions for at least 30 to 60 seconds to identify a baseline rate and rhythm. *Canadian guidelines state that a 60 second count will improve accuracy, however, a 30 second count during active labor may be more feasible.*

5. Count the FHR immediately after a contraction and for a minimum of 30 seconds to assess changes in baseline rate. If distinct changes such increases or decreases in the rate are noted, begin counting again to determine the change from baseline. For example, count for 6 seconds and multiply by 10 to calculate the beats per minute; repeat this process for consecutive intervals. Counting the FHR for multiple, brief intervals may provide a clearer picture of the FHR changes. *Canadian guidelines recommend* listening *for at least 60 seconds. Canadian guidelines state that a 60 second count will improve accuracy, however, a 30 second count during active labor may be more feasible.*

6. Indicate appropriate clinical responses and interventions on the basis of findings. Depending on the FHR and rhythm auscultated, interventions may include the following:
   a. Reposition the woman and reassess the FHR, if needed.
   b. Increase frequency of auscultation to clarify FHR characteristics (such as whether the FHR changes are increases or decreases).
   c. Auscultate with the next uterine contraction to further assess whether changes from the baseline are occurring, if it is not clear.
   d. Consider external EFM (to assess variability, presence/absence of increases (accelerations) or decreases (decelerations).
   e. Consider other assessment techniques (e.g., fetal acoustic or scalp stimulation) as needed to assess fetal well-being.
   f. Continue to promote maternal comfort and fetal oxygenation (e.g., position changes, anxiety reduction measures).
   g. Continue assessment with auscultation.
   h. Use a fetoscope to auscultate to validate irregular FHR rhythm (if using a Doppler device or ultrasonography).
   i. Notify the woman's obstetric care provider of FHR rhythm and recurrent decreases, if needed.

7. Record the FHR rate, rhythm, increases, decreases, clinical interventions (if any), and maternal-fetal response.

Criteria for Passing

Participants are required to meet all of the following criteria:

1. Choose the appropriate timing of auscultation in relation to uterine contractions.
2. Accurately assess and document baseline FHR and rhythm for two different audio cases of auscultated fetal heart sounds presented in this skill station.
3. Accurately document two appropriate responses/clinical interventions for the two FHR cases, which may include timing, method, and frequency of subsequent FHR assessment.

FSE AND IUPC PLACEMENT

This skill station focuses on the techniques of FSE and IUPC placement.

Objectives

The participant will be asked to complete the following:

1. Describe two relative contraindications and two potential risks to placing FSEs and IUPCs.
2. Demonstrate the correct sequence of steps for placing an FSE.
3. Demonstrate the correct sequence of steps for placing an IUPC and ensuring that it functions properly.

Principles of FSE and IUPC Placement

1. Placement of an FSE or IUPC requires skills and techniques of vaginal examination and EFM, as well as knowledge of indications, risks, limitations, and contraindications associated with the use of these devices.
2. Placing an FSE or IUPC is an invasive procedure; the practitioner should have knowledge

and understanding of the following aspects of intrapartum care:

- Maternal and fetal anatomy, as assessed by vaginal examination
- Intrapartum changes
- Indications for direct measurement of the fetal heart rate or uterine contractions
- Relative contraindications to direct, invasive monitoring, including chorioamnionitis, active maternal genital herpes infection, human immunodeficiency virus infection, and certain fetal presentations and conditions that preclude vaginal examinations such as placenta previa or undiagnosed vaginal bleeding
- Potential risks of direct, invasive monitoring, including hemorrhage, abruption, uterine perforation, and maternal or fetal infection

3. The spiral electrode usually is attached to the fetal scalp or buttock for direct measurement of the FHR by electrical activity. The electrode attaches approximately 2 mm into the presenting fetal part. The fetal lead detects the FHR electrical activity. The maternal reference electrode detects the maternal heart rate via her vaginal secretions or via placement of an external reference electrode. The external reference, when available, may be helpful when signal quality is poor.

4. An IUPC offers a direct method of measuring uterine activity during labor; it is the only objective method of measuring uterine intensity or strength. It is measured in millimeters of mercury (mm Hg).

Steps in Skill Performance

FSE Placement

1. Explain the procedure to the woman before application.
2. Wash hands. (Verbalize only for this skill station.)
3. Open electrode package and put on gloves. (Verbalize sterile technique.)

4. Remove wires from between the drive tube and the guide tube.
5. Pull electrode 1 inch back into the guide tube so it does not extend beyond the end of the guide (Figure 9-2).
6. Perform a vaginal examination to assess the presenting part. Feel for firm bone and avoid the fetus's face, sutures, fontanels, and genitalia (see Figures 9-3, 9-4a, 9-4b); maintain finger placement on the target area.
7. Place the guide tube between the two examining fingers and firmly place it against the fetal presenting part at a right angle.
8. Advance the drive tube until it touches the presenting part.
9. Maintain pressure against the presenting part and turn the tube clockwise (about 1½ times) until resistance is met.
10. Release the lock device and remove the guide tube.
11. Check placement of electrode before withdrawing examining fingers.
12. Connect FSE to leg plate. (Verbalize for this station.)
13. Plug cable into monitor. (Verbalize only for this skill station.)
14. Document placement of FSE. (Verbalize only for this skill station.)

FIGURE 9-2   Fetal Spiral Electrode Placement—Preparation

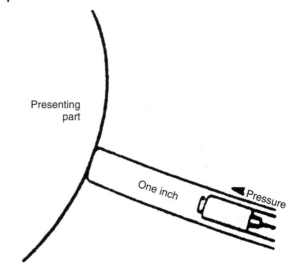

FIGURE 9-3   Fetal Spiral Electrode Placement

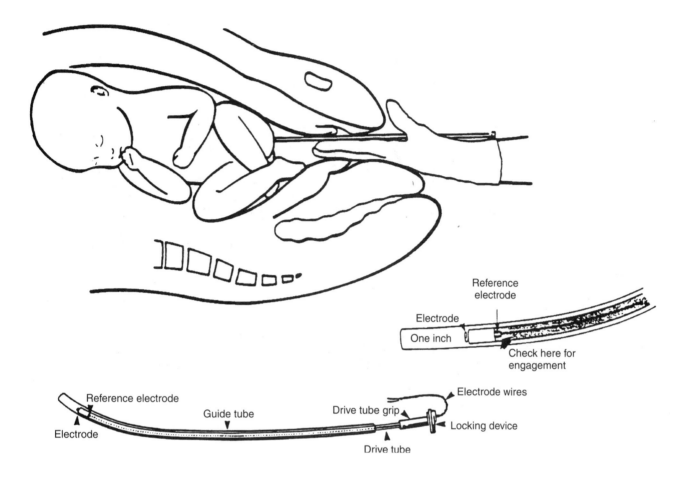

15. Remove the FSE. To detach the electrode, rotate the electrode counterclockwise until it is free from the fetal presenting part. Do not pull the electrode from the fetal skin. Do not pull wires apart to displace the electrode. Document that the electrode was removed intact.

IUPC Placement

1. Prepare IUPC according to the type of device and the manufacturer's instructions.
2. Wash hands.
3. Set up IUPC and put on gloves. (Verbalize sterile technique.)
a. Assemble equipment and attach IUPC to adaptor cable. (Verbalize only for this skill station.)
b. Calibrate to zero to assess normal atmospheric pressure if using sensor-tipped IUPC. Consult IUPC manufacturer's guidelines. (Verbalize only for this skill station.)
c. Flush IUPC with syringe and calibrate to zero to assess normal atmospheric pressure if using fluid-filled IUPC. (Verbalize only for this skill station.)
4. Determine cervical site for catheter insertion and gently displace presenting part, if needed.
5. Insert guide (containing IUPC) between examining fingers.
6. Ensure that catheter guide does not extend beyond fingers.
7. Insert IUPC through the guide tube until the catheter is between 30-cm and 45-cm markers identified on the catheter. Do not insert the IUPC into the uterus beyond the 45-cm mark. Do not force the IUPC. If resistance is met, stop advancing the IUPC, reposition fingers and IUPC, and continue insertion. If

FIGURE 9-4a and 9-4b   Fetal Spiral Electrode Placement—Cephalic (a) and Fetal Spiral Electrode Placement—Breech (b)

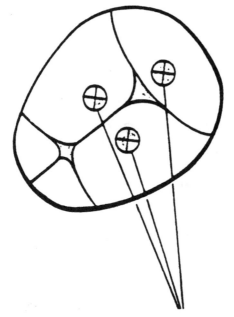

Electrode placement—
cephalic

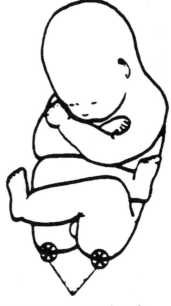

Electrode placement—breech
presentation

FIGURE 9-5   Intrauterine Pressure Catheter Placement

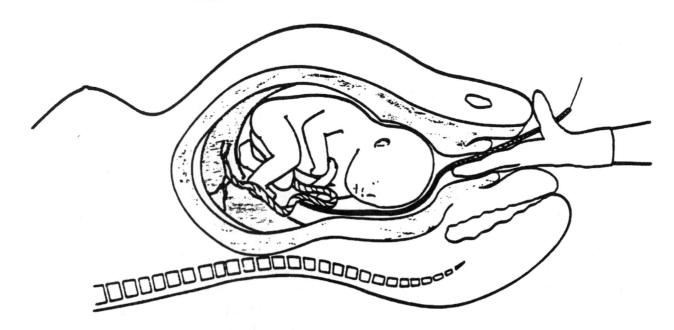

resistance is still met, discontinue insertion (Figure 9-5).

8. Attach to cable and ensure proper functioning. (Verbalize only for this skill station.)

9. Document placement of IUPC. (Verbalize only for this skill station.)

Criteria for Passing

Participants are required to meet all of the following criteria:

1. Describe two relative contraindications and two potential risks to placement of FSEs and IUPCs.

2. Demonstrate all the steps, in the correct sequence, for FSE and IUPC placement procedures (as described previously).

INTEGRATION OF FETAL HEART MONITORING KNOWLEDGE AND PRACTICE

This skill station focuses on integrating all the information gathered, including history, assessments, physiology, monitoring modes, interpretation, interventions, and evaluation. In the practice portion of this skill station, each participant will be given time to review and discuss patient histories and fetal monitor tracings. Verbal responses are appropriate for practice sessions; during testing, written responses to the fetal monitor tracings will be expected.

Objectives

The participant will be asked to complete the following:

1. Demonstrate appropriate interpretation of the fetal monitor tracing.

2. Demonstrate knowledge of the physiologic mechanisms for the observed patterns.

3. Demonstrate knowledge of instrumentation factors affecting interpretation of the fetal monitor tracing.

4. Demonstrate an understanding of how physiologic mechanisms and interpretation influence the decision-making process.

5. Describe appropriate interventions or management steps for each case scenario.

6. Demonstrate knowledge of evaluation of fetal response to selected interventions.

Principles for Integrating FHR Monitor Data into Practice

1. A systematic review of the fetal monitor tracing provides the basis for determining appropriate responses or interventions to be initiated.

2. The fetal monitor tracing should be interpreted in light of the maternal and fetal histories and data from physical assessments.

3. The physiology of pregnancy and labor is a dynamic process. Integration of physiologic-based data must accommodate changes in physiologic states. Each maternal-fetal unit presents along a physiologic continuum. The nursing process forms the basis for the progression from assessment to interpretation, integration, decision making, interventions, and evaluation.

4. Key physiologic goals and supportive actions are as follows:

   a. Support maternal coping and labor progress using the following principles:
      • Review labor plans and expectations with the woman, support persons, and family.
      • Maintain a calm environment.
      • Remain at the bedside as much as possible.
      • Minimize pain and anxiety with culturally appropriate touch, eye contact, and coached breathing.
      • Choose lower levels of technology when possible and avoid unnecessary interventions.

   b. Maximize uterine blood flow using the following interventions:
      • Maternal position change
      • Hydration
      • Medication administration
      • Anxiety/pain reduction

   c. Maximize umbilical circulation using the following interventions:

- Maternal position change
- Elevation of presenting fetal part
- Amnioinfusion

d. Maximize oxygenation using the following interventions:
  - Modified pushing
  - Maternal position change
  - Maternal supplemental oxygen administration
  - Breathing techniques
  - Correction or treatment of underlying disease

e. Reduce uterine activity using the following interventions:
  - Modified pushing
  - Maternal position change
  - Reduction/discontinuation of uterotonic drugs
  - Hydration
  - Medication/tocolytic administration

5. FHR patterns may be categorized as category I (normal), category II (indeterminate), or category III (abnormal). Although there is not always universal agreement on specific management for category II and III FHR patterns, there is a clear understanding that actions are indicated on the basis of the interpretation of certain fetal responses (e.g., variable decelerations, variability changes). Remember to respond to the likely physiologic etiology of the FHR characteristics.

6. Additional actions to be considered are based on evaluation of responses to interventions and may include further assessments (e.g., scalp stimulation), troubleshooting of equipment, notification of woman's obstetric care providers, and documentation.

7. Monitoring methods have improved over the years. However, every mode of fetal monitoring has certain limitations that may affect interpretation.

8. Evaluation includes reassessing maternal and fetal response to interventions to determine whether there is a need to continue, alter, or discontinue them on the basis of observed responses.

Steps in Skill Performance

1. Review pertinent patient history.
2. Interpret the monitor tracing for FHR baseline, variability, periodic and episodic changes, and classification of the tracing.
3. Interpret the uterine activity patterns.
4. Describe possible physiologic mechanisms for patterns (e.g., inadequate oxygen reserves; inadequate uterine, placental or cord blood flow; fetal response to nervous system stimulation or movement; cord compression).
5. Identify instrumentation factors that may affect interpretation of the tracings.
6. Describe intervention and management steps that may be taken on the basis of findings from the history, interpretation of data, and physiologic responses.
7. Evaluate maternal-fetal response to interventions.

Criterion for Passing

The participant is required to meet the following criterion:

1. Complete the written examination for this skill station, correctly answering 80% of the items.

COMMUNICATION OF FETAL HEART MONITORING DATA

In this skill station, participants demonstrate proficiency in communicating and documenting maternal-fetal assessment information and initiating the chain of command (chain of authority).

Objectives

The participant will be asked to complete the following:

1. Critique a scenario of an interprofessional communication, identifying important points that the clinician in the video omitted.

2. Accurately interpret an EFM tracing and appropriately document the interpretation. *Baseline FHR, FHR variability, periodic and episodic FHR changes, classification of the FHR pattern, and uterine activity must be identified and documented.*

3. Document a plan of action or appropriate clinical response that takes into account communication principles, the role and responsibility of the clinician as a patient advocate, and what to do when a provider's order or actions are not consistent with what the clinician believes to be in the best interest of the woman, her fetus, or both.

Principles of Communication

1. Communication is the process by which we understand others and endeavor to be understood by them.

2. Communication is dynamic, constantly changing in response to the environment and the many factors within it.

3. The clinician caring for a maternity patient should possess effective communication skills.

4. Whether communication is verbal, nonverbal, or recorded, it must be accurate, objective, and concise.

Steps in Skill Performance

Communication with the Primary Health Care Provider

1. Clearly state the identity and location (hospital name, unit or room number) name of the person initiating the communication, and name of the patient being discussed.

2. Clarify the purpose of the conversation or call and use a structured patient handoff technique such as SBAR (Situation-Background-Assessment-Recommendation) or CHAT (Context, History, Assessment, Tentative plan) to convey information (e.g., to report an update of progress, obtain an order, ask questions, state concerns, or request the presence of a primary health care provider).

3. Provide a clear, concise review of the patient's history and her status. More detail is needed if the primary health care provider is covering for someone else or does not know the patient well. If the primary health care provider requests actions that contradict hospital policy, advise that it is not possible to do so and offer an alternative, when possible. For example, say, "I am not permitted to rupture membranes, but Dr. Jones is here. Would you like to speak to Dr. Jones?"

4. If the primary health care provider requests an action that seems inappropriate for the situation, verbalize concerns along with rationale. If a conflict remains, inform the primary health care provider that the supervisor will be notified, thus initiating the chain of command (chain of authority).

5. Telephone orders should be in compliance with hospital protocol. Repeat the order back to the primary health care provider. Write legibly and include the date and time when the order was written. For example, "T.O. 4/15/07/ 8:35 a.m. Dr. Smith notified of request for pain medication for Ms. Thomas. Dr. Smith gave TO for Nubain 10 milligrams via slow IVP. Medication order repeated back to Dr. Smith; order verified."

6. Document in the patient record the time when the conversation with the primary health care provider occurred, the information given, and the purpose or outcome. For example, "Dr. Smith was notified of the patient's vaginal examination and EFM pattern." In this case, the patient's record will contain documentation of the EFM pattern and vaginal examination that coincides with what was reported to the physician. The notes contain only action information, not details about the conversation. For example, "Dr. Smith requested to come for birth." Each hospital has a protocol for documenting variances such as a quality assurance report form or incident report. Clinicians should be familiar with these protocols and forms.

Communication with the Woman in Labor and Her Support Person(s)

1. Explain events and procedures to the woman in labor in clear terms (at the level of the patient's understanding).
2. Ask whether the woman and her support person(s) have any questions, concerns, fears, or requests.
3. Listen and respond to concerns, fears, or requests. Answer questions and refer to other appropriate personnel when necessary.

Communication with Another Clinician

1. Clearly identify the patient(s) being discussed.
2. Convey urgent and stat requests or information directly and as clearly and as calmly as possible.
3. Provide complete and accurate patient care information and any additional pertinent information.
4. Convey strategies that were particularly successful or unsuccessful for patient care continuity.
5. Use hospital-approved reporting methodologies, as indicated.

Guidelines for Recording Fetal Heart Monitoring Information

1. When documenting auscultation information, include the rate and rhythm heard, as well as the presence or absence of decreases or increases.

2. Documentation of EFM data includes the mean baseline rate rounded to increments of 5 bpm (unless indeterminate), baseline variability, periodic or episodic FHR changes, accelerations, decelerations, interpretation of the FHR pattern, and uterine activity according to the capability of the equipment.
3. Documentation of uterine activity includes frequency, duration, and intensity of contractions, and uterine resting tone.
4. Documentation should reflect the trend of the FHR pattern over time.
5. Documentation also should describe the events so that they can be reasonably understood if the FHR tracing is mislabeled, lost, or incomplete.

Criteria for Passing

The participant is required to meet all of the following criteria:

1. List four important points that were omitted in the DVD communication scenario.
2. Accurately interpret an EFM tracing and appropriately document that interpretation. *Baseline FHR, FHR variability, periodic and episodic FHR changes, classification of the FHR pattern, and uterine activity must be identified and documented.*
3. Document a plan of action/appropriate clinical response that takes into account communication principles, the role and responsibility of the clinician as a patient advocate, and what to do when an obstetric provider's orders or other actions are not consistent with what is believed to be in the best interest of the woman, her fetus, or both.

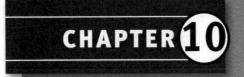

Case Study Exercises

Rebecca L. Cypher

This chapter provides case study exercises that are an adjunct to the content presented in the Intermediate and Advanced Fetal Monitoring courses. A practice case answer sheet is provided to facilitate analysis of the case studies and EFM tracings. For each case study exercise, readers are encouraged to (1) review the brief history and data provided, (2) analyze the EFM tracing, and (3) complete the practice case answer sheet. Answer keys for each exercise are provided at the end of the scenario. Readers should review their work and identify areas of strength and those areas requiring more practice or review related to electronic FHR monitoring interpretation.

Objectives

For each case study exercise, the participant will be able to do the following:

- Interpret the fetal heart rate (FHR) baseline and variability using National Institute of Child Health and Human Development (NICHD) terminology.
- Identify periodic and episodic FHR patterns to include accelerations, late decelerations, variable decelerations, early decelerations, and prolonged decelerations.
- Determine the frequency, duration, intensity, and resting tone for the contraction pattern.
- Describe the appropriate interventions for each case study.

AWHONN FETAL HEART MONITORING PROGRAM INTEGRATION OF FETAL HEART MONITORING KNOWLEDGE AND PRACTICE

PRACTICE CASE ANSWER SHEET

Case Study Exercise: _____

1. Baseline FHR:

2. Variability

   a. Absent (undetectable) _____
   b. Minimal (>0 but ≤ 5 bpm) _____
   c. Moderate (6–25 bpm) _____
   d. Marked (>25 bpm) _____
   e. Unable to determine _____

3. Contractions

   Frequency: _____
   Duration: _____
   Intensity: _____
   Resting tonus: _____

4. Accelerations and decelerations. When present, circle P if periodic or E if episodic.

Accelerations	P	E
Early decelerations	P	
Variable decelerations	P	E
Late decelerations	P	
Prolonged decelerations	P	E

5. Interpretation

   Category I ____
   Category II ____
   Category III ____

6. List possible underlying physiologic mechanisms or rationales for observed patterns.

7. List in order of priority the physiologic goal(s) for observed patterns.

8. List actions and interventions indicated based on overall interpretation (physiologic based, instrumentation based, and further assessments).

FIGURE 10-1   Skylar: Labor and Delivery EFM Tracing at 0345 Using Ultrasound and Tocodynamometer

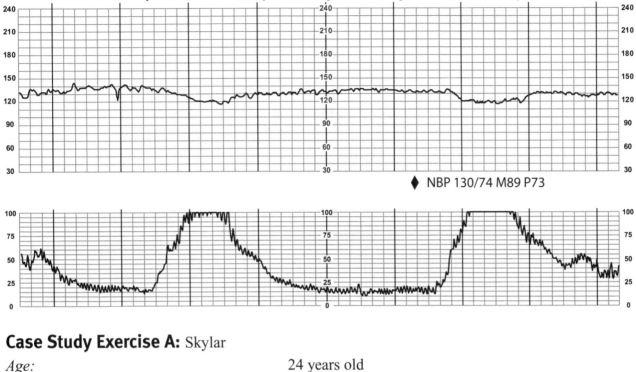

♦ NBP 130/74 M89 P73

Case Study Exercise A: Skylar

Age:	24 years old
Gravida/Para:	G10000
Gestational Age:	40 − 5/7 weeks
Medical History:	Unremarkable
Surgical History:	Lumpectomy for benign left breast mass
	Appendectomy
Psychosocial History:	Married
	Father of baby medically retired military veteran
Past Obstetric History:	Not applicable
Current Obstetric History:	Elevated 1-hour glucose tolerance test (GTT) = 174
	Declined 3-hour GTT and use of glucometer
	2nd trimester ultrasound consistent with last menstrual period (LMP), normal anatomy
	3rd trimester growth ultrasounds consistent with size and dates

Skylar presented to labor and delivery at 0030 for contractions with increasing intensity for 3 hours. Vaginal examination (VE) on admission revealed a cervix that was 4 cm dilated, 90% effaced, and a fetal vertex at 0 station. Her vital signs were as follows: temperature oral: 98.2° F (36.7° C); blood pressure: 132/87 mm Hg; pulse: 79 bpm; and respirations: 24 breaths per minute. At 0345, Skylar requested an epidural. VE prior to epidural placement revealed a cervix of 7 cm dilated, 100% effaced, and vertex at 0 station with an occiput posterior position.

PRACTICE CASE ANSWER SHEET

Case Study Exercise A: Skylar

1. Baseline FHR: **135 bpm**

2. Variability   Absent (undetectable)   _____
                      Minimal (>0 but ≤ 5 bpm)   **Remainder of tracing**
                      Moderate (6–25 bpm)   **First 2 minutes of tracing**
                      Marked (>25 bpm)   _____
                      Unable to determine   _____

3. Contractions   Frequency: **q 4 min**
                      Duration: **120–150 seconds**
                      Intensity: **Palpate**
                      Resting tone: **Palpate**

4. Accelerations and decelerations. When present, circle P if periodic or E if episodic.

Accelerations	P	E
Early decelerations	**P**	
Variable decelerations	P	E
Late decelerations	P	
Prolonged decelerations	P	E
None present		

5. Interpretation   **Category I**   First 2 minutes
                     Category II   Remainder of tracing
                     Category III

6. List possible underlying physiologic mechanisms or rationales for observed patterns.
   - Primigravida in active labor
   - Reflex vagal response related to the following:
     - Head compression
     - Persistent occiput posterior presentation
     - Possible cephalopelvic disproportion
   - Fetal behavioral state change (fetal sleep cycle)

7. List in order of priority the physiologic goal(s) for observed patterns.
   - Promote maternal comfort and labor progress.
   - Continue to promote oxygenation.
   - Continue to promote uteroplacental blood flow.

8. List actions and interventions indicated based on overall interpretation (physiologic based, instrumentation based, and further assessments).
   - Review previous tracings to evaluate variability and periodic/episodic changes
   - Palpate contractions to validate uterine monitoring data.
   - If minimal variability persists, assess FHR response to scalp stimulation, vibroacoustic stimulation, or manipulation of maternal abdomen to evaluate fetal oxygenation.
   - Continue to assess deceleration pattern and variability.
   - Change maternal position frequently to promote uteroplacental blood flow and encourage rotation of vertex to occiput anterior position.
   - Continue routine assessments and interventions for labor such as maternal comfort measures.
   - Keep provider notified of FHR pattern (decelerations and variability), interventions, and maternal-fetal response.

PRACTICE CASE ANSWER SHEET
Case Study Exercise: _____

1. Baseline FHR:

2. Variability   a. Absent (undetectable)   _____
     b. Minimal (>0 but ≤ 5 bpm)   _____
     c. Moderate (6–25 bpm)   _____
     d. Marked (>25 bpm)   _____
     e. Unable to determine   _____

3. Contractions   Frequency: _____
     Duration: _____
     Intensity: _____
     Resting tonus: _____

4. Accelerations and decelerations. When present, circle P if periodic or E if episodic.

Accelerations	P	E
Early decelerations	P	
Variable decelerations	P	E
Late decelerations	P	
Prolonged decelerations	P	E

5. Interpretation   Category I   ____
     Category II   ____
     Category III   ____

6. List possible underlying physiologic mechanisms or rationales for observed patterns.

7. List in order of priority the physiologic goal(s) for observed patterns.

8. List actions and interventions indicated based on overall interpretation (physiologic based, instrumentation based, and further assessments).

Case Study Exercise B : Margaret

Age:	23 years old
Gravida/Para:	G20010
Gestational Age:	37 − 4/7 weeks
Medical History:	Chronic hypertension requiring Labetolol 200 mg po bid
Surgical History:	Unremarkable
Psychosocial History:	Married; father of baby involved
Past Obstetric History:	Spontaneous abortion at 11 weeks
Current Obstetric History:	Twin gestation (dichorionic/diamniotic)
	Gestational diabetes mellitus A2 requiring insulin
	Mild preeclampsia

Margaret was admitted to labor and delivery at 0500 for labor induction because of worsening blood pressures (140–150s/90s mm Hg) and proteinuria (462 mg in 24-hour urine). VE on admission revealed a cervix that was 1 cm dilated and 50% effaced. The fetal vertex for twin A was at −1 station with Twin B in a transverse lie. Induction was started with a Foley bulb and low-dose oxytocin. Magnesium sulfate was started for seizure prophylaxis. Hourly fingerstick blood glucose samples were obtained, and values were within a normal range. Spontaneous rupture of membranes occurred at 1720. The fluid was clear, and the Foley bulb was removed.

The patient requested an epidural at 2100. VE after epidural placement revealed a cervix that was 4 cm dilated, 90% effaced, and a fetal vertex at 0 station. Oxytocin was infusing at 12 mU/minute. Margaret's vital signs were as follows: temperature oral: 97.8° F (36.5° C); blood pressure: 135–157/66–90 mm Hg; pulse: 107–120 bpm; and respirations 22 breaths per minute.

FIGURE 10-2 Margaret: Labor and Delivery EFM Tracing at 2135 Using Ultrasound and Tocodynamometer

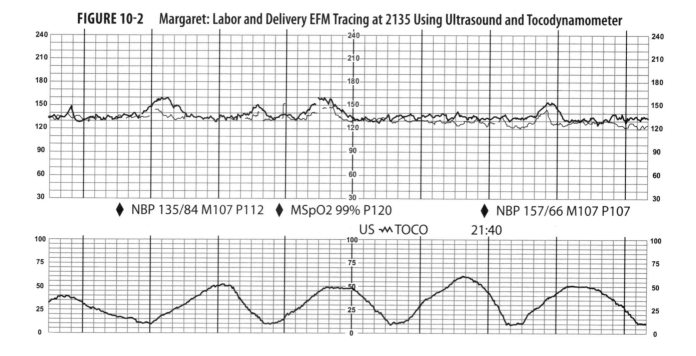

◆ NBP 135/84 M107 P112　◆ MSpO2 99% P120　　　◆ NBP 157/66 M107 P107

US ⌁ TOCO　　21:40

PRACTICE CASE ANSWER SHEET

Case Study Exercise B: Margaret

1. Baseline FHR: **Twin A (dark line): 135 bpm**
Twin B (light line): 130 bpm

2. Variability Absent (undetectable) _____
Minimal (>0 but ≤ 5 bpm) _____
Moderate (6–25 bpm) _____
Marked (>25 bpm) _____
Unable to determine _____

3. Contractions Frequency: **q 1 1/2-2 min**
Duration: **90–100 seconds**
Intensity: **Palpate**
Resting tone: **Palpate**

4. Accelerations and decelerations. When present, circle P if periodic or E if episodic.

Accelerations	P	**E (Twin A & B)**
Early decelerations	P	
Variable decelerations	P	E
Late decelerations	P	
Prolonged decelerations	P	E
None present		

5. Interpretation **Category I** _____
Category II _____
Category III _____

6. List possible underlying physiologic mechanisms or rationales for observed patterns.
  • Associated with adequate oxygenation at present
  • Spontaneous fetal movement or in response to environmental stimulus
  • Uterine contraction
  • Direct sympathetic stimulation of the fetus
  • Autonomic regulation of FHR

7. List in order of priority the physiologic goal(s) for observed patterns.
  • Maintain appropriate levels of uterine activity.
  • Promote maternal comfort and labor progress.
  • Maximize oxygenation.
  • Maximize uteroplacental blood flow.
  • Maximize umbilical circulation.

8. List actions and interventions indicated based on overall interpretation (physiologic based, instrumentation based, and further assessments).
   - Decrease oxytocin given adequate labor progress and contractions every 1½ to 2 minutes with less than 1 minute resting tone between them.
   - Continue to observe FHR patterns.
   - Maternal positioning to optimize oxygenation and maternal comfort.
   - Monitor maternal vital signs.
   - Palpate contractions to validate uterine monitoring data.
   - Continue routine assessments and interventions for care of the high-risk labor patient to include blood sugar monitoring, magnesium sulfate management, blood pressure evaluation, and maternal comfort and support.
   - Keep provider informed of FHR patterns (normal), interventions, and maternal-fetal response.

PRACTICE CASE ANSWER SHEET
Case Study Exercise: _____

1. Baseline FHR:

2. Variability   a. Absent (undetectable)   _____
         b. Minimal (>0 but ≤ 5 bpm)   _____
         c. Moderate (6–25 bpm)   _____
         d. Marked (>25 bpm)   _____
         e. Unable to determine   _____

3. Contractions   Frequency: _____
         Duration: _____
         Intensity: _____
         Resting tonus: _____

4. Accelerations and decelerations. When present, circle P if periodic or E if episodic.
     Accelerations   P   E
     Early decelerations   P
     Variable decelerations   P   E
     Late decelerations   P
     Prolonged decelerations   P   E

5. Interpretation   Category I   ____
         Category II   ____
         Category III   ____

6. List possible underlying physiologic mechanisms or rationales for observed patterns.

7. List in order of priority the physiologic goal(s) for observed patterns.

8. List actions and interventions indicated based on overall interpretation (physiologic based, instrumentation based, and further assessments).

Case Study Exercise C: Susan

Age:	41 years old
Gravida/Para:	G41112
Gestational Age:	28 − 2/7 weeks
Medical History:	Unremarkable
Surgical History:	Unremarkable
Psychosocial History:	Day care worker, married
	Smoker—one pack per day
Past Obstetric History:	Spontaneous vaginal birth at 38 − 3/7 weeks
	Spontaneous abortion at 13 − 1/7 weeks
	Preterm birth at 33 weeks (abruption)
Current Obstetric History:	Advanced maternal age: normal first trimester screening test
	Symmetric intrauterine growth restriction (IUGR)
	Primary cytomegalovirus (CMV) diagnosed on amniocentesis

Susan was admitted to the high-risk antepartum unit for severe IUGR with no interval growth between 25 and 28 weeks. The ultrasound revealed a fetus in the 3rd percentile for growth and an estimated fetal weight less than 575 grams. Doppler flow studies showed absent end diastolic flow, a worrisome finding. The amniotic fluid index was 2 cm (oligohydramnios). A sterile speculum examination ruled out ruptured membranes. VE revealed a cervix that was closed and long. The fetus was in a breech presentation. A biophysical profile was 6 out of 10 with points being taken off for decreased amniotic fluid and a nonreactive nonstress test. Antenatal steroids were administered.

FIGURE 10-3   Susan: Second Inpatient Hospital Day; EFM Tracing at 1530 Using Ultrasound and Tocodynamometer

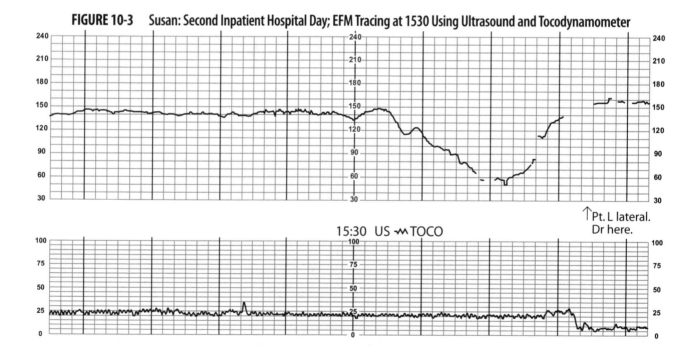

PRACTICE CASE ANSWER SHEET

Case Study Exercise C: Susan

1. Baseline FHR: **145 bpm**

2. Variability   Absent (undetectable)   _____

          Minimal (>0 but ≤ 5 bpm)   _____

          Moderate (6–25 bpm)   _____

          Marked (>25 bpm)   _____

          Unable to determine   _____

3. Contractions   Frequency: **None**

          Duration: **Not applicable**

          Intensity: **Not applicable**

          Resting tone: **Need to palpate**

4. Accelerations and decelerations. When present, circle P if periodic or E if episodic.

          Accelerations   P   E

          Early decelerations   P

          Variable decelerations   P   E

          Late decelerations   P

          Prolonged decelerations   P   **E**

          None present

5. Interpretation   Category I   _____

          Category II   _____

          Category III   _____

6. List possible underlying physiologic mechanisms or rationales for observed patterns.
   - Cord compression related to oligohydramnios or fetal movement
   - Uteroplacental insufficiency related to the following:
     o Maternal smoking
     o Hypotension from supine maternal positioning during monitoring session
     o Placental abnormalities from CMV

7. List in order of priority the physiologic goal(s) for observed patterns.
   - Maximize umbilical circulation.
   - Maximize oxygenation.
   - Maximize uteroplacental blood flow.

8. List actions and interventions indicated based on overall interpretation (physiologic based, instrumentation based, and further assessments).

- Position changes to promote uteroplacental blood flow and relieve cord compression.
- Palpate uterus to validate uterine monitoring data and adjust tocodynamometer to monitor contraction pattern if palpable.
- Assess maternal vital signs (blood pressure).
- Continue to assess deceleration pattern and variability.
- Provide reassurance to Susan and her family.
- Review previous tracings to evaluate variability and periodic/nonperiodic changes.
- Keep provider notified of FHR pattern (decelerations and variability), interventions, and maternal-fetal response.
- Evaluate maternal-fetal response to interventions.
- Continue routine assessments and interventions such as providing maternal comfort measures and keeping family informed of clinical situation.
- Prepare for birth if FHR pattern cannot be corrected.
- Alert neonatal team for possible birth.

PRACTICE CASE ANSWER SHEET
Case Study Exercise: _____

1. Baseline FHR:

2. Variability
- a. Absent (undetectable) _____
- b. Minimal (>0 but ≤ 5 bpm) _____
- c. Moderate (6–25 bpm) _____
- d. Marked (>25 bpm) _____
- e. Unable to determine _____

3. Contractions
- Frequency: _____
- Duration: _____
- Intensity: _____
- Resting tonus: _____

4. Accelerations and decelerations. When present, circle P if periodic or E if episodic.

Accelerations	P	E
Early decelerations	P	
Variable decelerations	P	E
Late decelerations	P	
Prolonged decelerations	P	E

5. Interpretation
- Category I ____
- Category II ____
- Category III ____

6. List possible underlying physiologic mechanisms or rationales for observed patterns.

7. List in order of priority the physiologic goal(s) for observed patterns.

8. List actions and interventions indicated based on overall interpretation (physiologic based, instrumentation based, and further assessments).

Case Study Exercise D: Lori

Age: 36 years old
Gravida/Para: G21001
Gestational Age: 41 − 1/7 weeks
Medical History: Unremarkable
Surgical History: Laparoscope for endometriosis
Psychosocial History: Unremarkable
Past Obstetric History: Previous cesarean birth for breech presentation
Current Obstetric History: Advanced maternal age—normal quad screen
                                     Low-lying placenta on ultrasound

Lori presented to OB triage at 0350 for q 3 to 5 minute contractions and bloody show. This was her third visit to triage in 24 hours. She was admitted for therapeutic rest using morphine sulfate. VE on admission revealed a cervix that was 1 cm dilated, 90% effaced, and fetal vertex at −3 station. Lori progressed to 4 cm dilated, 100% effaced, and a fetal vertex at −1 station by 0645. The membranes were artificially ruptured at this time for a large amount of clear fluid. Lori continued to contract q 3 to 4 minutes but had inadequate cervical change. Internal monitors were placed at 0915, and an oxytocin augmentation was started at 1000. Lori requested an epidural at 1230. The initial dosing rates of the epidural caused hypotension requiring two doses of ephedrine.

FIGURE 10-4   Lori: Labor and Delivery EFM Tracing at 1300 Using Fetal Spiral Electrode and Internal Monitoring

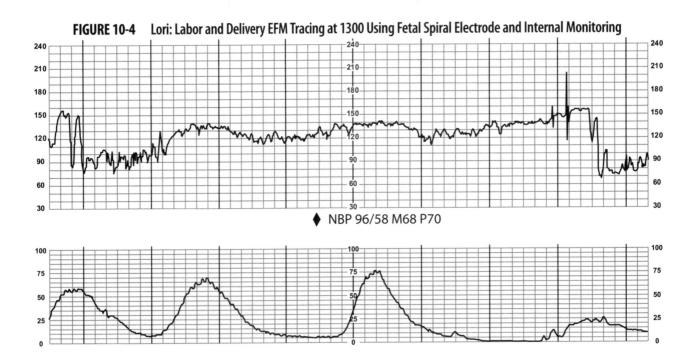

♦ NBP 96/58 M68 P70

PRACTICE CASE ANSWER SHEET

Case Study Exercise D: Lori

1. Baseline FHR: **140 bpm**
2. Variability   Absent (undetectable)   _____
                          Minimal (>0 but ≤ 5 bpm)   _____
                          Moderate (6–25 bpm)   _____
                          Marked (>25 bpm)   _____
                          Unable to determine   _____
3. Contractions   Frequency: **q 2 to 3 minutes**
                          Duration: **90–110 seconds**
                          Intensity: **55–75 mm Hg**
                          Resting tone: **5 mm Hg**

4. Accelerations and decelerations. When present, circle P if periodic or E if episodic.

Accelerations	P	E
Early decelerations	P	
Variable decelerations	P	E
Late decelerations	P	
Prolonged decelerations	P	E
None present		

5. Interpretation   Category I   _____
                         Category II   _____
                         Category III   _____

There is a mixed pattern of decelerations according to NICHD terminology. Definitions in the NICHD language emphasize the abruptness or gradualness of the onset of the deceleration. According to the definitions, the first, third, and last decelerations are variable, and the second deceleration is late. (The third deceleration reaches its nadir in less than 30 seconds.) Some participants may feel strongly that these are late decelerations based on the timing and the etiology (maternal hypotension). When interpreting the FHR pattern, it is important to evaluate the baseline variability, the evolution of the pattern over time, the overall clinical picture, and the fetal response to interventions.

6. List possible underlying physiologic mechanisms or rationales for observed patterns.
   • Uteroplacental insufficiency related to maternal hypotension
   • Decreased uteroplacental perfusion related to postmature placenta and abnormal placentation
   • Possible decreasing fetal reserves and hypoxia
   • Fetal behavioral state change (fetal sleep cycle)
   • Possible cord compression

7. List in order of priority the physiologic goal(s) for observed patterns.
   • Maximize oxygenation.
   • Maximize uteroplacental blood flow.
   • Reduce uterine activity.

8. List actions and interventions indicated based on overall interpretation (physiologic based, instrumentation based, and further assessments).
- Change maternal position to promote uteroplacental blood flow.
- Assess maternal vital signs (blood pressure):
  o Repeat ephedrine sulfate doses as ordered/indicated.
- Administer oxygen at 10 Liters/minute via a tight non-rebreather face mask.
- Give IV (intravenous) fluid bolus to increase maternal blood volume and increase placental perfusion.
- Turn off oxytocin and consider tocolytic medication if uterine activity is not reduced.
- Consider vaginal examination to evaluate labor progress.
- Continue to assess deceleration pattern and variability.
- Review previous tracings segments to evaluate variability and periodic/episodic changes.
- Notify provider of FHR pattern (decelerations and variability), interventions, and patient response.
- Evaluate FHR response to interventions.
- Palpate uterus to validate uterine monitoring data.
- Continue routine assessments and interventions for labor, such as maternal comfort measures.
- Prepare for birth if FHR pattern deteriorates.
- Alert neonatal team for possible emergent delivery.

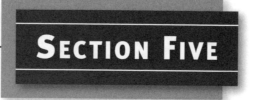

SECTION FIVE

Advanced Fetal Heart Monitoring Principles and Practices

1. Read This Book
2. Take the On-Line Test
3. Earn Continuing Nursing Education Credit

www.awhonn.org/fhm

AWHONN is accredited as a provider of continuing nursing education by the American Nurses Credentialing Center's Commission on Accreditation.

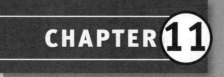

CHAPTER 11

Antenatal Fetal Assessment and Testing

Catharine M. Treanor

INTRODUCTION

Maternity care changed dramatically during the last half of the twentieth century, owing to the remarkable technologic and pharmacologic improvements in obstetric care and surveillance (Centers for Disease Control and Prevention, 2001). As a result, the fetal and neonatal mortality rate decreased more than fourfold during that time (CDC), and although the pace has slowed since the mid-1990s, the rate remains stable (Kochanek & Smith, 2004). Many techniques have been used to identify a fetus that may be at risk for hypoxic injury or death, but for various reasons, the ideal fetal screening test has not been developed to identify all factors that contribute to a risk for hypoxic injury or death (Manning, 1995). Furthermore, no single test is ideal for all high-risk fetuses (Vintzileos, 2000).

For most of the twentieth century, fetal well-being was determined by assessment and evaluation of the fetal heart rate (FHR), maternal perception of fetal movement, and several indirect and often unreliable maternal markers, including physical (e.g., fundal height), historical (e.g., risk assessment), or biochemical (e.g., estriol) characteristics (Manning, 1995). Since the 1970s the expansion of fetal research and the development of new technologies, such as electronic FHR monitoring and high-resolution sonography, has made information about fetal status more accessible (Vintzileos, 1995). For example, knowledge about fetal cardiovascular physiology and neurologic development has grown significantly. Fetal physiologic parameters that can now be assessed include (1) observing gross motor activities (e.g., breathing, tone), (2) determining activity state (e.g., quiet sleep, active sleep), (3) monitoring eye lens motion, (4) measuring urine production, and (5) observing systolic-to-diastolic blood flow (Manning). Today, these fetal assessment parameters can be observed, quantified, and compared with established norms (Vintzileos, 2000). In addition, fetal effects from maternal conditions, such as diabetes or hypertension, can be described so that it is now possible to differentiate maternal from fetal risk (Manning).

Throughout pregnancy, numerous pathophysiologic processes can place the fetus at risk for metabolic derangement, hypoxia, or death. Early identification of those phenomena is an important first step in fetal surveillance (Vintzileos, 2000). Perinatal deaths are most often associated with (1) congenital malformations and chromosomal abnormalities, (2) prematurity and low birth weight, and (3) the effects of maternal complications on the fetus/neonate (Kochanek & Smith, 2004). Neurologic injury is another potential and important adverse fetal outcome. Insights into the origin of cerebral palsy (CP) have dispelled the commonly held belief that most cases of CP arise from intrapartum events. Neurologic injury can occur during the antepartum, intrapartum, or neonatal period (MacLennan, 1999; Perlman, 2006). In a seminal publication, the American College of Obstetricians and Gynecologists (ACOG) and the American Academy of Pediatrics (AAP) identified that the pathway from hypoxic injury to a diagnosis of CP progresses through a series of pathopyhsiologic phases, including neonatal encephalopathy, a subset of CP (ACOG & AAP, 2003). Seventy percent of neonatal encephalopathy is secondary to an antepartum event; however, it is important to note that neonatal encephalopathy may or may not result in permanent neurologic compromise. Approximately 8% to 9% of cases of CP are attributed to intrapartum events (ACOG & AAP; Perlman).

FETAL ANTEPARTUM SURVEILLANCE METHODS

Antepartum testing modalities are based on fundamental physiologic principles and are used to identify the fetus at risk for hypoxia versus the normally oxygenated fetus (Boehm & Gabbe,

2002; Harris, 1999). The fetal response to an acute or chronic reduction in oxygen availability is a decline in activities regulated by the central nervous system (CNS), including heart rate reactivity, breathing, movement, and tone (Figure 11-1) (Manning, Harmon, Menticoglou, & Morrison, 1991). Oxygenated blood is shunted to the brain, heart, and adrenal glands; if the insult is prolonged or repetitive, growth restriction and/or oligohydramnios can develop. The purpose of antepartum testing is to validate fetal well-being or identify potentially hypoxemic fetuses by the presence or absence of one or more biophysical parameters and to intervene before permanent injury or death can occur. The efficacy of antepartum surveillance to predict perinatal outcomes for different patient populations has not been clearly established, but testing is usually indicated for conditions that place the fetus at risk for uteroplacental insufficiency and fetal demise. Evaluation of factors such as the potential for fetal and neonatal survival or risk of death, the severity of maternal disease, and the risk of iatrogenic prematurity due to false-

FIGURE 11-1 Fetal Responses to Acute and Chronic Hypoxemia and Effects on CNS-Regulated Activities

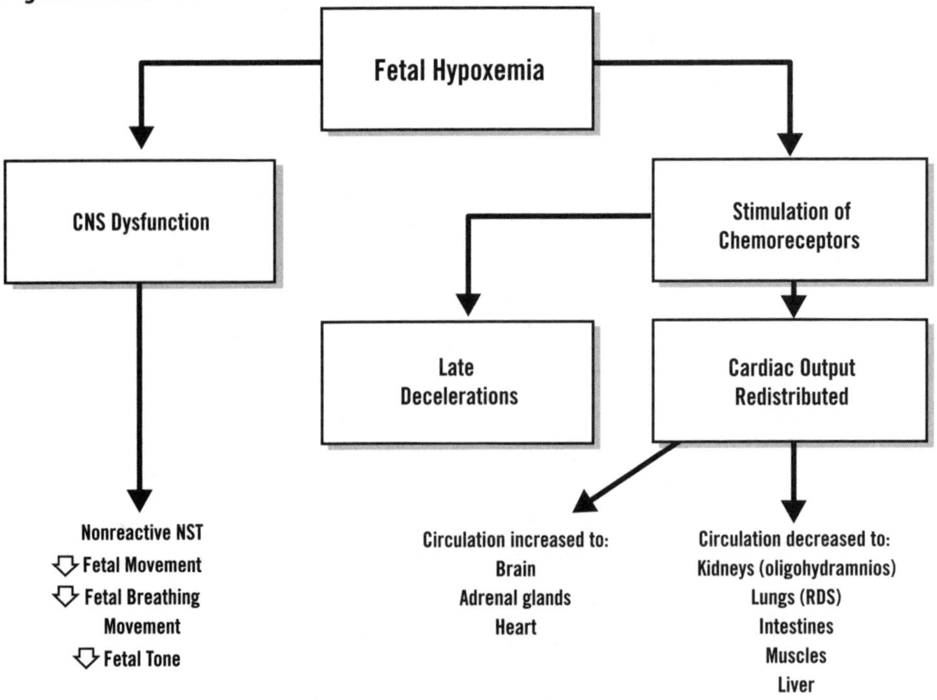

Adapted from: Manning, Harmon, Menticoglou, & Morrison, 1991.

positive test results should be undertaken to help determine when to begin fetal surveillance (ACOG, 1999).

FETAL MOVEMENT DETECTION

Maternal perception of fetal movement after approximately 16 to 20 weeks of gestation is one of the oldest, simplest, least expensive, and most widely used tests of fetal well-being. Counting fetal movements during the second half of pregnancy requires no monitoring devices and is both noninvasive and cost-effective (Velazquez & Rayburn, 2002). Although a variety of fetal movement counting (FMC, or kick counting) methods are used in clinical practice, the ideal number of fetal kicks or movement or optimal duration of FMC has not been defined (AAP & ACOG, 2007).

Development of Fetal Gross Body Movements

The fetus moves spontaneously by approximately the 7th to 8th week of gestational age. Maternal perception of fetal movement occurs between the 16th and 18th weeks of gestation (Blackburn, 2007). With neurologic maturation, fetal movement becomes more complex and coordinated (deVries, Visser, & Prechtl, 1982). Cycling between periods of high and low activity begins as early as 22 weeks (Groome, Owen, Singh, Neely, & Gaudier, 1992). Total weekly movements increase, reaching a maximum between the 26th and 32nd week (Blackburn). Between the 32nd and 38th week, fetal movements decrease and then should remain constant until term under normal circumstances (Olesen & Svare, 2004; Blackburn; Rayburn, 1990). Synchronization of fetal movement with fetal behavioral states (e.g., active sleep) begins early in the third trimester (Drogtrop, Ubels, & Nijhuis, 1990). Consequently, most healthy term fetuses exhibit coordinated movement patterns that correspond to specific behavioral states (Groome & Watson, 1992).

Maternal perception of fetal movement as a screening tool is based on the physiologic principle that compromised fetuses reduce activity in response to decreased oxygenation (Boehm & Gabbe, 2002). Decreases in maternally perceived fetal movements prior to fetal death have been reported (Pearson & Weaver, 1976; Sadovsky & Yaffe, 1973). Patrick, Campbell, Carmichael, Natale, and Richardson (1982) demonstrated a positive correlation between maternal perception and ultrasound-confirmed fetal movement. A comparison of ultrasound-detected fetal movements with maternally perceived fetal movements is presented in Table 11-1.

Fetal Movement Counting

Several different schemata for fetal movement counting (FMC) have been proposed for quantifying maternally perceived movements and for identifying potentially hypoxemic fetuses. FMC methods vary greatly according to the counting interval, number of movements considered reassuring, maternal activity during testing, and method of recording (Christensen & Rayburn, 1999), but all appear acceptable (ACOG, 1999). Typically, patients are instructed to count all fetal movements occurring in a specific time period and to contact the primary provider if a certain number of movements are not perceived during the prescribed counting interval (Rayburn, 1982). However, perhaps more valuable than any single proposed FMC guideline is the mother's perception of fetal activity in relation to previously perceived fetal movement levels (AAP & ACOG, 2007).

A suggested approach to assessing fetal well-being includes daily fetal movement counting after the 28th week of pregnancy (AAP & ACOG, 2007). Maternal perception of 10 distinct fetal movements within a 2-hour period is considered reassuring; once the number of movements is achieved within the time period, counts can be discontinued for that day (AAP & ACOG). Although the presence of fetal movement within a specified protocol is usually a reliable indicator

Table 11-1	Comparison of Maternally Perceived and Ultrasound-Visualized Movement Patterns			
MATERNAL PERCEPTION	**ULTRASOUND VISUALIZED**	**MOTION TYPE**	**DURATION (SEC)**	**INTENSITY**
Rollover, stretch	Whole fetal body	Rolling and stretching	3–30	Strong
Kick, jab, startle	Trunk and extremities	Simple or isolated	1–15	Strong
Flutter, weak kick	Lower extremities	Simple	<1	Weak
Hiccup	Chest wall and extremities	High frequency	<1	Weak

Adapted from Rayburn, 1982.

of fetal well-being, the absence of fetal movement may or may not be predictive of adverse fetal outcomes (Devoe et al., 1994; Gibby, 1988). Therefore, an insufficient fetal movement count should be followed by a biophysical means of fetal assessment such as a nonstress test (NST), biophysical profile (BPP), or modified BPP (AAP & ACOG).

Factors Influencing Fetal Movement

Fetal body movements and fetal movements perceived by the mother can be affected by several factors. When fetal movement is used to assess fetal well-being, one must be aware of how movement changes with gestational age and other factors. As previously mentioned, the number of movements increases between the 26th and 32nd week, decreases between the 32nd and 38th week, and then remains constant to term (Olesen & Svare, 2004; Blackburn, 2007; Rayburn, 1990). Contrary to common belief, the qualitative and quantitative measures of fetal movement do not decrease appreciably prior to labor and birth (Velazquez & Rayburn, 2002).

Fetal behavioral states (sleep-wake cycles) should also be considered when fetal movement is evaluated. Fetal sleep-wake cycles vary considerably but are well established by the third trimester (Nijhuis, Prechtl, Martin, & Bots, 1982). Fetal behavioral states are presented in Table 11-2. Studies in term fetuses indicate that the mean length of the quiet state is 23 minutes and the longest period of inactivity is 75 min-

utes (Timor-Tritsch, Dierker, Hertz, Deogan, & Rosen, 1978a; Patrick et al., 1982). Fetuses spend most of their time in quiet and active sleep cycles (Pillai & James, 1990).

Fetal movement tends to decrease during periods of heavy physical activity by the mother (Manders, Sonder, Mulder, & Visser, 1997); however, low-impact exercise had only mild transitory effects, and aerobic exercise had no significant impact on movement or kick response (Hatoum, Clapp, Newman, Dajani, & Amini, 1997). Chronic maternal anxiety and stress can also influence fetal movement. Mothers with high

Table 11-2	Comparison of Maternally Perceived and Ultrasound-Visualized Movement Patterns
BEHAVIORAL STATE	**DESCRIPTION**
1F (Quiet Sleep)	• Quiet sleep • Quiescent state • Diminished FHR variability
2F (Active Sleep)	• Active sleep • Frequent whole body movements • Moderate variability • FHR accelerations
3F (Quiet Awake)	• Absent body movement • No FHR accelerations
4F (Active Awake)	• Vigorous body movement • FHR acceleration

FHR, Fetal heart rate.
Adapted from Nijhuis et al., 1982.

anxiety scores tend to have fetuses who demonstrate significantly less movement than fetuses whose mothers have low anxiety scores (DiPietro, Costigan, & Gurewitsch, 2003; Groome, Swiber, Bentz, Holland, & Atterbury, 1995).

Several additional factors have been reported to affect fetal motor activity, including time of day, maternal tobacco and caffeine use, and glucose load (Devoe, Murray, Youssif, & Arnaud, 1993; Eller, Stramm, & Newman, 1992; Patrick, et al., 1982; Thaler, Goodman, & Dawes, 1980). However, gross fetal body movements are unaffected by maternal glucose levels, thus dispelling another commonly held belief that juice or a meal is necessary prior to FMC (Velazquez & Rayburn, 2002). Maternal perception of fetal movements can also be affected by maternal body size, anterior placental location, and polyhydramnios (Timor-Tritsch, Dierker, Hertz, & Rosen, 1979).

A vigorous, active fetus is a reassuring finding while the presence of decreased fetal movement in pregnancy complications of a chronic nature correlate with a higher likelihood of subsequent fetal death (ACOG, 1999; Christensen & Rayburn, 1999). However, FMC has not been shown to prevent fetal death (ACOG; Velazquez & Rayburn, 2002). Factors affecting the technique's effectiveness include a lack of FMC adherence, delayed follow-up, and/or inadequate follow-up (Gribbin & James, 2004). As a screening tool, FMC is appealing (Boehm & Gabbe, 2002), especially in high-risk pregnancies in which decreasing fetal movements are more often associated with chronic rather than acute compromise. FMC is of greatest value when there is long-standing placental insufficiency (Velazquez & Rayburn); however, its role in low-risk pregnancies requires further investigation. Research is needed to determine the ideal system for performing FMC, the optimal criteria for assessing the number of movements, the time needed for testing, the interval for repeat evaluation, gestational age at which to begin testing, and, ultimately, the efficacy of FMC to prevent fetal mortality.

Doppler-Detected Fetal Movement

The evolution of Doppler-based ultrasound technology led to advances and improvements in the processing of data between first- and second-generation electronic fetal monitors (Boehm, Fields, Hutchison, Bowen, & Vaughn, 1986). Today's fetal monitors (EFMs, also known in some European countries as cardiotocography or CTG) use a Doppler-based recording of the FHR, fetal activity, and uterine contractions to identify potentially hypoxemic fetuses (Garite, 2007; Johnson, 1994). How EFMs detect and differentiate between the fetal heart rate and fetal movement (actocardiotocography or ACTG) is an often asked question.

Doppler transducers transmit ultra-high-frequency sound waves to the moving heart valves; the sound waves are deflected back and converted into electrical signals. The raw signals are then processed by onboard algorithms that generate a baseline heart rate (Devoe, 1999). Doppler filtering systems further enable the transducer to record and distinguish low-frequency shifts from high-frequency shifts. These special band-pass filters allow for a more accurate detection of fetal movement (i.e., low-frequency shifts) from fetal cardiac activity (i.e., high-frequency shifts). Filtering systems are now incorporated into many EFMs, allowing for documentation of not only FHR and variability but also fetal movement (Devoe, 1999). Several studies indicate a strong positive correlation between movements recorded with Doppler-based systems and those observed with real-time ultrasound. Regardless of the movement detection algorithm, Doppler-based EFM detected more than 95% of all body movements lasting more than 5 seconds and 100% of multiple movements seen during sonography (Besinger & Johnson, 1989; DiPietro, Costigan, & Pressman, 1999; Lowery et al., 1997). In addition, up to 80% of maternally perceived movements are recorded with EFM, whereas fewer than 20% of Doppler-recorded movements are detected by the mother. The large discrepancy may result from the ability of the Doppler-based device to detect small or single movements or to detect movements lasting fewer than 20 seconds (Johnson, Jordan, & Paine, 1990; Lowery et al.).

The Cochrane Library (Pattison & McCowan, 1999) reviewed reports concerning the reliability of antepartum CTG in reducing perinatal morbidity and mortality as well as maternal mortality. Four randomized controlled trials (RCTs) with a combined study population of more than 1,500 women with high-risk pregnancies achieved the review criteria, but antenatal CTG had no effect on perinatal or maternal outcomes. Although in one study women with CTG experienced significantly fewer hospital admissions and shorter patient stays, the reviewers concluded there was insufficient evidence to show that the use of antenatal CTG reduced fetal mortality (Pattison & McCowan).

NONSTRESS TEST

Introduced during the 1970s, the nonstress test (NST) has become a cornerstone of antenatal fetal surveillance. The NST evolved from early evidence that FHR accelerations were associated with fetal well-being (Lee, DiLoreto, & O'Lane, 1975) and that, conversely, the absence of FHR reactivity (acceleration), was associated with an increased risk of perinatal mortality (Rochard et al., 1976). In a subsequent investigation, contraction stress tests (CSTs) were always negative when two accelerations were recorded, and the criteria for NST reactivity (i.e., two accelerations in 20 minutes) evolved from that report (Evertson, Gauthier, Schifrin, & Paul, 1979).

The NST is technically easy to perform (Nageotte, Towers, Asrat, Freeman, & Dorchester, 1994b); lacks contraindications (Devoe & Jones, 2002); requires fewer resources than the contraction stress test (CST) and biophysical profile (Keegan & Paul, 1980); and can be used in inpatient, outpatient, and home settings (Naef et al., 1994; Reece, Hagay, Garofalo, & Hobbins, 1992). The NST is widely accepted as the primary testing modality for pregnancies at risk for

fetal demise (Devoe & Jones). Evidence supporting the NST is based on multiple-time series rather than randomized controlled trials (Devoe & Jones) in view of the fact that the random allocation of pregnant women to antepartum fetal surveillance versus care that does not include fetal surveillance is unlikely in today's practice of obstetrics in the United States (ACOG, 1999). A critical review of NST testing standards and diagnostic values reveal a wide range of test sensitivity, specificity and predictive values suggesting the NST is better at identifying fetal well-being than fetal compromise, and that its inclusion in the care and management of high-risk patients has been associated with an apparent reduction in intrauterine fetal deaths (Devoe & Jones).

Physiology of the Nonstress Test

FHR accelerations that accompany fetal movement reflect CNS alertness and activity (Freeman, Garite, & Nageotte, 2003). Rabinowitz, Persitz, and Sadovsky (1983), using simultaneous ultrasound imaging, confirmed that fetal movements were virtually always present when fetal accelerations were observed. FHR reactivity reflects adequate oxygenation and normal autonomic nervous system (ANS) function (ACOG, 1999). Fetal movement and FHR accelerations are highly correlated. Typically, fetal movement increases in a linear fashion until approximately 32 weeks, when movement decreases due to the constraints of the intrauterine environment imposed by the growing fetus (Blackburn, 2007; DiPietro et al., 1999; Pillai & James, 1990). More than 95% of accelerations have a synchronous onset or begin immediately after movement (Freeman, 1975; Lee et al., 1975). The frequency and amplitude of accelerations increase with gestational age (Dawes, Houghton, Redman, & Visser, 1982; Groome et al., 1997a; Snijders, McLaren, & Nicolaides, 1990).

The FHR response is reflective of the nature of fetal movement. For example, a larger increase in heart rate occurs with complex movements than with isolated fetal movements (Johnson, 1994). Heart rate variation with fetal movement is an important criterion for behavior states and demonstrates normal ANS function (Dawes et al., 1982; Nijhuis et al., 1982). As FHR variability increases, so do the number of movements as well as the number and amplitude of accelerations (Dawes et al.). The presence of accelerations, fetal movement, and variability usually preclude acidemia (Krebs, Petres, Dunn, & Smith, 1982; Ribbert, Snijders, Nicolaides, & Visser, 1990; Vintzileos & Knuppel, 1994; Walkinshaw, Cameron, MacPhail, & Robson, 1992). However, the absence of accelerations may be related to hypoxia, or may be due to normal fetal sleep cycles, CNS depression resulting from medications, or congenital anomalies (Freeman et al., 2003). Therefore, the absence of accelerations requires further investigation when fetal well-being is assessed.

The effects of hypoxia on NST results are unclear because the sequence of the FHR changes in the transition from normal oxygenation to asphyxia is unclear. Progressive hypoxia may cause the loss-of-state changes before the FHR fails to accelerate (Visser, Bekedam, & Ribbert, 1990a). As fetal compromise continues, the rest cycles lengthen, eventually disappearing, and FHR variability and fetal movement decrease. Subsequently, accelerations become smoother and less frequent, and they finally disappear. Before fetal death, variability has been reported to decrease to fewer than 5 beats per minute (bpm), with absent movement and FHR accelerations (Visser, Sadovsky, & Nicolaides, 1990b).

Clinical Application of the Nonstress Test

A key limitation of early antenatal testing was that its use was limited primarily to inpatient settings and populations. Development of the NST, which allowed testing in the outpatient arena, quickly changed the antenatal testing experience. Formerly limited to hypertensive disorders, insulin-dependent diabetes, or other se-

vere medical conditions, the indications for testing quickly expanded to include postdates, complaints of decreased fetal movement, and women with a history of previous fetal death (Paul & Miller, 1995).

Test Procedure and Interpretation

Assist the woman to a physiologically appropriate position, such as sidelying or semi-Fowler's with a lateral tilt. Assess fetal position with Leopold's maneuvers and apply the fetal monitor. Continuously record the FHR and uterine activity for the duration of the test. A lateral tilt position is usually recommended when performing an NST (ACOG, 1999); however, maternal semi-Fowler's position can shorten time to complete testing and has been associated with more reactive NSTs than supine positioning (Nathan, Haberman, Burgess, & Minkoff, 2000). Aortocaval compression can occur, however, when the maternal head is elevated less than 45 degrees, and maternal symptoms of supine hypotension can occur before a drop in blood pressure is recorded. Therefore, maternal position during NST should be determined by the clinical situation; supine positioning with the head lower than 45 degrees should be avoided (Moffatt & van den Hof, 1997).

Historically, many criteria have been suggested for interpreting the NST; however, the currently accepted criteria for a reactive test is the presence of two accelerations (spontaneous or acoustically stimulated) within a 20-minute period for fetuses greater than 32 weeks' gestation (AAP & ACOG, 2007; Macones, Hankins, Spong, Hauth, & Moore, 2008). The FHR accelerations should peak at least 15 bpm above the baseline and last 15 seconds in duration from the beginning to the end of the acceleration (baseline to baseline). The peak in amplitude does not have to be sustained at 15 bpm above baseline; rather, the total duration of the increase in heart rate must be at least 15 seconds (ACOG, 1999; Macones, et al., 2008). The monitoring period may be extended to 40 minutes to accommodate normal fetal sleep-wake cycles (AAP & ACOG, 2007; ACOG).

Castillo and associates (1989) recommended lower-amplitude criteria for fetuses less than 32 weeks gestation to reduce the confounding affect of gestational age. In 1997, the NICHD workgroup on FHR monitoring concurred that a minimal threshold for acceleration should reflect gestational age norms, and this was reaffirmed in 2008. In fetuses less than 32 weeks gestation, accelerations are defined as abrupt FHR increases peaking at least 10 bpm above the baseline, and lasting at least 10 seconds (Macones, et al., 2008). Therefore a reactive NST in a fetus under 32 weeks gestation exhibits at least two 10 bpm x 10 second accelerations in a 20-minute period.

The NST is interpreted as reactive or nonreactive (Figure 11-2a & b). A reactive NST meets the stated gestational age criteria with or without maternal perception of fetal movement. Documentation of fetal movement is not necessary (Freeman et al., 2003). A nonreactive NST is defined as fewer than two accelerations meeting the above criteria during a 40-minute period (AAP &

ACOG, 2007; ACOG, 1999). A nonreactive NST typically requires additional follow-up with testing such as ultrasound or BPP (Devoe, 1999).

Variable Decelerations during a Nonstress Test

Variable decelerations occur in as many as half of NSTs (Meis et al., 1986) and have been associated with umbilical cord compression (O'Leary, Andrinopoulos, & Giordano, 1980). Perinatal outcomes following NSTs with variable decelerations may vary depending on the depth, duration, and frequency of FHR changes and the overall reactivity of the NST. A reactive NST accompanied by intermittent variable decelerations lasting less than 30 seconds is not typically indicative of fetal compromise and usually requires no intervention in the absence of other conditions or cause for concern (ACOG, 1999). However "nonreassuring" intrapartum FHR patterns occured more often after a NST with three or more variable decelerations of more than 15 seconds duration (Glantz & D'Amico, 2001;

Figure 11-2a   Reactive NST

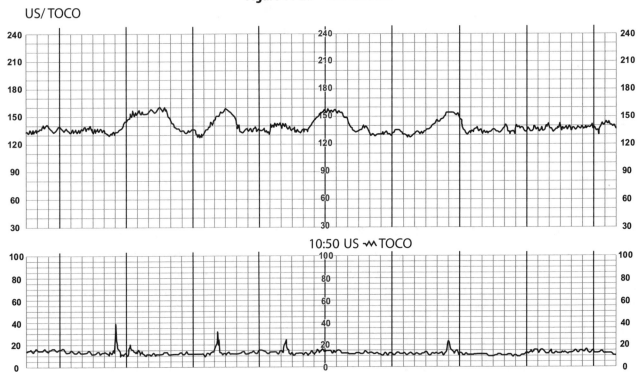

Figure 11-2b   Nonreactive NST

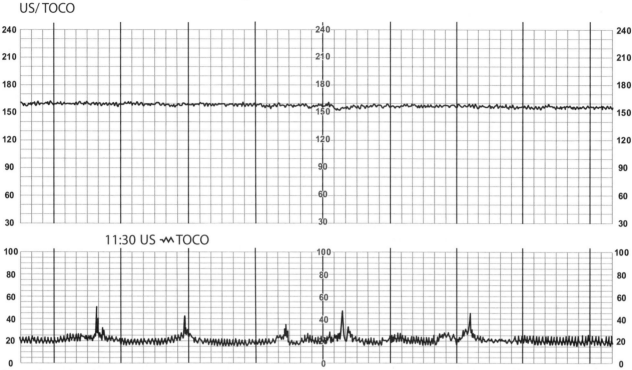

O'Leary et al.). NSTs with repetitive prolonged decelerations are associated with a greater risk of "nonreassuring" FHR patterns; cord complications (e.g., multiple nuchal or occult), and meconium (Jaschevatzky et al., 1998). Oligohydramnios has been reported to be present in study groups in which NSTs revealed variable decelerations (Glantz & D'Amico; Hoskins, Frieden, & Young, 1991). The risk of cesarean birth for alterations in FHR patterns has been shown to increase progressively with the worsening severity of antepartum decelerations and decreasing amniotic fluid volume (Hoskins et al.). Therefore, further evaluation is recommended when repetitive variable decelerations occur during an NST.

Efficacy of Nonstress Tests

A reactive NST with normal amniotic fluid volume is indicative of fetal well-being in 99% of pregnancies (Shalev, Zalel, & Weiner, 1993;

Vintzileos et al., 1987) and has a false-negative rate (e.g., stillbirth of a nonanomalous fetus or neonate within 1 week of a reactive NST) of less than 1% (Miller, Rabello, & Paul, 1996). However, a nonreactive NST is much less reliable in predicting adverse perinatal outcomes, and false-positive rates (e.g., normal newborn after a nonreactive NST) of greater than 90% have been reported (Miller-Slade et al., 1991; Mills, James, & Slade, 1990). Many factors can affect the accuracy of the NST and contribute to the high rate of false-positive results; of those, a significant influence is gestational age. Antenatal testing may begin for patients at risk for stillbirth at 32–34 weeks gestation and may be indicated at 26–28 weeks depending on the clinical circumstances. False-positive results occur in more than 15% of NST's performed before 32 weeks gestation (AAP & ACOG, 2007). The large proportion of nonreactive tests in premature fetuses is concerning because of the risk for potentially unnecessary intervention with false-positive tests.

Several conditions other than hypoxemia can reduce heart rate reactivity or interfere with fetal movement and should be considered when interpreting NSTs (Manning, 1995). During quiet sleep, the FHR tracing may have nonreactive features (e.g., diminished FHR variability, reduced fetal movement), but with a state change, the FHR can become reactive (Groome et al., 1999; Nijhuis et al., 1982). At term, the fetus is in a quiet sleep state approximately 30% of the time (Groome et al., 1999). Thus, extending the observation period until a fetus becomes more active can reduce the incidence of nonreactive NSTs (Ware & Devoe, 1994). Maternal cigarette smoking and chronic maternal stress affect the FHR, fetal movement, and NST results (Groome et al., 1995; Thaler, Goodman, & Dawes, 1980). Ingestion of substances such as caffeine, cocaine, morphine, sedatives, and alcohol has also been associated with false-positive NST results (Devoe et al., 1993; Kopecky et al., 2000; Rizk, Atterbury, & Groome, 1996; Vintzileos et al., 1987). In addition, poor maternal nutritional status can decrease FHR reactivity (Onyeije & Divon, 2001).

FETAL STIMULATION

Various methods of fetal stimulation have been proposed to improve the reliability of antepartum surveillance and to differentiate nonreactive NSTs caused by hypoxia from those associated with fetal sleep states or narcosis. Three methods of fetal stimulation have been reviewed by the Cochrane Collaboration, including vibroacoustic stimulation (VAS), fetal manipulation, and glucose administration. Fetal manipulation (e.g., abdominal rocking) has been used during nonreactive NSTs in two trials, with no demonstrated effect on the efficacy of antepartum testing (Tan & Sabapathy, 2001a). Glucose administration increases fetal breathing, but oral (e.g., orange juice) or intravenous glucose administration did not decrease the incidence of nonreactive NSTs in two trials with fewer than 1,000 participants (Tan & Sabapathy, 2001b). The reviewers concluded that there was no benefit to antepartum surveillance from either fetal manipulation or glucose administration, and further research with both methods was recommended (Tan & Sabapathy, 2001a, 2001b).

Vibroacoustic Stimulation

Fetal hearing begins at approximately 24 to 25 weeks gestation, and auditory-provoked responses can be recorded as early as 25 to 26 weeks. External environmental sounds are audible to the fetus; high-frequency sounds are attenuated, but low-frequency sounds are not (Blackburn, 2007). Fetal response to sound has been studied since the 1920s. The first reported evidence of VAS-induced FHR accelerations and movement was by Sontag and Wallace (1936). Walker, Grimwade, and Wood (1971) reported a substantial increase in the number, amplitude, and duration of VAS stimulated FHR accelerations. Subsequent VAS studies demonstrated a decrease in the number of falsely abnormal FHR pattern interpretations and shortened NST testing time without adversely affecting perinatal outcomes (Sarno & Bruner, 1990; Serafini et al., 1984; Smith, Phelan, Paul, & Broussard, 1985; Smith, Phelan, Platt, Broussard, & Paul, 1986). The expected fetal responses to VAS are FHR accelerations and increased gross body movements (Clark, Sabey, & Jolley, 1989; Sarno, Ahn, Phelan, & Paul, 1990). Although some differences in specific FHR responses have been reported (Gagnon, Hunse, & Patrick, 1988; Jensen & Flottorp, 1982), a single startle response and acceleration of the FHR in response to VAS is associated with a functional brainstem, regardless of gestational age (Groome, Mooney, Holland, Smith, & Atterbury, 1997b).

The fetal response to sound has been tested using different sound intensities, frequencies, and durations. The VAS significantly increases the baseline intrauterine sound level, exposing the fetus to a sound intensity similar to the takeoff of a jet airplane (Smith, 1995). The primary device used to generate a stimulus for VAS is an artificial larynx (Clark et al., 1989; Miller-Slade, et al.,

1991; Sarno et al., 1990; Yao et al., 1990). The commercially available device produces 82 decibels at 1-meter air (Sarno et al.). Although the long-term sequelae of VAS stimulation on hearing or cognition are not clearly understood, fetuses clinically exposed to VAS have had no reported adverse effects when the children reached 4 years of age (Nyman, Barr, & Westgren, 1992). Different stimulus durations have been used, including 1-, 2-, 3-, and 5-second durations (Clark et al.; Saraço lu, Göl, Sahin, Türkkani, & Oztopçu, 1999; Sarno et al.). A significant increase in the amplitude and duration of accelerations has been associated with 3- and 5-second stimuli durations (Pietrantoni et al., 1991).

Several investigations have explored the reliability of antepartum testing with VAS compared with other surveillance methods. Significantly more visualized or palpated fetal movements occurred after VAS than without stimulation; and evoked accelerations were associated with more than 99% of reactive NSTs (Marden, McDuffie, Allen, & Abitz, 1997) and 100% of negative CSTs (Read & Miller, 1977). Compared with standard NSTs, acoustic stimulation reduced the incidence of false-positive tests (Clark et al., 1989; Saraço lu et al., 1999; Serafini et al., 1984; Smith et al., 1986), and an impaired or absent response was a better predictor of perinatal outcomes than NSTs alone (Saraço lu et al.; Trudinger & Boylan, 1980). In addition, VAS reduced the incidence of nonreactive NSTs by as much as 50% and decreased the average test duration by 10 to 20 minutes (Clark et al.; Miller-Slade et al., 1990; Saraço lu et al.).

Test Procedure and Interpretation

A commercially available artificial larynx may be used to perform acoustic stimulation when indicated. The procedure includes positioning the artificial larynx on the maternal abdomen near the fetal head and applying the stimulus for 1 second (ACOG, 1999). If the NST remains nonreactive, acoustic stimulation may be repeated at

1-minute intervals up to three times, progressively increasing the stimuli time to 3 seconds (ACOG). A reactive NST using VAS is considered a valid indicator of fetal well-being (ACOG). However, if the NST is still nonreactive following VAS, the test should be followed with a BPP or CST (Druzin, Smith, Gabbe, & Reed, 2007).

No differences in perinatal outcome (e.g., meconium-stained amniotic fluid, Apgar scores < 7) have been reported following NSTs with spontaneous or stimulated accelerations (Sarno et al., 1990; Serafini et al., 1984; Smith, Phelan, Nguyen, Jacobs, & Paul, 1988). A Cochrane Collaboration review of the literature concerning fetal vibroacoustic stimulation tests revealed that VAS reduced the incidence of nonreactive antepartum NSTs and reduced the overall testing time (Tan & Smyth, 2001). The reviewers were unable to draw conclusions about the efficacy of VAS because the prevalence of perinatal morbidity and mortality in the reviewed studies was too small. In addition, the reviewers observed that there is a paucity of literature concerning fetal hearing and neurologic development after sound stimulation and that little is known about maternal anxiety and maternal satisfaction regarding testing. The reviewers concluded that VAS offered benefits by reducing the incidence of nonreactive NSTs as well as the time to complete testing, but future research was recommended to define the optimal stimulus intensity, frequency, duration, and position and to determine the efficacy, reliability, safety, and perinatal outcomes associated with VAS (Tan & Smyth).

CONTRACTION STRESS TEST AND THE OXYTOCIN CHALLENGE TEST

The CST was the first antepartum surveillance method developed following the advent of electronic FHR monitoring and quickly became a primary fetal evaluation technique, replacing technically more difficult and prognostically less accurate biochemical (estriol) analyses. As an antepartum test, the CST evolved from animal studies in which the flow of oxygenated blood into the intervillous space ceased during uterine contractions stronger than 30 mm Hg; this, in turn, resulted in transient reductions of fetal oxygen pressure (PO_2) and caused late decelerations of the FHR. The mechanism for late decelerations during antepartum evaluation of a potentially chronically stressed fetus is the same as that of an acutely stressed fetus during labor (see Chapter 5) (Olofsson, Thuring-Jönsson, & Marsál, 1996).

The CST is based on the principle of gradually developing uteroplacental insufficiency (Lagrew, 1995). Fetal acidemia is more likely to occur with chronic uteroplacental insufficiency and may not cause obvious changes in the fetal response during periods without uterine activity. However, in a chronically stressed fetus, the additional acute stress of even small contractions can result in hypoxemia and late decelerations (Lagrew; Paul & Miller, 1995).

Over time, the chronically stressed fetus can also develop oligohydramnios, thus reducing the normal volume of amniotic fluid that surrounds and protects the umbilical cord. Therefore, the cord may be vulnerable, and if it is compressed during uterine contractions, variable decelerations may appear on the FHR tracing (ACOG, 1999).

Clinical Application of the Contraction Stress Test

As a primary means of fetal surveillance, the CST has a low incidence of unexpected fetal death within 1 week of negative test results (Freeman et al., 2003). Nevertheless, Freeman et al. cite a number of concerns associated with its use as a primary surveillance technique, including:

- High false-positive rate
- Frequent equivocal test results
- Time needed to perform the test
- Cost
- Inconvenience compared with other testing techniques.

The development of the NST, BPP, and modified BPP has replaced the CST in many practice settings (Freeman et al., 2003). Relative contraindications to the CST are conditions associated with an increased risk of preterm labor and delivery, preterm rupture of membranes, previous classical uterine incision or history of extensive uterine surgery, previous uterine rupture, known placenta previa or other uterine bleeding (AAP & ACOG, 2007; ACOG, 1999).

Uterine Contractions

Antepartum evaluation using the CST requires uterine activity that mimics the stress of early labor. The minimal number of contractions needed to adequately assess fetal health has not been clearly established, but the criteria for evaluation of the CST were extrapolated from studies performed in the 1970s (Lagrew, 1995; Paul & Miller, 1995). A primary limitation of external uterine monitoring is that only the frequency and duration of contractions—and not the intensity of contractions—can be assessed. However, the important assessment parameter for the CST is the FHR response to uterine contractions, regardless of the intensity.

Test Procedure

The CST is administered with the woman in the lateral recumbent (or semi-Fowler's) position, and the FHR and uterine activity are monitored for at least 10 minutes with external Doppler ultrasound and tocotransducers (ACOG, 1999). During the initial period of monitoring, if three or more spontaneous contractions lasting at least 40 seconds occur in a 10-minute period, additional uterine stimulation is unnecessary (AAP & ACOG 2007; ACOG). Intravenous (IV) oxytocin infusion or breast stimulation may be used to stimulate contractions if none are present within the first 10 to 20 minutes. The use of IV oxytocin for a CST, referred to as an oxytocin challenge test (OCT), is initiated at 0.5 to 1 mUnits per minute and increased every 15 to 20 minutes until at least three contractions occur in 10 minutes (AAP & ACOG).

An alternative method for a CST is breast stimulation (ACOG, 1999). The procedure is as follows: one nipple is massaged gently through clothing for 2 minutes or until a contraction begins. If the contraction criteria are not met, the patient rests for 5 minutes and the alternate nipple is stimulated. If breast stimulation is unsuccessful (contractions have not begun), an OCT can be initiated using the technique described earlier (AAP & ACOG, 2007; ACOG). Although breast stimulation has been associated with tachysystole (Schellpfeffer, Hoyle, & Johnson, 1985), similar rates of tachysystole, positive CST results, and successful tests with both IV oxytocin and breast stimulation methods have been reported in the literature (Lipitz, Barkai, Rabinovici, & Mashiach, 1987; Oki, Keegan, Freeman, & Dorchester, 1987).

Interpretation

CST interpretation is based on the presence or absence of FHR decelerations and FHR reactivity in response to uterine contractions (Figure 11-3a, b, c, d, e). According to AAP and ACOG (2007), CST interpretation criteria can be categorized as follows:

- Negative: No late or significant variable decelerations are identified (Figure 11-3a).
- Positive: Late decelerations are identified with 50% or more of contractions, even if the contraction frequency is less than three in 10 minutes (Figure 11-3b).
- Equivocal—Suspicious: Intermittent late (late decelerations with fewer than 50% of contractions) or significant variable decelerations are observed (Figure 11-3c).
- Equivocal—"Hyperstimulatory": Uterine contractions occur more frequently than every 2 minutes or last longer than 90 seconds with accompanying late decelerations (Figure 11-3d).
- Equivocal—Unsatisfactory: Fewer than three contractions occur within 10 minutes, or a tracing quality that cannot be interpreted (Figure 11-3e).

A negative CST is noted in 80% to 90% of tests. In the absence of clinical deterioration, the interval between CSTs is generally 7 days, although more frequent evaluation (including NST or BPP) may be indicated for conditions such as postterm pregnancy, diabetes, intrauterine growth restriction, or hypertension (ACOG, 1999; Huddleston, 2002). Isolated or recurrent variable deceleration may occur as a result of oligohydramnios and subsequent cord compression. The presence of variable decelerations should prompt consideration for ultrasound evaluation of the amniotic fluid volume and umbilical cord localization (Devoe, 1999). Equivocal results usually necessitate repeating the CST within 24 hours unless the woman is post term or other indications for delivery are present. Management of women with positive CST results should be individualized and based on evaluation of the woman's total clinical picture (ACOG). Positive CSTs correlate with intrauterine growth restriction, increased incidence of late decelerations in labor, and low 5-minute Apgar scores (Lagrew, 1995).

Efficacy of the Contraction Stress Test

A negative CST is highly reliable and correlates with good fetal outcomes (Lagrew, 1995). However, a significant limitation of the CST is its high false-positive rate (positive test findings in a person without disease), which can result in unnecessary intervention (Druzin et al., 2007). False-positive rates greater than 30% have been reported following CST (Gauthier, Evertson, & Paul, 1979; Shalev et al., 1993). Therefore, follow-up of positive CST results should be individualized and based on evaluation of the woman's total clinical picture (ACOG, 1999).

FETAL BIOPHYSICAL PROFILE

In response to the high proportion of false-positive NST and CST results, Manning, Platt, and Sipos (1980) proposed an assessment of fetal well-being that combined NST results with multiple physiologic parameters observed with real-time ultrasound. The BPP was based on previous reports that fetal activities such as breathing, decreased with hypoxia or narcosis (Manning & Platt, 1979). Furthermore, the BPP was based on the theory

Figure 11-3a   Negative OCT

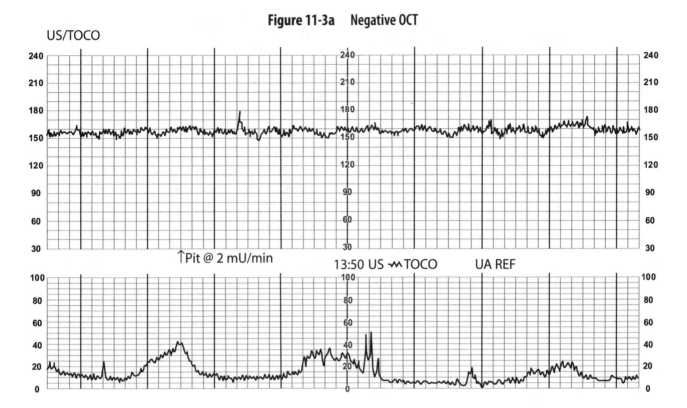

↑Pit @ 2 mU/min   13:50 US ᨀ TOCO   UA REF

Figure 11-3b   Positive CST

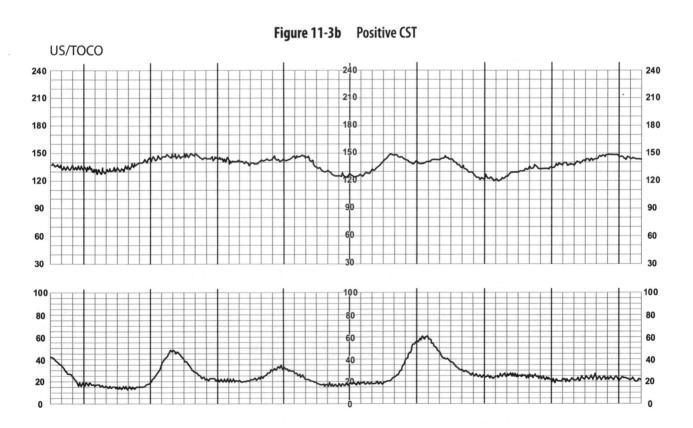

Figure 11-3c   Equivocal/Suspicious CST

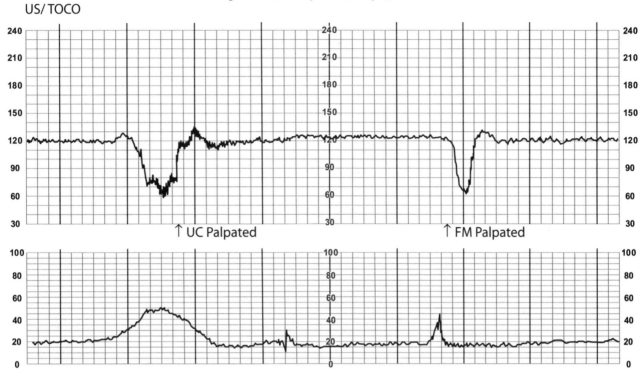

US/ TOCO

↑ UC Palpated   ↑ FM Palpated

Figure 11-3d   Equivocal-"Hyperstimulatory" OCT

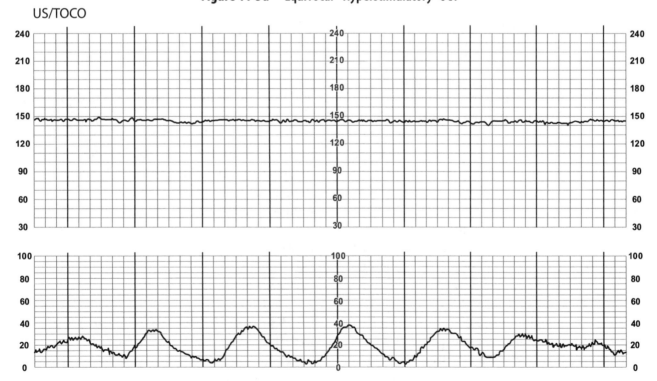

US/TOCO

Figure 11-3e   Unsatisfactory CST

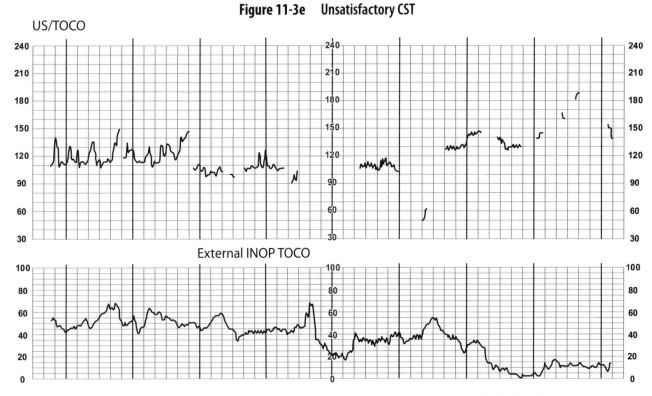

that acute and chronic hypoxia cause the reduction or cessation of fetal activities in a particular order, so that the absence of one or more parameters could represent the degree of fetal hypoxic stress (Manning, Morrison, Lange, & Harman, 1982).

The BPP provided improved prognostic information over other antepartum FHR tests because fetal physiologic parameters associated with both chronic (amniotic fluid volume, gross body movements, and tone) and acute (heart rate reactivity and breathing movements) hypoxia were evaluated (Manning et al., 1980). Thus, the BPP includes the assessment of the following five components: (1) fetal breathing movement, (2) gross body movement, (3) fetal tone, (4) amniotic fluid volume, and (5) FHR reactivity (NST).

The fetal activities observed during the BPP result from complex processes within the CNS and ANS, and the presence of each suggests normal neurologic function and adequate oxygenation (Vintzileos et al., 1987). Fetal activities decrease or cease as a means of reducing energy and oxygen consumption as fetal hypoxemia worsens,

and it occurs in the reverse order of normal neurologic development (Table 11-3). Fetal activities that appear earliest in pregnancy (i.e., tone and movement) are usually the last to be affected; conversely, activities last to develop (i.e., breathing and FHR reactivity) are usually the first to be suppressed (Vintzileos & Knuppel, 1994). The presence of fetal activities (FHR accelerations, breathing, movement, and tone) indicates normal central oxygenation (Manning et al., 1993) depending on gestational age, whereas the clinical significance of absent activities is more difficult to determine because factors other than hypoxia can cause CNS depression (e.g., sedatives, narcotics, anesthetics) (Manning et al., 1982; Vintzileos, Campbell, Ingardia, & Nochimson, 1983).

Clinical Application of the Biophysical Profile

Multiple studies have been undertaken worldwide to develop the scoring criteria, interpretation, and proposed management for BPP (Manning et al., 1980; Vintzileos et al., 1983). In

Table 11-3	Embryology of the CNS Centers Responsible for Fetal Activities		
ACTIVITY	CNS CENTER	GESTATIONAL AGE OF DEVELOPMENT	HYPOXIA*
Tone	Cortex—subcortical	7.5–8.5 weeks	↑
Movement	Cortex—nuclei	9.0 weeks	
Breathing	Ventral surface, 4th ventricle	20–21 weeks	
Fetal heart rate	Posterior hypothalamus, medulla	28--32 weeks	

CNS, Central nervous system.
*The arrow indicates the order in which hypoxia affects fetal activities.
Adapted from: Manning, 1995; Vintzileos & Knuppel, 1994.

Table 11-4	Biophysical Profile Scoring	
BIOPHYSICAL VARIABLE	NORMAL SCORE (SCORE = 2 POINTS)	ABNORMAL (SCORE = 0 POINTS)
Fetal Breathing Movements	At least 1 episode of FBM of at least 30 sec duration in 30 min	Absent FBM or no episodes > 30 sec in 30 min
Gross Body Movement	At least 3 discrete body/limb movements in 30 min (episodes of active continuous movement considered as single movement)	2 or fewer episodes of body/ limb movements in 30 min
Fetal Tone	At least 1 episode of active extension with return to flexion of fetal limb(s) or truck. Opening and closing of hand is considered normal tone	Either slow extension with return to partial flexion or movement of limb in full extension. Absent movement
Reactive FHR	At least 2 episodes of FHR accelerations of ≥15 beats/min and of least 15 sec duration associated with fetal movement in 30 min	<2 episodes of accelerations of FHR or accelerations <15 bpm in 30 min
Qualitative AFV	At least 1 pocket of AF that measures at least 2 cm in 2 perpendicular planes	Either no AF pockets or a pocket <2 cm in 2 perpendicular planes

AF, Amniotic fluid; bpm, beats per minute; FHR, fetal heart rate; V, volume.
Source: Manning, F. (1995). Dynamic ultrasound-based fetal assessment: The fetal biophysical profile score. *Clinical Obstetrics and Gynecology, 38*(1), 35. Copyright 1995 by J.B. Lippincott Company. Reprinted with permission.

initial descriptions, an NST was performed first, and if nonreactive after 20 minutes, the FHR was monitored for an additional 20 minutes (Vintzileos & Knuppel, 1994). An ultrasound examination followed, and a score was assigned for each parameter detected during a 30-minute observation period. The scoring criteria for BPPs are listed in Table 11-4 (Manning, 1995).

Test Procedure and Interpretation

During a real-time sonogram, the biophysical variables are monitored simultaneously until the normal criteria for each have been observed, or for a total observation period of 30 minutes. A system for BPP interpretation and management is summarized in Table 11-5. The average time to complete the BPP is 10 to 20 minutes when performed by an experienced sonographer (Manning et al., 1981, 1982). Normal fetal gross body movement is classified by at least three rolling movements of the extremities or trunk (Vintzileos et al., 1987), and fetal tone is defined by extension of the extremities with return to flexion or by opening and closing of the fetal hand (Manning et al., 1980).

Fetal breathing is the continuous movement of the chest or abdominal walls lasting at least

Table 11-5	Biophysical Profile Interpretation and Suggested Management	
SCORE	**INTERPRETATION**	**MANAGEMENT**
8-10	Reassuring	• Consider increased frequency of testing or delivery if oligo-hydramnios is present
6	Equivocal	• Term fetus – consider delivery • Preterm fetus – retest within 12 – 24 hours • Consider increased frequency of testing or delivery if oligo-hydramnios is present
4 or less	Non-reassuring	• Further evaluation is indicated • Consider delivery

Adapted from AAP & ACOG, 2007

30 seconds, with breath-to-breath intervals shorter than 6 seconds. Amniotic fluid volume is determined by the presence of at least one pocket of fluid measuring 2 cm or more in the vertical axis (Manning, 1995; Vintzileos & Knuppel, 1994). The NST may be performed before or after observation and assessment of the ultrasound components of the BPP (Manning; Vintzileos et al., 1987).

The usual interval between BPP examinations is 1 week (Manning et al., 1991), but more frequent testing may be used for specific high-risk conditions. In addition, the optimal gestational age at which to initiate antepartum surveillance with the BPP has not been established, and recommendations range from 24 to 25 weeks (Manning, 1995) to 32 to 34 weeks (ACOG, 1999; Miller et al., 1996). As is the case with most antepartum testing methods, the interpretation of the BPP score is based on consideration of the maternal and fetal clinical situation, and a management approach based on specific pregnancy complications is also recommended (Vintzileos & Knuppel, 1994).

Efficacy of the Biophysical Profile

A BPP score of 10/10 is associated with normal fetal oxygenation and development more than 99.9% of the time (ACOG, 1999). In con-

trast, a significant inverse relationship exists between a worsening fetal cord pH and the absence of FHR reactivity, fetal breathing, movement, and tone—in that order (Vintzileos & Knuppel, 1994). However, there is less conformity regarding the predictive accuracy of abnormal results because of differences in study methodologies, participants, and sample size and a lack of standard criteria for BPP interpretation and divergent outcome definitions across studies. Although multiple cohort and case-controlled studies of the BPP have reported encouraging results, the BPP has been studied in only a small number of RCTs (Lalor, Fawole, Alfirevic & Neilson, 2007). Therefore, BPP scores between normal (8/10 or 10/10) and the most abnormal (0/10) require further testing and consideration when making management plans for follow-up care (Boehm & Gabbe, 2002).

Nursing Role in Biophysical Profile Testing

The BPP was developed in an antepartum testing center where the majority of ultrasound examinations were performed by nurses with special education (Manning et al., 1981). An increasing number of nurses have completed additional training to conduct a fetal assessment with real-time Doppler sonography, and the BPP interpretation by specially trained nurses has been shown to be equal to or better than that of medical subspecialists (Gegor, Paine, Costigan, & Johnson, 1994). The BPP is an ultrasound examination of limited scope that may be performed by nurses who have completed additional education and who can demonstrate competence to perform limited obstetric ultrasound (Association of Women's Health, Obstetric and Neonatal Nurses [AWHONN], 1994). Furthermore, nurses should verify that performing limited obstetric ultrasound is within their scope of practice as defined by state or provincial licensing bodies and is consistent with individual facility regulations (AWHONN, 1998). Nurses who use specialized skills such as sonography are professionally responsible for documentation of specialized training used to determine initial competence, are responsible for maintenance of competence, and may participate in establishing local policies and procedures (Gegor et al., 1994; Raines, 1996).

Modified Biophysical Profile

Amniotic fluid volume may reflect a normal decline near or beyond term or may be indicative of fetal hypoxia. Hypoxic fetuses demonstrate a physiologic redistribution or "shunting" of cardiac output to allow for greater oxygenation of the heart, brain, and adrenals while decreasing blood flow to other organs, such as the kidneys, gut, and skeletal systems (Manning, 1995). That response may be followed by a decrease in renal function and then a decrease in fetal urine, which is the primary component of amniotic fluid in the third trimester. Thus, oligohydramnios can reflect long-term uteroplacental function, acute or chronic fetal asphyxia, and an increased risk for adverse perinatal outcomes (Chauhan et al., 2004). Those concepts led to the development of the so-called modified BPP, which combines the NST and an ultrasound-obtained amniotic fluid volume index as a test of uteroplacental function (Nageotte, Towers, Asrat, & Freeman, 1994a). The amniotic fluid index (AFI) represents the sum of the measurements (in centimeters) of the deepest umbilical cord–free pockets of amniotic fluid in all four abdominal quadrants (ACOG, 1999).

The modified BPP consists of an NST and a measurement of AFI as indicators of short-term fetal well-being and long-term placental function, respectively (ACOG, 1999). A modified BPP is considered normal when the NST is reactive and the AFI is greater than 5 cm (ACOG). The modified BPP has the advantage of requiring less time to complete, and it is associated with similar perinatal outcomes when compared with antepartum tests (Nageotte et al., 1994b; Shah, Brown, Salyer, Fleischer, & Boehm, 1989).

DOPPLER ULTRASOUND VELOCIMETRY OF THE UMBILICAL ARTERY

Doppler ultrasound velocimetry of the umbilical artery is a noninvasive technique used to assess resistance to blood flow within the placenta (AAP & ACOG, 2007). It is easy to perform and has been the subject of more RCTs than any other test evaluating fetal well-being (Boehm & Gabbe, 2002). Doppler ultrasound waves are transmitted at one frequency and reflected back to the transducer at a different frequency. When directed at blood vessels, the frequency of the reflected sound is determined by the direction and velocity of the blood cells. (Druzin et al., 2007). This frequency change is called a "Doppler shift." Changes in blood flow represent systolic and diastolic shifts that occur during the cardiac cycle (Woods, Glantz, Pittinaro, & Giffi, 2007). The Doppler test result, or S/D ratio, represents the ratio between the velocity of blood flow during systole and diastole and is a reflection of placental vascular resistance to flow (Druzin et al.; Woods et al.). The **S** represents the peak systolic velocity, and the **D** represents the velocity of flow at the end of diastole (Woods et al.). As resistance increases, diastolic flow decreases and the S/D ratio increases (AAP & ACOG).

The umbilical artery velocimetry appears to correlate best with fetal outcomes and is based on the physiologic principle that with increasing gestational age there is a decrease in placental resistance and a decrease in the systolic to diastolic ratio (Boehm & Gabbe, 2002). S/D ratios are high early in pregnancy and decrease with advancing gestational age. An S/D ratio greater than 3 beyond 30 weeks' gestation is considered abnormal (Druzin et al., 2007). At the most extreme end of the spectrum, abnormal results are absent end-diastolic flow and reverse flow, respectively (Figure 11-4). When placental resistance remains elevated, there may be no blood flow during diastole (absent end-diastolic flow); in the worst case, flow may even be reversed (reverse flow). In these cases the fetus may be se-

Figure 11-4 Examples of Umbilical Doppler Flow Results

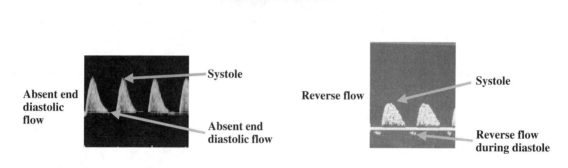

verely compromised. Further testing for fetal well-being is indicated (Woods et al., 2007). Both absent end-diastolic flow and reverse flow are associated with an increased risk of perinatal morbidity and mortality; however, reverse flow is even more indicative of a poor outcome (Druzin et al.).

Umbilical artery Doppler velocimetry is not recommended as an independent testing modality (Boehm & Gabbe, 2002), and, in fact, a large number of studies have shown that blood flow investigation is of little value in low-risk pregnancies (Westergaard, Langhoff, Lingman, & Marsai, 2001). However, when used in high-risk pregnancies, especially intrauterine growth restriction, the use of Doppler velocimetry significantly lowered perinatal mortality by 34% (Westergaard et al.). Studies have also shown that additional antenatal testing is unnecessary in suspected growth restriction when the Doppler result is normal. Conversely, abnormal Doppler findings are helpful in identifying a growth-restricted fetus at risk for a poor outcome where implementation of antenatal testing is advisable to monitor fetal well-being (Boehm & Gabbe).

SUMMARY

A great deal remains unknown about the benefits and risks of antepartum surveillance. Adverse perinatal outcomes are infrequent, which is an important factor in the overall positive pre-

dictive ability of each of the antepartum tests described in this chapter. The indications for testing vary among studies, but testing is usually reserved for maternal or fetal conditions associated with risks for uteroplacental insufficiency and stillbirth. Numerous lists of indications for antepartum testing have been proposed, although the efficacy of any test to predict long-term perinatal outcomes for complicated or normal pregnancies has not been determined. There is, however, a recognized need among clinicians for practice guidelines derived from evidence-based research. Condition-specific fetal testing that takes into account the underlying pathophysiology has been proposed (Kontopoulos & Vintzileos, 2004).

The optimal gestational age at which testing should begin continues to be the subject of research, and prematurity has confounding effects on the predictive value of surveillance. Different protocols for testing, including the intervals between tests and management of nonreactive results, have been recommended, but the ideal scheme has not yet been identified.

The use of low- and high-technology fetal assessment methods has led to a decrease in perinatal death and complications in pregnancies with identified risk factors for uteroplacental insufficiency. One goal of fetal testing is to reduce the frequency of preventable stillbirths secondary to hypoxic insults; however, half of all unexpected fetal deaths occur in women with low-risk pregnancies without identifiable risk factors that would make them candidates for antepartum fetal testing. Although antepartum surveillance is yet of unproven value, it is a widely integrated and accepted clinical practice and has been consistently associated with substantially lower rates of fetal death in both untested (presumably lower-risk) pregnancies and pregnancies with similar complicating factors that were managed before the advent of currently employed techniques of antepartum surveillance.

Research aimed at improving existing tests and technologies, and developing new technologies is ongoing. Computerized systems for interpreting antepartum FHR tracings and BPPs have been developed and may improve the prognostic ability of current antepartum tests while reducing the time needed for completion (Bracero, Morgan, & Byrne, 1999). Nurses' responsibilities and roles are expanding in the care of high-risk pregnant women. Ongoing assessment and evaluation, patient care, education, research, and application of evidence-based interventions can improve the outcomes for both women and their newborns.

REFERENCES

American Academy of Pediatrics (AAP) & American College of Obstetricians and Gynecologists (ACOG). (2007). *Guidelines for perinatal care* (6th ed.). Elk Grove Village, IL: Authors.

American College of Obstetricians and Gynecologists (ACOG). (1999). *Antepartum fetal surveillance* (Practice Bulletin No. 9). Washington, DC: Author.

American College of Obstetricians and Gynecologists (ACOG) & American Academy of Pediatrics (AAP). (2003). *Neonatal encephalopathy and cerebral palsy: Defining the pathogenesis and pathophysiology.* Washington, DC: Author.

Association of Women's Health, Obstetric and Neonatal Nurses (AWHONN). (2005). *Advanced fetal monitoring course.* Washington DC: Author.

Association of Women's Health, Obstetric and Neonatal Nurses (AWHONN). (1994). *Clinical competencies and education guide: Limited ultrasound examinations in obstetric and gynecologic/infertility settings.* Washington, DC: Author.

Association of Women's Health, Obstetric and Neonatal Nursing (1998). Achieving consistent quality care. Washington, DC: Author.

Baser, I., Johnson, T. R., & Paine, L. L. (1992). Coupling of fetal movement and fetal heart rate accelerations as an indicator of fetal health. *Obstetrics and Gynecology, 80*(1), 62–66.

Besinger, R. E., & Johnson, T. R. (1989). Doppler recordings of fetal movement: Clinical correlation with real-time ultrasound. *Obstetrics and Gynecology, 74*(2), 277–280.

Blackburn, S. (2007). Neurologic, muscular, and sensory systems. In S. Tucker Blackburn (Ed.), *Maternal, fetal, & neonatal physiology: A clinical perspective* (3rd ed., pp. 542–597). St. Louis: Saunders.

Boehm, F. H., Fields, L. M., Hutchison, J. M., Bowen, A. W., & Vaughn, W. K. (1986). The indirectly obtained fetal heart rate: Comparison of first and second generation electronic fetal monitors. *American Journal of Obstetrics and Gynecology, 155*(1), 10–14.

Boehm, F. H., & Gabbe, S. G. (2002). Putting it all together. *Clinical Obstetrics, 45*(4), 1063–1068.

Bracero, L. A., Morgan, S., & Byrne, D. W. (1999). Comparison of visual and computerized interpretation of nonstress test results in a randomized controlled trial. *American Journal of Obstetrics and Gynecology, 181*(5 Pt. 1), 1254–1258.

Castillo, R. A., Devoe, L. D., Arthur, M., Searle, N., Metheny, W. P., & Ruedrich, D. A. (1989). The preterm nonstress test: Effects of gestational age and length of study. *American Journal of Obstetrics and Gynecology, 160*(1), 172–175.

Centers for Disease Control and Prevention (CDC) & National Center for Health Statistics (NCHS). (2001). Infant mortality rates, fetal mortality rates, and perinatal mortality rates, according to race: United States, selected years 1950–99. Deaths: Final data for 1999. In *National vital statistics reports*, 49, Table 23. Retrieved December 13, 2007. http://origin.cdc.gov/nchs/data/hus/tables/2001/01hus023.pdf.

Chauhan, S. P., Doherty, D. D., Magann, E. F., Cahanding, F., Moreno, F., & Klausen, J. H. (2004). Amniotic fluid index vs. single deepest pockets technique during modified biophysical profile: A randomized clinical trial. *American Journal of Obstetrics and Gynecology, 191*(2), 661–668.

Christensen, F. C., & Rayburn, W. F. (1999). Fetal movement counts. *Obstetrics and Gynecology Clinics of North America, 26*(4), 607–621.

Clark, S. L., Sabey, P., & Jolley, K. (1989). Nonstress testing with acoustic stimulation and amniotic fluid volume assessment: 5973 tests without unexpected fetal death. *American Journal of Obstetrics and Gynecology, 160*(3), 694–697.

Dawes, G. S., Houghton, C. R., Redman, C. W., & Visser, G. H. (1982). Pattern of normal fetal heart rate. *British Journal of Obstetrics and Gynaecology, 89*(4), 276–284.

Devoe, L. D. (1999). Nonstress testing and contraction stress testing. *Obstetrics and Gynecology Clinics of North America, 26*(4), 535–556.

Devoe, L., Boehm, F., Paul, R., Frigoletto, F., Penso, C., Goldenberg, R., et al. (1994). Clinical experience with the Hewlett-Packard M-1350A fetal monitor: Correlation of Doppler-detected fetal body movements with fetal heart rate parameters and perinatal outcome. *American Journal of Obstetrics and Gynecology, 170*(2), 650–655.

Devoe, L. D., & Jones, C. R. (2002). Nonstress test: Evidence-based use in high-risk pregnancy. *Clinical Obstetrics and Gynecology, 45*(4), 986–992.

Devoe, L. D., Murray, C., Youssif, A., & Arnaud, M. (1993). Maternal caffeine consumption and fetal behavior in normal third-trimester pregnancy. *American Journal of Obstetrics and Gynecology, 168*(4), 1105–1112.

deVries, J. I., Visser, G. H., & Prechtl, H. F. (1982). The emergence of fetal behavior: I. Qualitative aspects. *Early Human Development, 7*(4), 301–322.

DiPietro, J. A., Costigan, K. A., & Gurewitsch, E. D. (2003). Fetal response to induced maternal stress. *Early Human Development, 74*(2), 125–138.

DiPietro, J. A., Costigan, K. A., & Pressman, E. K. (1999). Fetal movement detection: Comparison of the Toitu actograph with ultrasound from 20 weeks gestation. *Journal of Maternal–Fetal Medicine, 8*(6), 237–242.

Drogtrop, A. P., Ubels, R., & Nijhuis, J. G. (1990). The association between fetal body movements, eye movements, and heart rate patterns in pregnancies between 25 and 30 weeks of gestation. *Early Human Development, 23*(1), 67–73.

Druzin, M. L., Smith, J. F., Gabbe, S. G., & Reed, K. L. (2007). Antepartum fetal evaluation. In S. G. Gabbe, J. R. Neibyl, & J. L. Simpson (Eds.). *Obstetrics: Normal and problem pregnancies* (5th ed., pp. 267- 301). New York: Churchill Livingstone.

Eller, D. P., Stramm, S. L., & Newman, R. B. (1992). The effect of maternal intravenous glucose administration on fetal activity. *American Journal of Obstetrics and Gynecology, 167*(4 Pt. 1), 1071–1074.

Evertson, L. R., Gauthier, R. J., Schifrin, B. S., & Paul, R. H. (1979). Antepartum fetal heart rate testing. I. Evolution of the nonstress test. *American Journal of Obstetrics and Gynecology, 133*(1), 29–33.

Freeman, R. K. (1975). The use of the oxytocin challenge test for antepartum clinical evaluation of uteroplacental respiratory function. *American Journal of Obstetrics and Gynecology, 121*(4), 481–489.

Freeman, R. K., Garite, T. J., & Nageotte, M. P. (2003). *Fetal heart rate monitoring* (3rd ed.). Baltimore: Williams & Wilkins.

Gagnon, R., Hunse, C., & Patrick, J. (1988). Fetal responses to vibratory acoustic stimulation: Influence of basal heart rate. *American Journal of Obstetrics and Gynecology, 159*(4), 835–839.

Garite, T. (2007). Intrapartum fetal evaluation. In S. Gabbe, J. Niebyl, & J. Simpson (Eds.), *Obstetrics: Normal and problem pregnancies* (5th ed., pp. 365-395). Philadelphia: Churchill Livingstone.

Gauthier, R. J., Evertson, L. R., & Paul, R. H. (1979). Antepartum fetal heart rate testing. II. Intrapartum fetal heart rate observation and newborn outcome following a positive contraction stress test. *American Journal of Obstetrics and Gynecology, 133*(1), 34–39.

Gegor, C. L., Paine, L. L, Costigan, K., & Johnson, T. R. (1994). Interpretation of biophysical profiles by nurses and physicians. *Journal of Obstetric, Gynecologic, and Neonatal Nursing, 23*(5), 405–410.

Gibby, N. W. (1988). Relationship between fetal movement charting and anxiety in low-risk pregnant women. *Journal of Nurse-Midwifery, 33*(4), 185–188.

Glantz, C., & D'Amico, M. L. (2001). Lack of relationship between variable decelerations during reactive nonstress tests and oligohydramnios. *American Journal of Perinatology, 18*(3), 129–135.

Gribbin, C., & James, D. (2004). Assessing fetal health. *Best Practice and Research. Clinical Obstetrics & Gynaecology, 18*(3), 411–424.

Groome, L. J., Mooney, D. M., Holland, S. B., Bentz, L. S., Atterbury, J. L., & Dykman, R. A. (1997a). The heart rate deceleratory response in low-risk human fetuses: Effect of stimulus intensity on response topography. *Developmental Psychobiology, 30*(2), 103–113.

Groome, L. J., Mooney, D. M., Holland, S. B., Smith, L. A., & Atterbury, J. L. (1997b). Heart rate response in individual human fetuses to stimulation with a low-intensity sound. *Journal of Maternal–Fetal Investigation, 7*, 105–110.

Groome, L. J., Owen, J., Singh, K. P., Neely, C. L., & Gaudier, F. L. (1992). Spontaneous movement of the human fetus at 18–22 weeks of gestation: Evidence of early organization of the active rest cycle. *Journal of Maternal–Fetal Investigation, 2*, 27–32.

Groome, L. J., Swiber, M. J., Bentz, L. S., Holland, S. B., & Atterbury, J. L. (1995). Maternal anxiety during pregnancy: Effect on fetal behavior at 38 to 40 weeks of gestation. *Journal of Developmental and Behavioral Pediatrics, 16*, 391–396.

Groome, L. J., Swiber, M. J., Holland, S. B., Bentz, L. S., Atterbury, J. L., & Trimm, R. F., III. (1999). Spontaneous motor activity in the perinatal infant before and after birth: Stability in individual differences. *Developmental Psychobiology, 35*, 15–34.

Groome, L. J., & Watson, J. E. (1992). Assessment of in utero neurobehavioral development. I. Fetal behavioral states. *Journal of Maternal–Fetal Investigation, 2*, 183–194.

Harris, J. L. (1999). Physiologic basis of antenatal testing. *Current Opinion in Obstetrics and Gynecology, 11*(6), 571–575.

Hatoum, N., Clapp, J. F., III, Newman, M. R., Dajani, N., & Amini, S. B. (1997). Effects of maternal exercise on fetal activity in late gestation. *Journal of Maternal-Fetal Medicine, 6*(3), 134–139.

Hoskins, I. A., Frieden, F. J., & Young, B. K. (1991). Variable decelerations in reactive nonstress tests with decreased amniotic fluid index predict fetal compromise. *American Journal of Obstetrics and Gynecology, 165*(4 Pt. 1), 1094–1098.

Huddleston, J. F. (2002). Continued utility of the contraction stress test? *Clinical Obstetrics and Gynecology, 45*(4), 1005–1014.

Jaschevatzky, O. E., Marom, D., Ostrovsky, P., Ellenbogen, A., Anderman, S., & Ballas, S. (1998). Significance of sporadic deceleration during antepartum testing in term pregnancies. *American Journal of Perinatology, 15*(5), 291–294.

Jensen, O. H., & Flottorp, G. (1982). A method for controlled sound stimulation of the human fetus. *Scandinavian Audiology, 11*(3), 145–150.

Johnson, T. R. (1994). Maternal perception and Doppler detection of fetal movement. *Clinics in Perinatology, 21*(4), 765–777.

Johnson, T. R., Jordan, E. T., & Paine, L. L. (1990). Doppler recordings of fetal movement. II. Comparison with maternal perception. *Obstetrics and Gynecology, 76*(1), 42–43.

Keegan, K. A., Jr., & Paul, R. H. (1980). Antepartum fetal heart rate testing. IV. The nonstress as a primary approach. *American Journal of Obstetrics and Gynecology, 136*(1), 75–80.

Kochanek, K. D., & Smith, B. L. (2004). Deaths: Preliminary data for 2002 (National Vital Statistics Report). Hyattsville, MD: National Center for Health Statistics. Retrieved December 13, 2007. http://www.cdc.gov/nchs/data/nvsr52/nvsr52_13.pdf.

Kontopoulos, E.V., & Vintzileos, A. M. (2004). Condition-specific antepartum fetal testing. *American Journal of Obstetrics and Gynecology, 191*(5), 1546–1551.

Kopecky, E. A., Ryan, M. L., Barrett, J. F., Seaward, P. G., Ryan, G., Koren, G., et al. (2000). Fetal response to maternally administered morphine. *American Journal of Obstetrics and Gynecology, 183*(2), 424–430.

Krebs, H. B., Petres, R. E., Dunn, L. J., & Smith, P. J. (1982). Intrapartum fetal heart rate monitoring: VI. Prognostic significance of accelerations. *American Journal of Obstetrics and Gynecology, 142*(3), 297–305.

Lagrew, D. C., Jr. (1995). The contraction stress test. *Clinical Obstetrics and Gynecology, 38*(1), 11–25.

Lalor, J. G., Fawole, B., Alfirevic, Z., & Devane, D. (2007). Biophysical profile for fetal assessment in high risk pregnancies. *Cochrane Database of Systematic Reviews, 4,* CD000038. http://www.cochrane.org/reviews/en/ab000038.html

Lee, C. Y., DiLoreto, P. C., & O'Lane, J. M. (1975). A study of fetal heart rate acceleration patterns. *Obstetrics and Gynecology, 45*(2), 142–146.

Lipitz, S., Barkai, E., Rabinovici, J., & Mashiach, S. (1987). Breast stimulation test and oxytocin challenge test in fetal surveillance: A prospective randomized study. *American Journal of Obstetrics and Gynecology, 157,* 1178–1181.

Lowery, C. L., Russell, W. A., Jr., Baggot, P. J., Wilson, J. D., Walts, R. C., Bentz, L. S., et al. (1997). Time quantified detection of fetal movements using a new fetal movement algorithm. *American Journal of Perinatology, 14*(1), 7–12.

MacLennan, A. (1999). A template for defining a causal relation between acute intrapartum events and cerebral palsy: International consensus statement. *British Medical Journal, 319,* 1054–1059.

Macones, G. A., Hankins, G. D., Spong, C. Y., Hauth, J. D., & Moore, T. (2008). The 2008 National Institute of Child Health Human Development workshop report on electronic fetal monitoring: Update on definitions, interpretations, and research guidelines. *Obstetrics & Gynecology, 112,* 661-666, and *Journal of Obstetric, Gynecologic, and Neonatal Nursing, 37,* 510-515.

Manders, M. A., Sonder, G. J., Mulder, E. J., & Visser, G. H. (1997). The effects of maternal exercise on fetal heart rate and movement patterns. *Early Human Development, 48*(3), 237–247.

Manning, F. A. (1995). Dynamic ultrasound-based fetal assessment: The fetal biophysical profile score. *Clinical Obstetrics and Gynecology, 38*(1), 26–44.

Manning, F. A., Baskett, T. F., Morrison, I., & Lange, I. (1981). Fetal biophysical profile scoring: A prospective study in 1,184 high-risk patients. *American Journal of Obstetrics and Gynecology, 140*(3), 289–294.

Manning, F. A., Harman, C. R., Menticoglou, S., & Morrison, I. (1991). Assessment of fetal well-being with ultrasound. *Obstetrics and Gynecology Clinics of North America, 18*(4), 891–905.

Manning, F. A., Morrison, I., Lange, I. R., & Harman, C. (1982). Antepartum determination of fetal health: Composite biophysical profile scoring. *Clinics in Perinatology, 9*(2), 285–296.

Manning, F. A., & Platt, L. D. (1979). Maternal hypoxemia fetal breathing movements. *Obstetrics and Gynecology, 53*(6), 758–760.

Manning, F. A., Platt, L. D., & Sipos, L. (1980). Antepartum fetal evaluation: Development of a fetal biophysical profile. *American Journal of Obstetrics and Gynecology, 136*(6), 787–795.

Manning, F. A., Snijders, R., Harman, C. R., Nicolaides, K., Menticoglou, S., & Morrison, I. (1993). Fetal biophysical profile score. VI. Correlation with antepartum umbilical venous fetal pH. *American Journal of Obstetrics and Gynecology, 169*(4), 755–763.

Marden, D., McDuffie, R. S., Jr., Allen, R., & Abitz, D. (1997). A randomized controlled trial of a new fetal acoustic stimulation test for fetal well-being. *American Journal of Obstetrics and Gynecology, 176*(6), 1386–1388.

Meis, P. J., Ureda, J. R., Swain, M., Kelly, R. T., Penry, M., & Sharp, P. (1986). Variable decelerations during nonstress tests are not a sign of fetal compromise. *American Journal of Obstetrics and Gynecology, 154*(3), 586–590.

Miller, D. A., Rabello, Y. A., & Paul, R. H. (1996). The modified biophysical profile: Antepartum testing in the 1990s. *American Journal of Obstetrics and Gynecology, 174*(3), 812–817.

Miller-Slade, D., Gloeb, D. J., Bailey, S., Bendell, A., Interlandi, E., Kline-Kaye, V., et al. (1991). Acoustic stimulation-induced fetal response compared to traditional nonstress testing. *Journal of Obstetric, Gynecologic, and Neonatal Nursing, 20*(2), 160–167.

Mills, M. S., James, D. K., & Slade, S. (1990). Two-tier approach to the biophysical assessment of the fetus. *American Journal of Obstetrics and Gynecology, 163*(1 Pt. 1), 12–17.

Moffatt, F. W., & van den Hof, M. (1997). Semi-Fowler's positioning, lateral tilts, and their effects on nonstress tests. *Journal of Obstetric, Gynecologic, and Neonatal Nursing, 26*(5), 551–557.

Naef, R. W., III, Morrison, J. C., Washburne, J. F., McLaughlin, B. N., Perry, K. G., Jr., & Roberts, W. E. (1994). Assessment of fetal well-being using the nonstress test in the home setting. *Obstetrics and Gynecology, 84*(3), 424–426.

Nageotte, M. P., Towers, C. V., Asrat, T., & Freeman, R. K. (1994a). Perinatal outcome with the modified biophysical profile. *American Journal of Obstetrics and Gynecology, 170*(6), 1672–1676.

Nageotte, M. P., Towers, C. V., Asrat, T., Freeman, R. K., & Dorchester, W. (1994b). The value of a negative antepartum test: Contraction stress test and modified biophysical profile. *Obstetrics and Gynecology, 84*(2), 231–234.

Nathan, E. B., Haberman, S., Burgess, T., & Minkoff, H. (2000). The relationship of maternal position to the results of brief nonstress tests: A randomized clinical trial. *American Journal of Obstetrics and Gynecology, 182*(5), 1070–1072.

National Institute of Child Health and Human Development Research Planning Workshop. (1997). Electronic fetal heart rate monitoring: Research guidelines for interpretation. *Journal of Obstetrics, Gynecology and Neonatal Nursing, 26*(6), 635–640.

Nijhuis, J. G., Prechtl, H. F., Martin, C. B., Jr., & Bots, R. S. (1982). Are there behavioral states in the human fetus? *Early Human Development, 6*(2), 177–195.

Nyman, M., Barr, M., & Westgren, M. (1992). A four-year follow-up of hearing and development in children exposed in utero to vibro-acoustic stimulation. *British Journal of Obstetrics and Gynaecology, 99*(8), 685–688.

Oki, E. Y., Keegan, K. A., Freeman, R. K., & Dorchester, W. L. (1987). The breast-stimulation contraction stress test. *Journal of Reproductive Medicine, 32*(12), 919–932.

O'Leary, J. A., Andrinopoulos, G. C., & Giordano, P. C. (1980). Variable decelerations and the nonstress test: An indication of cord compromise. *American Journal of Obstetrics and Gynecology, 137*(6), 704–706.

Olesen, A. G., & Svare, J. A. (2004). Decreased fetal movements: Background, assessment and clinical management. *Acta Obstetricia et Gynecologica Scandinavica, 83*(9), 818–826.

Olofsson, P., Thuring-Jönsson, A. & Marsál, K. (1996). Uterine and umbilical circulation during the oxytocin challenge test. *Ultrasound in Obstetrics and Gynecology, 8*(4), 247–251.

Onyeije, C. I., & Divon, M. Y. (2001). The impact of maternal ketonuria on fetal test results in the setting of postterm pregnancy. *American Journal of Obstetrics and Gynecology, 184*(4), 713–718.

Patrick, J., Campbell, K., Carmichael, L., Natale, R., & Richardson, B. (1982). Patterns of gross fetal body movements over 24-hr observation intervals during the last 10 weeks of pregnancy. *American Journal of Obstetrics and Gynecology, 142*(4), 363–371.

Pattison, N., & McCowan, L. (1999). Cardiotocography for antepartum fetal assessment. *Cochrane Database of Systematic Reviews, 1*, CD001068.

Paul, R., & Miller, D. A. (1995). Nonstress test. *Clinical Obstetrics and Gynecology, 38*(1), 3–10.

Pearson, J. F., & Weaver, J. B. (1976). Fetal activity and fetal wellbeing: An evaluation. *British Medical Journal, 1*(6021), 1305–1307.

Perlman, J. M. (2006). Intrapartum asphyxia and cerebral palsy: Is there a link? *Clinics in Perinatology, 33*(2), 335–353.

Pietrantoni, M., Angel, J. L., Parsons, M. T., McClain, L., Arango, H. A., & Spellacy, W. N. (1991). Human fetal response to vibroacoustic stimulation as a function of stimulus duration. *Obstetrics and Gynecology, 78*(5 Pt. 1), 807–811.

Pillai, M., & James, D. (1990). Are the behavioral states of the newborn comparable to those of the fetus? *Early Human Development, 22*(1), 39–49.

Rabinowitz, R., Persitz, E., & Sadovsky, E. (1983). The relation between fetal heart rate accelerations and fetal movements. *Obstetrics and Gynecology, 61*(1), 16–18.

Raines, D. A. (1996). Fetal surveillance: Issues and implications. *Journal of Obstetric, Gynecologic, and Neonatal Nursing, 25*(7), 559–564.

Rayburn, W. F. (1982). Antepartum fetal assessment: Monitoring fetal activity. *Clinics in Perinatology, 9*, 1–14.

Rayburn, W. F. (1990). Fetal body movement monitoring. *Obstetrics and Gynecology Clinics of North America, 17*(1), 95–110.

Read, J. A., & Miller, F. C. (1977). Fetal heart rate acceleration in response to acoustic stimulation as a measure of fetal well-being. *American Journal of Obstetrics and Gynecology, 129*(5), 512–517.

Reece, E. A., Hagay, Z., Garafalo, J., & Hobbins, J. C. (1992). A controlled trial of self-nonstress test versus assisted nonstress test in the evaluation of fetal well-being. *American Journal of Obstetrics and Gynecology, 166*(2), 489–492.

Ribbert, L. S., Snijders, R. J., Nicolaides, R. H., & Visser, G. H. (1990). Relationship of fetal biophysical profile and blood gas values at cordocentesis in severely growth-restricted fetuses. *American Journal of Obstetrics and Gynecology, 163*(2), 569–571.

Rizk, B., Atterbury, J. L., & Groome, L. J. (1996). Reproductive risks of cocaine. *Human Reproduction Update, 2*(1), 43–55.

Rochard, F., Schifrin, B. S., Goupil, F., Legrand, H., Blottiere, J., & Sureau, C. (1976). Nonstressed fetal heart rate monitoring in the antepartum period. *American Journal of Obstetrics and Gynecology, 126*(6), 699–706.

Sadovsky, E., & Yaffe, H. (1973). Daily fetal movement recording and fetal prognosis. *Obstetrics and Gynecology, 41*(6), 845–850.

Saraço lu, F., Göl, K., Sahin, I., Türkkani, B., & Oztopçu, C. (1999). The predictive value of fetal acoustic stimulation. *Journal of Perinatology, 19*(2), 103–105.

Sarno, A. P., Ahn, M. O., Phelan, J. P., & Paul, R. H. (1990). Fetal acoustic stimulation in the early intrapartum period as a predictor of subsequent of fetal condition. *American Journal of Obstetrics and Gynecology, 162*(3), 762–767.

Sarno, A. P. Jr., & Bruner, J. P. (1990). Fetal acoustic stimulation as a possible adjunct to diagnostic ultrasound: A preliminary report. *Obstetrics and Gynecology, 76*(4), 668–690.

Schellpfeffer, M. A., Hoyle, D., & Johnson, J. W. (1985). Antepartal uterine hypercontractility secondary to nipple stimulation. *Obstetrics and Gynecology, 65*(4), 588–591.

Serafini, P., Lindsay, M. B., Nagey, D. A., Pupkin, M. J., Tseng, P., & Crenshaw, C., Jr. (1984). Antepartum fetal heart rate response to sound stimulation: The acoustic stimulation test. *American Journal of Obstetrics and Gynecology, 148*(1), 41–45.

Shah, D. M., Brown, J. E., Salyer, S. L., Fleischer, A. C., & Boehm, F. H. (1989). A modified scheme for biophysical profile scoring. *American Journal of Obstetrics and Gynecology, 160*(3), 586–591.

Shalev, E., Zalel, Y., & Weiner, E. (1993). A comparison of the nonstress test, oxytocin challenge test, Doppler velocimetry, and biophysical profile in predicting umbilical vein pH in growth-retarded fetuses. *International Journal of Gynaecology and Obstetrics, 43*(1), 15–19.

Smith, C. V. (1995). Vibroacoustic stimulation. *Clinical Obstetrics and Gynecology, 38*(1), 68–77.

Smith, C. V., Phelan, J. P., Nguyen, H. N., Jacobs, N., & Paul, R. H. (1988). Continuing experience with the fetal acoustic stimulation test. *Journal of Reproductive Medicine, 33*(4), 365–368.

Smith, C. V., Phelan, J. P., Paul, R. H., & Broussard, P. M. (1985). Fetal acoustic stimulation testing: A retrospective analysis of the fetal acoustic stimulation test. *American Journal of Obstetrics and Gynecology, 153*(5), 567–569.

Smith, C. V., Phelan, J. P., Platt, L. D., Broussard, P., & Paul, R. H. (1986). Fetal acoustic stimulation testing. II. A randomized clinical comparison with the nonstress test. *American Journal of Obstetrics and Gynecology, 155*(1), 131–134.

Snijders, R. J., McLaren, R., & Nicolaides, K. H. (1990). Computer-assisted analysis of fetal heart rate patterns at 20–41 weeks' gestation. *Fetal Diagnosis and Therapy, 5*(2), 79–83.

Sontag, L. W., & Wallace, R. E. (1936). Changes in the rate of human fetal heart rate response to vibratory stimuli. *American Journal of Diseases of Children, 51*, 383.

Tan, K. H., & Sabapathy, A. (2001a). Fetal manipulation for facilitating tests of fetal wellbeing. *Cochrane Database of Systematic Reviews, 4*, CD003396.

Tan, K. H., & Sabapathy, A. (2001b). Maternal glucose administration for facilitating tests of fetal well-being. *Cochrane Database of Systematic Reviews, 4*, CD003397.

Tan, K. H., & Smyth, R. (2001c). Fetal vibroacoustic stimulation for facilitation of tests of fetal well-being. *Cochrane Database of Systematic Reviews, 4*, CD002963.

Thaler, I., Goodman, J. D., & Dawes, G. S. (1980). Effects of maternal cigarette smoking on fetal breathing and fetal movements. *American Journal of Obstetrics and Gynecology, 138*(3), 282–287.

Timor-Tritsch, I. E., Dierker, L. J., Hertz, R. H., Deogan, N. C., & Rosen, M. G. (1978a). Studies of antepartum behavioral state in the human fetus at term. *American Journal of Obstetrics and Gynecology, 132*(5), 524–528.

Timor-Tritsch, I. E., Dierker, L. J. Jr., Hertz, R. H., & Rosen, M. G. (1979). Fetal movement: A brief review. *Clinical Obstetrics and Gynecology, 22*(3), 583–592.

Trudinger, B. J., & Boylan, P. (1980). Antepartum fetal heart rate monitoring: Value of sound stimulation. *Obstetrics and Gynecology, 55*(2), 265–268.

Velazquez, M., & Rayburn, W. F. (2002). Antenatal evaluation of the fetus using fetal movement monitoring. *Clinical Obstetrics and Gynecology, 45*(4), 993–1004.

Vintzileos, A. M. (1995). Antepartum fetal surveillance. *Clinical Obstetrics and Gynecology, 38*(1), 1–2.

Vintzileos, A. M. (2000). Antenatal assessment for the detection of fetal asphyxia: An evidenced-based approach using indication-specific testing. *Annals of the New York Academy of Sciences, 900,* 137–150.

Vintzileos, A. M., Campbell, W. A., Ingardia, C. J., & Nochimson, D. J. (1983). The fetal biophysical profile and its predictive value. *Obstetrics and Gynecology, 62*(3), 271–278.

Vintzileos, A. M., Gaffney, S. E., Salinger, L. M., Kontopoulos, V. G., Campbell, W. A., & Nochimson, D. J. (1987). The relationships among the fetal biophysical profile, umbilical cord pH, and Apgar scores. *American Journal of Obstetrics and Gynecology, 157*(3), 627–631.

Vintzileos, A. M., & Knuppel, R. A. (1994). Multiple parameter biophysical testing in the prediction of fetal acid-base status. *Clinics in Perinatology, 21*(4), 823–848.

Visser, G. H., Bekedam, D. J., & Ribbert, L. S. (1990a). Changes in antepartum heart rate patterns with progressive deterioration of the fetal condition. *International Journal of Biomedical Computing, 25*(4), 239–246.

Visser, G. H., Sadovsky, G., & Nicolaides, K. H. (1990b). Antepartum heart rate patterns in small-for-gestational-age third-trimester fetuses: Correlations with blood gas values obtained at cordocentesis. *American Journal of Obstetrics and Gynecology, 162*(3), 698–703.

Walker, D., Grimwade, J., & Wood, C. (1971). Intrapartum noise: A component of the fetal environment. *American Journal of Obstetrics and Gynecology, 109*(1), 92–95

Walkinshaw, S., Cameron, H., MacPhail, S., & Robson, S. (1992). The prediction of fetal compromise and acidosis by biophysical profile scoring in the small for gestational age fetus. *Journal of Perinatal Medicine, 20*(3), 227–232.

Ware, D. J., & Devoe, L. D. (1994). The nonstress test: Reassessment of the "gold standard." *Clinics in Perinatology, 21*(4), 779–796.

Westergaard, H. B., Langhoff-Roos, J., Lingman, G., Marsál, K., & Kreiner, S. (2001). A critical appraisal of the use of umbilical artery Doppler ultrasound in high-risk pregnancies: Use of meta-analysis in evidence-based obstetrics. *Ultrasound in Obstetrics and Gynecology, 17*(6), 466–467.

Woods, J., Glantz, J., Pittinaro, D. & Giffi, C. (2007). Doppler artery velocimetry: Umbilical artery and middle cerebral artery. In J. Woods, J. Glantz, D. Pittinaro, & C. Giffi (Eds.), *Principles of fetal heart rate monitoring* (3rd ed., pp. 251-265), Rochester, NY: University of Rochester.

Yao, Q. W., Jakobsson, J., Nyman, M., Rabaeus, H., Till, O., & Westgren, M. (1990). Fetal response to different intensity levels of vibroacoustic stimulation. *Obstetrics and Gynecology, 75*(2), 206–209.

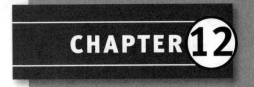

CHAPTER 12

Fetal Arrhythmias

Joanne D. Barnes

INTRODUCTION

The literature describes three main types of rhythm disturbance encountered in the fetus:

1. Irregular heart rhythms and extrasystole
2. Tachycardias
3. Bradycardias (Kleinman & Nehgme, 2004; Sharland, 2001)

The most common disturbance is an irregular heart rhythm, and this is usually benign (Kleinman & Nehgme, 2004; Sharland, 2001). Irregular beats can occur secondary to isolated atrial or ventricular premature beats, producing a perceived heart rhythm irregularity or skipped beats (Kleinman & Nehgme). A premature atrial signal can also be conducted to the ventricles, resulting in ventricular contraction; if it occurs early in diastole, the signal may not be conducted at all, resulting in skipped beats (Crossman & Brenner, 1999; Kleinman & Nehgme).

Fetal arrhythmias are rarely seen, occurring in 1% to 3% of pregnancies (Strasburger, et al., 2007). Clinicians should be able to recognize that a rhythm disturbance may be present. Any rhythm disturbance has the potential to decrease fetal cardiac output as alterations from the normal ECG cycle are produced. When a woman is in labor, a rhythm disturbance may present an additional stressor on the fetus above and beyond the normal reductions in blood flow that occur with contractions. In some cases this can present a challenge to fetal reserve and fetal tolerance of labor. Perinatal clinicians may detect a rhythm disturbance during a routine prenatal visit, during a nonstress test (NST), or when the patient presents in labor. Clinicians caring for childbearing women should be knowledgeable about the etiology of different patterns, available treatment options, and potential outcomes and should anticipate questions that the woman and her family may ask.

DEFINITION

The term "arrhythmia" is described as "any irregularity of the fetal cardiac rhythm or any regular rhythm that remains outside the general range of 100-160 bpm [beats per minute]" (Kleinman, Nehgme, & Copel, 2004, p. 465). Arrhythmias fall into two broad categories. They are associated with the following:

1. Variations in the R-R intervals. There may be normal P waves that occur in a regular fashion preceding each QRS complex.
2. Disordered impulse formation, impulse conduction, or a combination of both. There will be an abnormal P-QRS relationship as evidenced by early or absent P waves; widened, bizarre-looking QRS complexes; or both.

Specific arrhythmias are typically named according to the anatomic site of aberrant impulse formation, conduction, or both and may be unassociated with uterine activity.

FETAL CARDIAC DEVELOPMENT AND FUNCTION

Three separate but related concepts are significant to any discussion of arrhythmias:

1. Cardiac development
2. The differences in the adaptive mechanisms of the fetal and adult hearts
3. Conduction physiology

An understanding of these concepts is important when discussing specific arrhythmias and the fetus' ability to withstand the changes in cardiac output that may be produced.

Cardiac Development

The fetal cardiovascular system, including the heart, blood vessels, and cells, all originate from the mesenchymal germ layers (Blackburn, 2007; Moore & Persaud, 2003). The mesenchymal cells form a tube that by the third week of development begins to beat under the control of a primitive pacemaker (Blackburn; Moore & Persaud).

During the fourth week, the tube forms a loop (Blackburn, 2007; Moore & Persaud, 2003). Soon after, differentiation of the heart regions begins, and the atrial septum begins to form from the roof of the atrium downward. During the sixth week, the pulmonary arteries begin to form, and both the atrial and ventricular septa continue to develop. By the end of the sixth week, the valves are forming and the coronary circulation has been established. If there are alterations in any of these processes, lesions may develop and continue to evolve during the rest of gestation (Blackburn; Moore & Persaud).

The development of the fetal cardiac conduction system also progresses over time. The sinoatrial (SA) node develops from the sinus venosus musculature during the fifth week of gestation (Blackburn, 2007; Moore & Persaud, 2003). The SA node is then incorporated into the wall of the right atrium and will eventually lie near the entrance of the superior vena cava (Blackburn).

After the SA node is incorporated into the wall of the right atrium, cells from part of the SA node combine with cells from the atrioventricular (AV)

canal to form the AV node and bundle of His. The bundle of His continues to develop into the right and left bundle branches and the Purkinje fibers, which are distributed throughout the ventricles (Blackburn, 2007; Moore & Persaud, 2003). By the end of this process, there is neurogenic control of the heart, and the conduction system represents the pathway for communication of electrical impulses between the atria and the ventricles (Blackburn; Moore & Persaud).

Electrical activity actually begins before the contractile apparatus of the fetal heart completely differentiates. Sympathetic innervation via the first thoracic sympathetic ganglia is usually present by day 10. The fetal cardiac muscle and the arterioles of the fetal circulation have direct sympathetic innervation. Parasympathetic innervation is present by day 80 of gestation and originates from the cardiac ganglia located on the surface and in the outflow tract of the fetal heart. Sensory innervation of the fetal heart originates from the distal ganglia of the vagus nerve, although there is little clinical evidence to show at what stage of development this begins to function (Kirby, 2004). The right and left branches of the vagus nerve innervate both the SA and the AV nodes. Early in gestation, the sympathetic nervous system has the major influence on the fetal heart rate (FHR). Parasympathetic influence on the heart increases gradually during the latter part of gestation (Pickoff, 2004).

Differences between Fetal and Adult Cardiac Functioning

The fetal heart is less able than the adult heart to alter the forces of cardiac contraction because of a number of factors, including decreased contractile mass, differences in calcium transport, differences in the pressures within the heart, and rate-dependent cardiac output. The fetal heart has approximately half the contractile mass of the adult heart because there are fewer sarcomeres, the smallest contractile units within heart muscle. Sarcomeres are arranged into myofibrils, which, in the fetus, are also fewer in number and more randomly arranged. Calcium transport into and out of the muscle cells is also limited in the fetus, resulting in cardiac muscle that is less compliant. These three factors limit the fetus' ability to alter stroke volume or the force of cardiac contractions (Blackburn, 2007).

As discussed in Chapter 2, cardiac pressures and contributions to cardiac output also differ in the fetus when compared with the adult. Right-sided pressure is higher in the fetus, and right-sided output accounts for two-thirds of the entire fetal cardiac output as a result of the shunting of blood through the patent foramen ovale and ductus arteriosus (Blackburn, 2007). The less compliant fetal myocardium and combined right and left contribution to cardiac output result in a fetus that cannot, for all practical purposes, alter its stroke volume to meet increased demand. Therefore, fetal cardiac output is rate–dependent, and the fetus is dependent on maintaining a heart rate in the normal range to maintain adequate cardiac output and tissue perfusion (Blackburn).

Cardiac Physiology

When fetal arrhythmias are studied, it is important to understand normal cardiac conduction physiology and electrocardiogram (ECG) patterns. Many arrhythmias result from alterations in normal conduction patterns that are reflected as abnormal-appearing ECGs.

Cardiac cells possess unique characteristics. *Automaticity* refers to the ability of cardiac cells to contract spontaneously. *Excitability* is the readiness and ability of cardiac cells to respond to electrical stimuli. *Conductivity* is the ability to conduct an electrical stimulus between different cardiac cells. Excitability and conductivity occur through polarization and depolarization of the cellular membrane.

Cardiac cells at rest are charged. Sodium is found primarily outside the cell, whereas potassium is found inside the cell, resulting in an overall negatively charged cell, called "polarization." When stimulated by an electrical impulse, sodium rushes into the cell and potassium is forced out of the cell. This process is called "depolarization." Following depolarization is a phase known as the "refractory period," when the cell cannot respond to further electrical stimulation. (The refractory period is differentiated into two parts, absolute and relative.) After depolarization and the refractory period, the cell reverts backs to its polarized, resting state (Bianchi, Crombleholme, & D'Alton, 2000; Tanel & Rhodes, 2001). This sequence of polarization, depolarization, and refractory period is responsible for the typical ECG pattern (Figure 12-1).

As with adult hearts, the depolarization and repolarization of the fetal cardiac muscle cells create electrical activity that can be recorded. This activity is controlled by the conduction system, composed of the SA node, AV node, the bundle of His, and Purkinje fibers. The typical cardiac impulse begins at the SA node, known as the "pacemaker of the heart." Firing of the SA node first generates an atrial contraction, which is responsible for approximately 30% of cardiac output. The impulse is then conducted down to the AV node, where it is slowed, enabling completion of atrial depolarization and contraction. As a result of atrial contraction, the ventricles fill with blood. The impulse then travels down the Bundle of His to the left and right bundle branches and through the Purkinje fibers to the ventricular muscle cells, stimulating ventricular depolarization and contraction (Table 12-1).

Each part of the conduction system has an intrinsic rate. This rate is slower when contraction impulses are generated further down the system. The SA node in a fetus has an intrinsic rate of 110 to 160 bpm, the normal fetal heart range. If the SA

FIGURE 12-1 Polarization/Depolarization Cycle

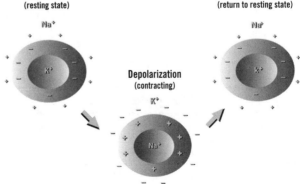

Polarization
(resting state)

Repolarization
(return to resting state)

Depolarization
(contracting)

node fails and the AV node assumes the role of fetal pacemaker, the intrinsic rate falls to 50 to 70 bpm. If the AV node fails, the Bundle of His, also called the AV junction, becomes the fetal pacemaker with an intrinsic rate of 40 bpm. This junctional rate is incompatible with continued fetal life because it is too low to maintain cardiac output.

A frequent method of monitoring cardiac conduction activity is by ECG (Kleinman, Nehgme, & Copel, 2004). The typical ECG has three sections: the P wave, QRS complex, and T wave. Each section corresponds to distinct cardiac events (Table 12-1):

1. The P wave, which is reflective of atrial depolarization and contraction (This is followed by a spike representing atrial repolarization, which is lost within the QRS complex.)
2. The QRS complex, which is indicative of ventricular depolarization and contraction
3. The T wave, representing ventricular repolarization and ventricular relaxation

The ECG is an important tool for assessing arrhythmias because it provides valuable information concerning the FHR and the relationships between atrial and ventricular events. It can also help identify the origin or mechanism of a variety of abnormal FHR rhythms (Kleinman et al., 2004; Shaffer & Wiggins, 1998) (Figure 12-2; Table 12-1).

FIGURE 12-2   Cardiac Conduction System and Normal ECG

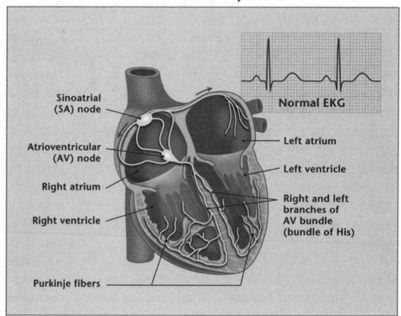

Table 12-1	ECG

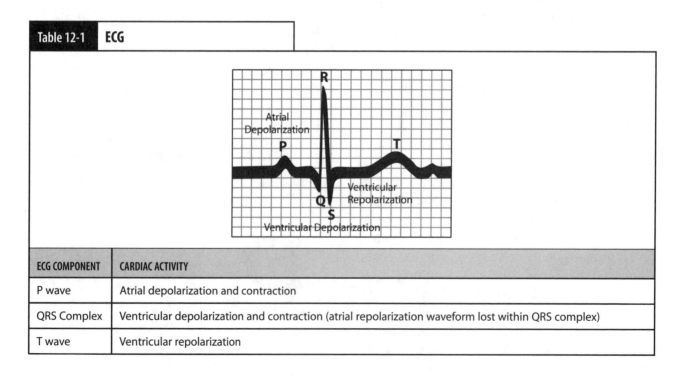

ECG COMPONENT	CARDIAC ACTIVITY
P wave	Atrial depolarization and contraction
QRS Complex	Ventricular depolarization and contraction (atrial repolarization waveform lost within QRS complex)
T wave	Ventricular repolarization

ETIOLOGIES OF FETAL RHYTHM DISTURBANCES

Fetal heart rhythm disturbances can develop in a number of ways, including conduction system defects, congenital heart defects, and infections. Conduction system defects such as AV block can develop as a result of abnormalities in development or from maternal collagen vascular diseases resulting in structural defects (Bianchi et al., 2000; Kleinman & Nehgme, 2004; Seferovi et al., 2006; Strasburger, 2000). Conduction defects can develop early in cardiac development when the cardiac tube loops to form the four-chamber heart. In the case of maternal collagen diseases such as lupus and fetal second- or third-degree AV block, maternal anti-Ro/SSA and/or anti-La/SSB antibodies cross the placenta and deposits of immunoglobulin and complement form in the atrial and ventricular myocardium. Inflammatory reaction to these deposits results in fibrosis, calcification and, eventually, interruption of the conduction through the AV node (Jaeggi et al., 2004; Seferovi et al.; Trines & Hornberger, 2004).

Congenital heart defects may also result in fetal arrhythmias, although the relationship varies according to the specific defect. For example, supraventricular tachycardia (SVT), the most frequently seen arrhythmia, is rarely associated with congenital heart defects. Atrial flutter is associated with congenital heart defects in approximately 20% of cases. However, complete heart block is associated with congenital heart defects in 50% of cases (Kleinman & Nehgme, 2004).

DIAGNOSIS OF FETAL ARRHYTHMIAS

Fetal arrhythmias may first be recognized during routine fetal assessment via fetal monitoring, either by auscultation or electronic fetal monitoring (EFM). When auscultation is used an irregular rhythm may be heard. EFM data usually associated with fetal assessment, such as baseline, variability, and presence of accelerations or decelerations, may be obscured, depending on the frequency and type of arrhythmia. In these instances, recognition of unusual FHR characteristics should be reported promptly.

Fetal Echocardiogram

A useful diagnostic tool to assess fetal arrhythmias is the fetal echocardiogram (echoCG). If a sustained rhythm disturbance is recognized, this diagnostic technique is recommended for direct imaging of cardiac wall motion to assess for rhythm, cardiac structure, cardiac function, and fetal well-being and to determine whether hydrops is present. Color flow mapping is often used in conjunction with the echoCG to identify abnormal shifts in blood flow as a result of specific arrhythmias (Jaeggi & Nii, 2005; Kleinman & Nehgme, 2004; Larmay & Strasburger, 2004; Pedra et al., 2002).

Fetal Magnetocardiography

Fetal magnetocardiography (FMCG) is a noninvasive diagnostic tool used to analyze electrophysical changes of the heart as early as 20 weeks' gestation. Compared with other common methods, FMCG provides more information that can be used to influence therapeutic decisions and thus contribute to optimal prenatal and postnatal management. FMCG can define fetal cardiac conduction and rhythm disturbances more precisely (Strasburger, 2005). It can provide information about the QRS and QT intervals, FHR variability, and T wave abnormalities (Strasburger). If no arrhythmias are found after the cardiac study with FMCG, further follow-up provides no added benefit. Limitations in using this diagnostic tool include the presence of a maternal pacemaker or other devices such as clips on cerebral aneurysms (Kumar & O'Brien, 2004).

M-Mode EchoCG

M-mode echoCG uses real-time imaging techniques to observe and time electromechanical events of the fetus' cardiac activity (Kleinman, 2004; Strasburger, 2005). M-mode imaging is helpful in the evaluation of contractility in abnormalities that affect heart wall motion by looking at the timing of atrial and ventricular events in the cardiac conduction cycle. The analysis of the AV contraction sequence can provide an accurate picture of the precise cardiac rhythm (Kleinman et al.; Strasburger). It is also useful in determining the degree of atrial hypertrophy associated with SVT and in defining those infants with AV block who will require pacing after birth (Strasburger, 2005). Some factors may limit the data from the M-mode echoCG. These factors include poor resolution due to maternal obesity, oligohydramnios, and rib shadowing; and difficulty obtaining a reproducible view due to fetal movement and position changes in utero (Comani et al., 2004). M-mode echoCG may be used in conjunction with other diagnostic techniques, including pulse-wave Doppler, when more information is required to arrive at a diagnosis (Jaeggi & Nii, 2005). In addition, M-mode echoCG may not be available at many institutions, necessitating a referral to a regional center (Kleinman et al.; Larmay & Strasburger, 2004).

Pulsed Doppler EchoCG

Pulsed Doppler echoCG provides information about electromechanical events as well as views of the heart chambers and the great vessels. The use of pulsed Doppler echoCG has been found to enhance the ability to detect cardiac malformations in utero (Jaeggi & Masaki, 2005; Strasburger, 2005). This technique is useful in determining atrial rate and flow reversal, ventricular rate and cardiac output, and AV contraction sequence (Strasburger, 2000). When used simultaneously with M-mode echoCG, blood flow velocities in the superior vena cava and ascending aorta, which can be determined with pulse Doppler echoCG, can provide additional information regarding atrial and ventricular events (Jaeggi & Nii, 2005; Strasburger). This additional information can provide the parents with reassurance about the fetal heart, even though the incidence of structural heart defects causing arrhythmic patterns is relatively low.

These techniques are not without limitations, however. Image resolution, fetal position, and the complexity of the specific arrhythmia may limit the information obtained when these modalities are used (Carvalho et al., 2007).

MORE COMMON CLINICALLY SIGNIFICANT FETAL ARRHYTHMIAS

Tachyarrhythmias: Sinus Tachycardia and SVT

Sinus Tachycardia

Tachycardia in the fetus is defined as a baseline rate over 160 bpm (Macones, Hankins, Spong, Hauth, & Moore, 2008). Tachycardias are the second most common type of fetal arrhythmia (Kleinman & Nehgme, 2004) and may originate from within or outside of the SA node. Sinus tachycardia is considered a sinus node variant and is defined as an FHR greater than 160 bpm sustained for greater than 10 minutes (Figure 12-3). Sinus tachycardia is generally considered benign when the rate is less than 180 bpm and moderate FHR variability is present. Sinus tachycardia warrants further evaluation when the FHR is sustained at greater than 180 bpm (Jaeggi & Nii, 2005; Sharland, 2001; Strasburger, 2000). The most common causes of sinus tachycardia include the following:

1. Responses to continuous fetal activity
2. Maternal fever
3. Use of beta-sympathomimetic medications, such as terbutaline (Jaeggi & Nii)
4. Use of parasympatholytic medications, such as atropine, hydralazine (Apresoline), or hydroxyzine hydrochloride (Atarax) (Kleinman et al., 2004; Strasburger)
5. Underlying conditions, such as infections (Jaeggi & Nii); fetal hypoxia or myocarditis (Jaeggi & Nii; Strasburger); or maternal drug ingestion or hormone or catecholamine transfer (Pickoff, 2004)
6. Maternal hyperthyroidism (Strasburger et al., 2007).

The tachycardic fetal ECG will display normal P waves occurring in routine fashion preceding each QRS complex (Figure 12-3). In contrast to

FIGURE 12-3   Sinus Tachycardia (Fetal Spiral Electrode and Tocodynamometer)

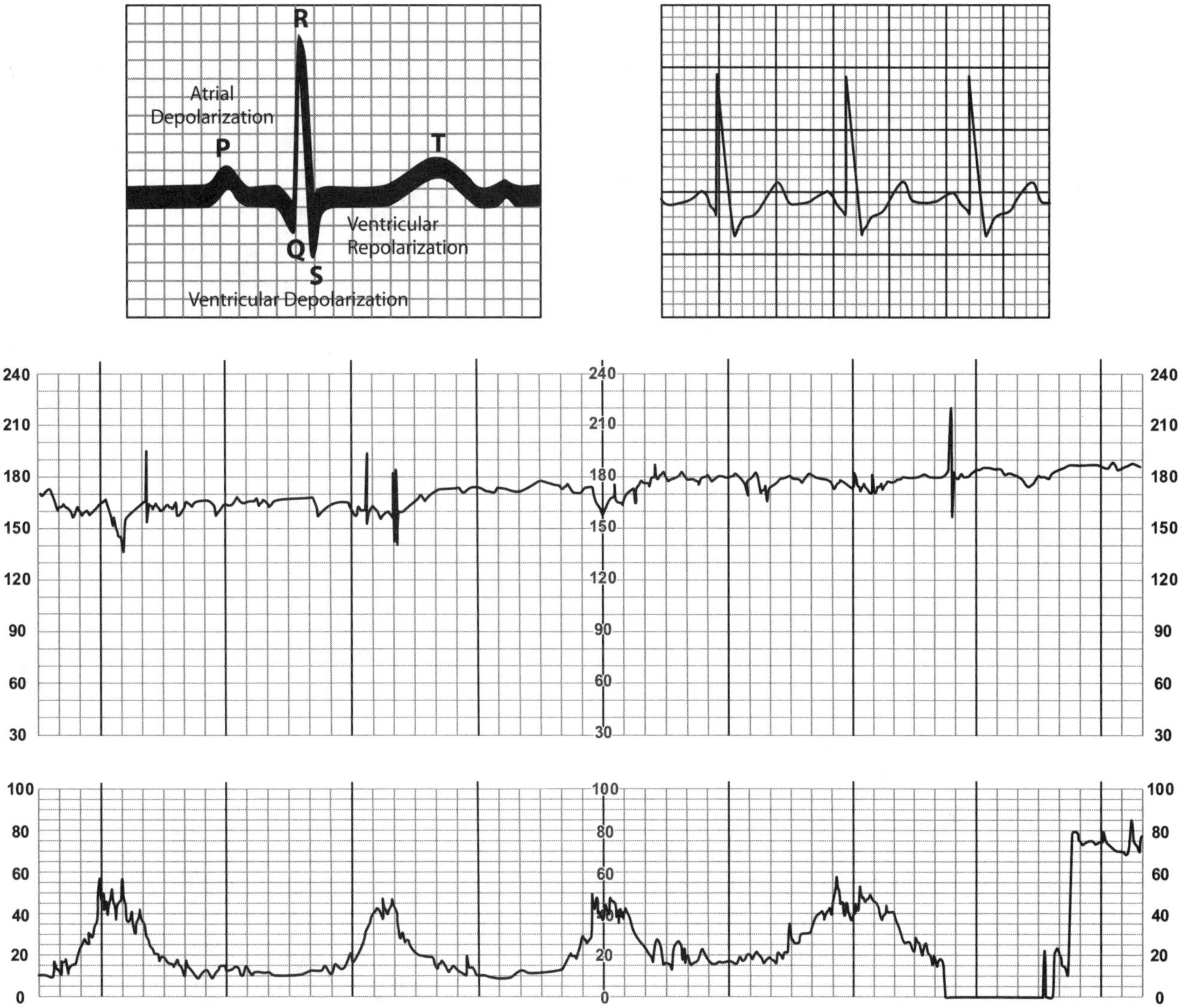

other tachycardias, sinus tachycardia may display moderate variability within the baseline rate (Jaeggi & Nii, 2005). Sinus tachycardia generally does not exceed 200 to 210 bpm (Jaeggi & Nii; Strasburger, 2000). However, when it does exceed 210 bpm, the rapid rate makes it difficult to differentiate from other types of tachycardia (Strasburger).

Interventions

When sinus tachycardia is noted, the clinician should evaluate maternal hydration status and assess the woman for fever and other signs and symptoms of infection. Correction of any identifiable underlying etiology is appropriate whenever possible, as is close surveillance of the

FHR tracing for maintenance of moderate variability. The primary provider should also be notified of findings.

Supraventricular Tachycardia

SVT is one of the few fetal arrhythmias with cause for concern (Figure 12-4). It is also the second most frequent cause of fetal tachycardia, after maternal infection (Strasburger, 2005). SVT usually presents after 15 weeks' gestation; it is most commonly seen at 30 to 32 weeks' gestation (Cuneo & Strasburger, 2000; Menihan & Kopel, 2008; Strasburger, 2005; Strasburger et al., 2007). SVT is a sustained, rapid, regular atrial arrhythmia. The rate may range from 210 to 320 bpm, but SVT rates are typically between

FIGURE 12-4 Supraventricular Tachycardia (Ultrasound and Tocodynamometer)

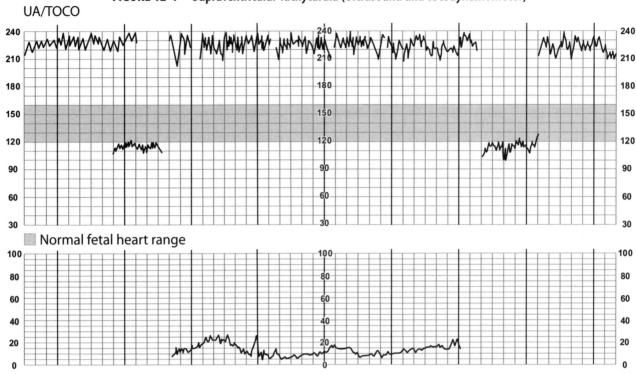

UA/TOCO

Normal fetal heart range

240 and 260 bpm (Kleinman & Nehgme, 2004; Larmay & Strasburger, 2004).

Multiple electrical impulse pathways exist for the development of SVT. Reentrant or reciprocating SVT occurs when a circular depolarization cycle has been established between an ectopic atrial pacemaker and the AV node. An automatic SVT results from the development of an irritable ectopic focus that has assumed the role of pacemaker. Atrial flutter or fibrillation or PACs can also produce SVT (Kleinman & Nehgme, 2004; Larmay & Strasburger, 2004; Strasburger, 2005; Strasburger, et al., 2007). Most fetal SVTs are reentrant in nature (Kleinman & Nehgme; Strasburger, 2005; Strasburger et al., 2007), meaning that more than one pathway conducts the impulse. The electrical impulse is carried over a secondary pathway, but the reentry of the impulse occurs over a primary pathway, creating the circular conduction pattern (Figure 12-5). On ECG, the P wave may be lost within the T wave of the previous complexes, and the QRS spike may be narrowed or widened, depending on the specific electrical pathway (Figure 12-4). The EFM tracings may exhibit half counting of these high rates.

FIGURE 12-5 Ectopic Circular Pathway of Supraventricular Tachycardia

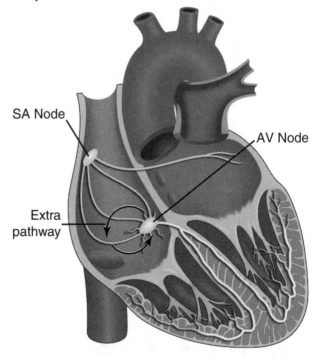

SVT may be paroxysmal (occurring suddenly in waves or spasms) or continuous (Strasburger, 2005). In general, SVT has absent variability because of a fixed R-R interval, especially at rates

greater than 240 bpm (Menihan & Kopel, 2008; Strasburger, 2005).

The rapid heart rate that occurs with SVT increases the workload of the fetal heart. It also increases cardiac oxygen demand. The rapid rate results in decreased stroke volume because of decreased filling time, and cardiac output is therefore diminished. Depending on gestational age and the persistence of the SVT, the fetus may not be able to meet its oxygen demands, resulting in the development of congestive heart failure because the heart fails as a pump. In addition, there is an increased hemolysis of red blood cells, further reducing oxygen delivery (Strasburger, 2000, 2005; Tanel & Rhodes, 2001). Nonimmunologic hydrops fetalis—the development of generalized edema in the abdomen, scalp, liver, and spleen—and fetal death may result (Strasburger, 2000, 2005).

The rate and progression of the hydrops depend on the severity of the hemodynamic compromise, as well as gestational age (Strasburger, 2000). The unborn, untreated fetus may develop cardiac failure and ischemic cerebral disease. Often, the fetus will demonstrate evidence of pericardial or pleural effusion, cardiomegaly, polyhydramnios, scalp edema, or ascites, all of which are suggestive of congestive heart failure (Strasburger, 2005).

Treatment

The treatment of SVT can be highly effective and improve fetal outcome. Treatment recommendations range from observation only, to prenatal medication therapy, to planned early birth of the affected fetus. Recommendations depend on whether the SVT is intermittent or sustained, the gestational age of the fetus, the presence or absence of hydrops, and parental wishes (Jaeggi & Masaki, 2005; Joglar & Page, 2001; Kleinman & Nehgme, 2004; Larmay & Strasburger, 2004; Sharland, 2001; Strasburger, 2000; Tulzer, 2000).

Observation is often used when the pregnancy is close to term, the tachycardic episodes are short lived, and there is no evidence of fetal hydrops. Decision making regarding medical management of SVT should weigh the risks of pre-

maturity against the risks of cardiac failure and poor oxygen delivery in utero. Generally, birth is recommended for term fetuses without hydrops. However, if the term fetus has hydrops, the fetus is usually treated in utero, and birth usually then occurs after the SVT has converted. If the fetus is preterm, intrauterine conversion therapy is usually initiated along with assessment of fetal lung maturity. In these cases, the risks of preterm birth and its associated complications should be weighed against the risks of a continued cardiac arrhythmia and its associated complications (Kleinman & Nehgme, 2004; Strasburger, 2005). If the lungs are deemed mature and the conversion of the SVT has been achieved, birth should proceed. However, if the lungs are immature, intrauterine conversion therapy is recommended along with steroid therapy. After the lungs are mature and conversion is achieved, birth should be considered (Sharland, 2001; Strasburger, 2000; Tanel & Rhodes, 2001).

In nonhydropic fetuses, digoxin therapy is the first-line medication choice. Initially, digoxin is administered intravenously because oral administration can result in erratic absorption rates as a result of delayed gastric emptying during pregnancy (Strasburger, 2000; Strasburger, et al., 2007). After adequate digitalization with intravenous (IV) digoxin has been accomplished and the fetus has converted to normal sinus rhythm, the mother can be switched to the oral form for maintenance, which is continued until birth (Kleinman & Nehgme, 2004). It is important to note that the dosage of digoxin may need to be as much as 100% higher (twice the normal dose) than is required in the adult, nonpregnant patient (Larmay & Strasburger, 2004; Strasburger, et al., 2007). It is recommended that frequent maternal digoxin levels be drawn; the therapeutic range is 0.8 to 2.0 ng/mL (Kleinman & Nehgme; Larmay & Strasburger).

The hydropic fetus with SVT remains a therapeutic challenge. Digoxin alone may be ineffective because the transfer of digoxin from the mother to the fetus is poor; adequate fetal blood levels may not be achieved even with near toxic maternal blood levels (Jaeggi & Nii, 2005). In these cases, switching to or adding additional medications, such as adenosine, amiodarone, sotalol, and flecainide, may be necessary (Campbell, Best, Eswaran, & Lowery, 2006; Kleinman & Nehgme, 2004; Larmay & Strasburger, 2004; Oudijk et al., 2003; Strasburger, et al., 2007). Kleinman and Nehgme recommend a protocol whereby propranolol is added as the second-line medication and flecainide is third line. Oudijk et al. (2002) do not recommend use of verapamil because it may increase mortality.

Sotalol is one of the newer medications used for fetal SVT. It is a Class III cardiac medication that has beta-blocker effects normally seen in Class II agents, as well as the potassium channel blocker effect of the Class III cardiac medications. If sotalol is used, it is important to discontinue propranolol and flecainide for 72 hours to allow clearance of these medications from the system; digoxin may be continued (Kleinman & Nehgme, 2004). If SVT continues after these medications, amiodarone can be considered. However, sotalol must be discontinued for 96 hours and the dosage of digoxin halved prior to beginning amiodarone therapy (Kleinman & Nehgme).

There have also been cases in which medications have been injected directly into the fetus, using the intramuscular, intraperitoneal, and umbilical vein routes. In these studies, there have been reports of increased conversion rates back to normal sinus rhythm (Singh, 2004; Strasburger et al., 2007). Use of fetal routes may require repetitive invasive procedures, potentially exposing both the woman and her fetus to subsequent problems, such as infection and hemorrhage. Strasburger (2000) advocates direct intramuscular injection of the fetus rather than using the umbilical cord for this purpose if a more direct fetal route is deemed necessary.

Bradyarrhythmias: Sinus Bradycardia and Atrioventricular Blocks

Bradycardia is defined as a baseline FHR below 110 bpm (Macones et al., 2008). Intermittent periods of bradycardia are considered benign when accompanied by moderate variability (Menihan & Kopel, 2008). Although transient FHRs less than 110 bpm may be normal, sustained bradycardia requires further assessment and evaluation. The eventual prognosis is dependent on the cause of the bradycardia, the ventricular rate, and the presence or absence of structural cardiac abnormalities (Wren, 2006).

Sinus Bradycardia

Sinus bradycardia is a FHR less than 110 bpm sustained for more than 10 minutes (Figure 12-6). The fetal ECG displays normal P waves occurring in routine relationship preceding each QRS complex (Figure 12-6). Sinus bradycardia is evaluated in relation to the entire clinical picture and may reflect an abnormal fetal or maternal condition, such as maternal or fetal compromise (Menihan & Kopel, 2008); increased vagal tone (Simpson, 2008; Strasburger, 2000); maternal hypothermia (Simpson); medications, such as beta-blocking agents (Strasburger); fetal hypothyroidism (Kleinman & Nehgme, 2004); placental insufficiency (Kleinman & Nehgme); intrauterine growth restriction (Strasburger); increased pressure on the uterus, such as that produced as a result of fetal hydrops (Strasburger); or prolonged QT syndrome (Larmay & Strasburger, 2004; Strasburger).

Interventions

Management of sinus bradycardia includes identification of any underlying etiology and determination of fetal well-being. If moderate variability is present and no underlying pathology is identified, continued observation is warranted and intervention may not be necessary; however, the primary provider should be notified of the FHR findings. Management of an identified underlying pathology will depend on the specific problem and whether or not fetal well-being can be confirmed.

Atrioventricular Blocks

AV blocks are categorized according to the severity of the block. The three degrees of AV block are first, second, and third (complete). In all blocks, impulse conduction through the AV node is abnormal.

All impulses are conducted through the AV node in first-degree block, but a delay in im-

FIGURE 12-6   Sinus Bradycardia (Fetal Scalp Electrode and Tocodynamometer)

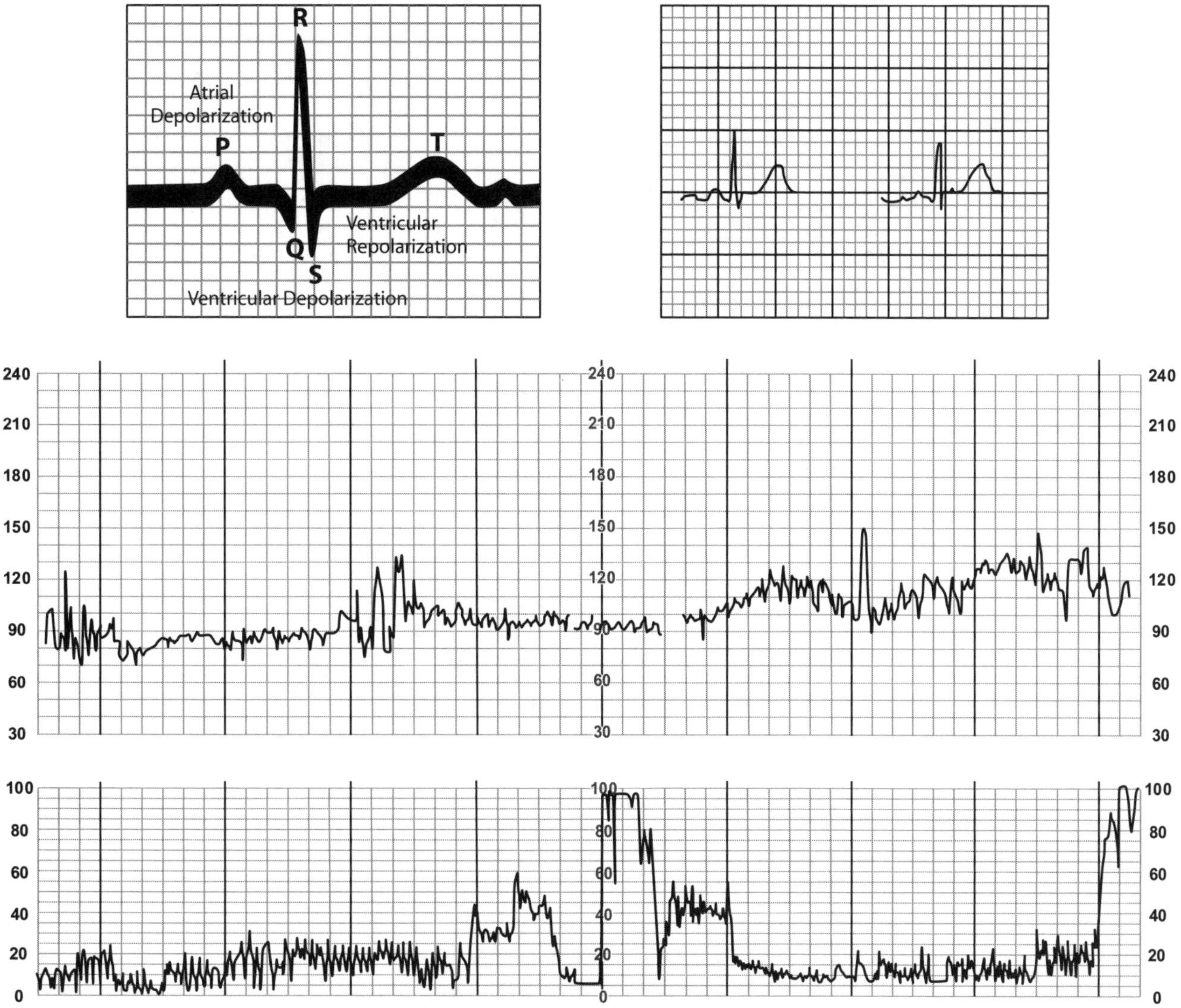

pulse conduction produces prolonged P-R intervals (Jaeggi & Nii, 2005; Kleinman & Nehgme, 2004). First-degree blocks are difficult to recognize in the fetus because the FHR is within normal range. They may be due to structural anomalies, although diagnosis of such an anomaly may be difficult (Kleinman & Nehgme; Strasburger, 2005).

Second-degree AV block represents intermittent failure of conduction of some of the atrial impulses through the AV node and may be manifested as occasional loss of conduction through the AV node or as several consecutive dropped beats (Jaeggi & Masaki, 2005; Kleinman & Nehgme, 2004). This may occur in association with a rapid atrial rate caused by SVT, atrial flutter or atrial fibrillation, or in association with conduction system disease. When associated with conduction system disease, second-degree block may progress to third-degree, or complete, heart block (Kleinman & Nehgme).

Maternal collagen vascular disease and fetal cardiac structural defects are two causes of second-degree block (Kleinman & Nehgme, 2004; Strasburger, 2000). The relationship between maternal collagen disease and AV block centers on the anti-SSA/Ro or anti-SSB/La antibodies developed by the mother. These antibodies cross the placenta, binding to fetal cardiac tissue, including the AV node and the atrial and ventricular myocardium (Kleinman et al., 2004). An inflammatory reaction occurs, leading to fibrosis, calcification,

FIGURE 12-7   Third-degree Atrioventricular Block (Ultrasound and Tocodynamometer)

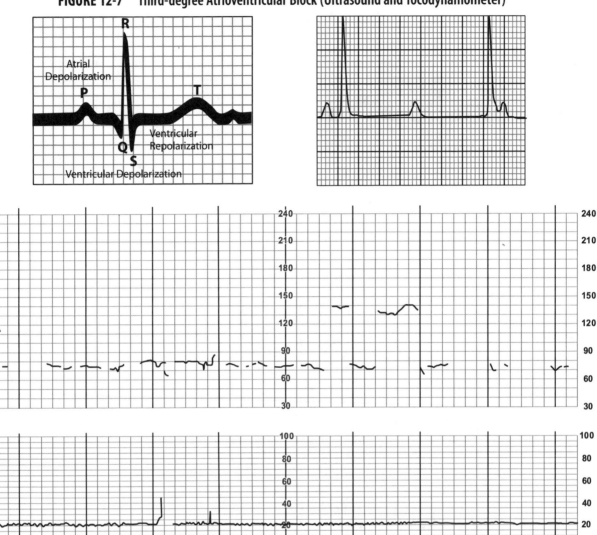

and eventual interruption of the fetal conduction pathway, producing the AV block (Kleinman et al., 2004; Larmay & Strasburger, 2004; Strasburger, 2000; Strasburger et al., 2007).

Third-degree, or complete, AV block may also be seen in the fetus (Figure 12-7). Third-degree heart block represents the complete absence of conduction of the impulse from the SA node through the AV node. There is a complete dissociation between the atrial and ventricular contractions, creating P waves that have no relationship to the QRS complexes. As a result, there is a higher atrial rate (within the normal range as atrial contraction is stimulated by the SA node) and a much slower ventricular rate (Jaeggi & Nii, 2005; Kleinman & Nehgme, 2004; Strasburger,

2005; Wren, 2006). This ventricular rate is initiated by an ectopic focus below the level of the block (Wren).

Third-degree blocks are caused by fetal cardiac structural defects, fetal cytomegalovirus infection, antiphospholipid antibody syndrome, or the presence of maternal anti-SSA/Ro or anti-SSB/La antibodies, which are present with maternal lupus (Kleinman & Nehgme, 2004; Kleinman et al., 2004; Strasburger, 2000). These antibodies cross the placenta and destroy the fetal cardiac conductive tissues, specifically the AV node (Kleinman et al., 2004; Larmay & Strasburger, 2004; Tanel & Rhodes, 2001; Wren, 2006). Maternal rheumatoid arthritis and other collagen diseases have also been associated with fetal third-degree heart block (Kleinman & Nehgme; Larmay & Strasburger).

In up to approximately 50% of fetuses with third-degree heart block, congenital heart disease is also present (Bianchi et al., 2000; Jaeggi & Nii, 2005; Strasburger, 2000). Third-degree AV block also may be associated with regurgitation of the mitral or tricuspid valves, damage to the His-Purkinje tissues, inflammation of the AV node and bundle of His, or damage to the fetal myocardium, all leading to congestive cardiomyopathy (Strasburger; Tulzer, 2000).

Treatment

Treatment of second- and third-degree AV block is essentially the same. If the patient has high anti-SSA/Ro or anti-SSB/La titers, use of steroids that cross the placenta (dexamethasone or betamethasone) may improve fetal cardiac function or prevent further manifestations of the disease process, such as cardiomyopathy (Jaeggi et al., 2004; Strasburger et al., 2007). Steroids are withheld if there is a specific contraindication for their use (Jaeggi & Nii, 2005; Kleinman & Nehgme, 2004). Other therapies are directed toward increasing the FHR with a beta-sympathomimetic such as terbutaline or salbutamol (Bianchi et al., 2000; Jaeggi et al., 2004). Jaeggi and Nii (2005) have reported success using dexamethasone and adding a beta-stimulant if the FHR remains below 55 bpm. Other therapies, such as maternal administration of immunoglobulin or early pacing of the fetus in utero, are not recommended because no successful outcomes have been achieved to date (Kleinman et al., 2004; Schmolling et al., 2000; Vautier-Rit et al., 2000; Vlagsma, Hallensleben, & Meijboom, 2001).

Hydropic fetuses are more difficult to manage. Overall the prognosis is not favorable, and current treatment modalities have not improved outcomes for these babies (Kleinman & Nehgme, 2004; Sharland, 2001; Strasburger, 2005). Factors such as a baseline FHR above 55 bpm, absence of structural defects, and absence of hydrops improve the prognosis (Jaeggi & Nii, 2005; Strasburger, 2005).

After birth, fetal epicardial or endocardial leads can be placed temporarily to pace the heart (Larmay & Strasburger, 2004). Following temporary pacing, permanent pacemaker implantation should be investigated. Permanent pacemaker implantation is usually required in neonates with structural cardiac disease and in approximately 50% of patients with isolated AV block. The recommended criteria for pacemaker application in neonates with isolated block include (1) symptomatic fetus or neonate, (2) resting heart rate less than 50 to 55 bpm, and (3) presence of wide complex escape rhythms (Larmay & Strasburger; Strasburger et al., 2007).

LESS COMMON FETAL ARRHYTHMIAS

Other types of fetal arrhythmias are occasionally seen. Rhythm disturbances are classified based on their origin and are referred to as atrial, supraventricular, atrioventricular, or ventricular arrhythmias. An irregular pattern or "skipped beats" may be observed with ultrasonography or a fetoscope. The underlying causes, fetal responses, and sequelae vary according to the specific type of arrhythmia. The fetal rhythm disturbances that clinicians are most likely to see (SVT and AV blocks, also known as junctional rhythms) have been discussed. This section will cover other atrial and ventricular fetal arrhythmias sometimes seen in clinical practice.

Atrial Arrhythmias

Premature atrial contractions (PACs), atrial flutter, and atrial fibrillation originate from an atrial pacemaker other than the SA node and demonstrate changes in electrical activity on the fetal ECG.

Premature Atrial Contractions

Premature atrial contractions (PACs) (Figure 12-8) may be associated with redundancy or an aneurysm of the flap covering the foramen ovale; maternal caffeine, nicotine or alcohol use; or maternal hyperthyroidism (Larmay & Strasburger, 2004; Strasburger, 2000; Strasburger, et al., 2007). PACs are characterized by an early atrial contraction. They exhibit a premature P wave and may be followed by a normal QRS complex (Figure 12-8). PACs can be either conducted or nonconducted. They are said to be conducted if the impulse is carried down the conduction system, producing a subsequent ventricular contraction. Nonconducted PACs occur with the discharge of an ectopic atrial focus that is too premature to move through the AV node. Because it partially penetrates the AV junction, the premature depolarization is followed by a pause (called a compensatory pause) until the AV node recovers sufficiently to conduct the next sinus node-initiated impulse (Strasburger, 2000) (Figure 12-8).

PACs also can occur in patterns described by the frequency of PAC occurrence. *Bigeminy* oc-

curs when premature atrial contractions alternate with normal sinus beats. The pattern will be one normal beat (normal P-QRS relationship) followed by one premature beat or PAC (Kleinman & Nehgme, 2004). *Trigeminy* occurs when there is a premature atrial contraction every third beat. The pattern will be two normal beats (normal P-QRS relationship) and one premature beat or PAC. In either case, the fetal tracing will show vertical spikes with upward and downward strokes. The upward stroke represents the PAC, and the downward stroke represents the compensatory pause. The baseline FHR will be seen intermittently between these upward and downward strokes. Treatment is geared toward the avoidance of caffeine products and beta-sympa-

FIGURE 12-8   Premature Atrial Contractions (Fetal Scalp Electrode and Tocodynamometer)

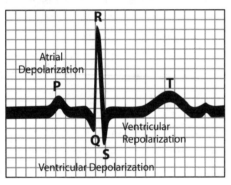
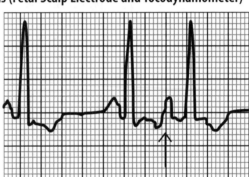
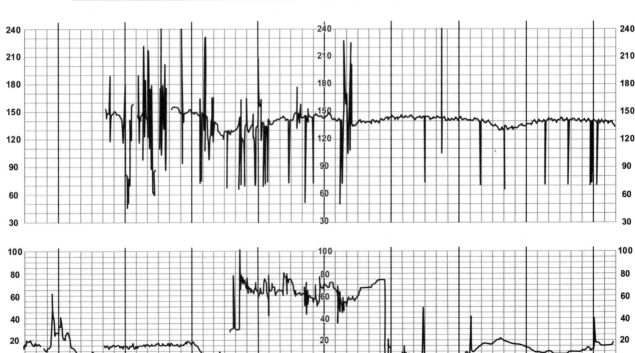

thomimetics (Larmay & Strasburger; Strasburger et al., 2007).

Atrial Flutter

There is a strong association between atrial flutter and SVT because atrial flutter is also due to the reentry of impulses around a circular pathway (Strasburger, 2005). However, instead of involving the AV node as seen with SVT, the reentrant pathway in atrial flutter is found within the atrial wall. The ECG reading will usually display regularly recurring sawtoothed atrial activity instead of the normal P wave. Atrial rates can approach 300 to 500 bpm in the fetus and 300 to 360 bpm in the neonate (Kleinman & Nehgme, 2004;

Strasburger et al., 2007). Because of the significantly increased atrial rate, the AV node slows or blocks some of these impulses, resulting in ventricular rates between 190 and 240 bpm (Kleinman et al., 2004; Larmay & Strasburger, 2004; Strasburger, 2000). In addition, the fetal tracing may show half counting of the FHR, as with SVT (Figure 12-9). This arrhythmia may be due to atrial dilatation, as occurs with some atrial structural defects, including deformity of the tricuspid valve; mitral regurgitation; atrial septal defects; hypoplastic left heart; chromosomal abnormalities; cardiomyopathy; or reentrant SVT (Kleinman et al., 2004; Larmay & Strasburger; Strasburger et al., 2007).

FIGURE 12-9   Atrial Flutter (Ultrasound and Tocodynamometer)

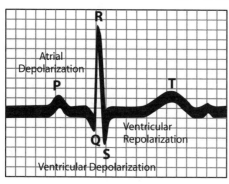
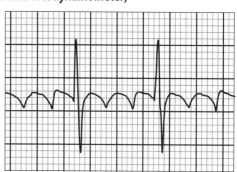
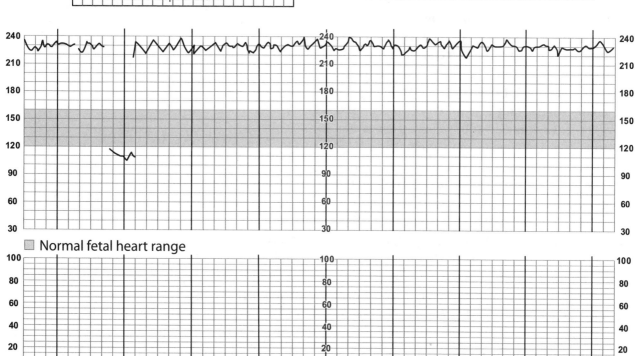

Atrial Fibrillation

Atrial fibrillation occurs even less frequently than atrial flutter (Kleinman & Nehgme, 2004; Strasburger, 2000). Atrial fibrillation may be associated with fetomaternal hemorrhage, Wolff-Parkinson-White (WPW) syndrome, or cardiac structural abnormalities, with the latter contributing most often to the high mortality rate. As with atrial flutter, many of these impulses are blocked at the AV node, resulting in ventricular rates that vary from 60 to 200 bpm. The ECG will often show low-amplitude irregular atrial activity with QRS complexes of various sizes.

Treatment of Atrial Flutter and Fibrillation

With atrial arrhythmias, as with SVT, the administration of digoxin or propranolol is used initially in the antepartum period to control ventricular response of the fetal heart (Kleinman & Nehgme, 2004; Schmolling et al., 2000; Strasburger, 2000; Vautier-Rit et al., 2000; Vlagsma et al., 2001). After an adequate ventricular response is accomplished with digoxin, it is maintained (Kleinman & Nehgme). If digoxin is not effective in converting the arrhythmia, Class I medications such as flecainide or procainamide slow the flutter rate, favoring AV node conduction (Joglar & Page, 2001; Kleinman & Nehgme; Tanel & Rhodes, 2001). Class III medications such as sotalol or amiodarone can also be used to convert atrial flutter (Cuneo & Strasburger, 2000; Kleinman & Nehgme; Larmay & Strasburger, 2004; Oudijk et al., 2000; Schmolling et al., 2000; Strasburger, 2005; Tanel & Rhodes, 2001; Vautier-Rit et al.; Vlagsma et al.). Although amiodarone has a long half-life, it has been associated with fetal cretinism and, as a result, is often not recommended (Schmolling et al., 2000; Vautier-Rit et al.; Vlagsma et al.). Some studies have suggested that sotalol should be the first-line agent for fetuses with atrial flutter (Oudijk et al., 2000). Verapamil is not recommended because it relies on an immature myocardium to allow for passage of calcium to the fetal heart (Joglar & Page; Kleinman et al., 2004).

Treatment for atrial fibrillation is similar to that for atrial flutter. However, because of the difficulty in converting this pattern to a normal sinus rhythm using digoxin alone, other more potent cardiac medications, as noted previously, may be needed in place of digoxin.

Premature Ventricular Contractions

Premature ventricular contractions (PVCs) are caused by stimulation of an ectopic ventricular focus, producing ventricular contractions that are independent of those originating in the atrium. There may be a compensatory pause after the PVC, during which time the ventricles will not respond to stimuli originating from the SA node. On the ECG, the PVC will be displayed as a bizarre, wide QRS complex without a P wave. The T wave can be in a direction opposite that of the QRS complex (Figure 12-10). The fetal monitor tracing will show a vertical spike with each PVC. Similar to PACs, PVCs can occur as *bigeminy* (occurring every second beat), *trigeminy* (occurring every third beat), or at random intervals. The fetal heart baseline may be obscured if the PVCs are occurring frequently (Figure 12-10).

Fetal PVCs are rare. They can be caused by cardiac anomalies; fetal hydrops; cardiomyopathies; myocarditis; digitalis toxicity; and maternal use of caffeine, nicotine, alcohol, or cocaine. In rare instances, hyperkalemia caused by maternal hyperemesis may also produce fetal PVCs (Strasburger, et al., 2007; Kleinman & Nehgme, 2004; Larmay & Strasburger, 2004).

CONSEQUENCES OF FETAL ARRHYTHMIAS

Fetal arrhythmias affect fetuses along a continuum from no apparent effect to the development of dilated cardiomyopathy, fetal hydrops, and progression to fetal death. The prognosis depends on a variety of factors, including the associated pathology, the type of arrhythmia, the FHR (because this determines cardiac output), how quickly the arrhythmia is diagnosed, and fetal response to treatment. Presence or absence of fetal hydrops is often the determining factor when considering treatment options.

FIGURE 12-10 Premature Ventricular Contractions (Fetal Scalp Electrode and Tocodynamometer)

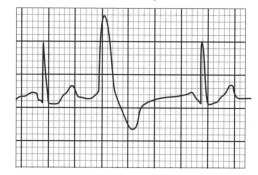

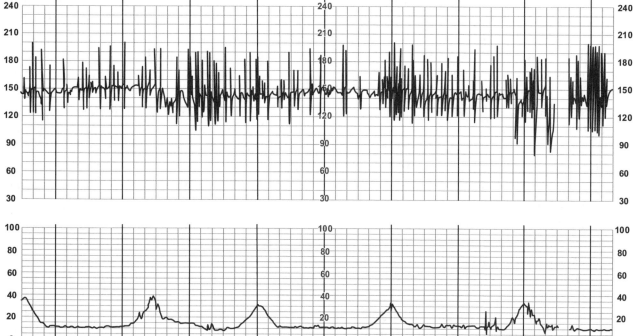

"Cardiomyopathy" is a broad term that can be subdivided into specific categories, including dilated cardiomyopathy, which is characterized by ventricular dilation and impaired contractility (Fujioka & Kitaura, 2001; Sivasankaran, Sharland, & Simpson, 2005). Dilated cardiomyopathy can be due to infectious agents, such as rubella, coxsackie B, cytomegalovirus, parvovirus, herpes, and toxoplasmosis, or may be associated with heart block, SVT, or PVCs (Fujioka & Kitaura; Jaeggi & Nii, 2005; Pedra et al., 2002; Strasburger, 2000). Therapies include specific antibiotics and antivirals, fetal administration of IVIG and/or administration of corticosteroids (Pedra et al., 2002).

Cardiomyopathy also may result from complications of pregnancy such as twin-twin transfusion. In this syndrome, there are vascular anastomoses between the placentas, producing an unbalanced transfusion of blood from the donor twin to the recipient (Harkness & Crombleholme, 2005; Huber & Hecher, 2004; Jain & Fisk, 2004; Rao, Sairam, & Shehata, 2004; Wee & Fisk, 2002). One twin becomes hypervolemic while the other twin becomes hypovolemic. The hypervolemic twin manifests with fluid overload, polyuria, polyhydramnios, hypertension, myocardial hypertrophy, and hemorrhagic infarctions in the kidneys. The hypovolemic twin manifests with growth restriction, decreased renal perfusion, oliguria, oligohydramnios, and renal hypoperfusion (Harkness & Crombleholme; Huber & Hecher; Jain & Fisk) Both twins may develop congenital heart disease and/or congestive heart failure and die in utero if untreated (Harkness & Crombleholme; Jain & Fisk; Pedra et al., 2002; Wee & Fisk).

Fetal hydrops is defined as edema in two or more fetal compartments (anasarca) such as the abdomen, scalp, skin, liver, and spleen. Pericardial and/or pleural effusion may also occur; it is the manifestation of fetal congestive heart failure (Hamdan & Cassady, 2006; Kleinman & Nehgme, 2004; Strasburger, 2000). It is hypothesized that the development of fetal hydrops is related to alterations in the pressures within the heart. Normally, the pressures in the right atrium are greater than those found in the left atrium, one of the factors responsible for maintaining a patent foramen ovale. With some arrhythmias—specifically SVT, atrial flutter, and AV blocks—the pressure in the left atrium is increased. This produces an increased back pressure, resulting in increased pressure in the right atrium, and eventually in the venous system. Increased venous pressures cause interstitial fluid accumulation, producing edema and effusion. To complicate the situation, hepatic synthesis of albumin may be compromised as a result of the decreased hepatic circulation, further contributing to edema formation (Hamdan & Cassady; Kleinman & Nehgme; Larmay & Strasburger, 2004). As a result of increased venous pressure, there is a secondary increase in aldosterone, renin, norepinephrine, and angiotensin I; this produces vasoconstriction, further worsening the edema (Hamdan & Cassady).

Fetal death is related to the severity of the edema and associated conditions such as cardiac anomalies. Most cases report a 60% to 90% mortality, although there have been improvements in these figures in some recent reports (Hamdan & Cassady, 2006). With SVT, fetal mortality can range between 8% and 30%. These numbers do not tell the entire story, however. To save the fetus's life, birth may be the only option. In these cases, the difficulties associated with premature

birth must be overcome. In general, the earlier the hydrops occurs in gestation, the poorer the prognosis (Hamdan & Cassady).

TREATMENT ISSUES

Treatment of fetal arrhythmias is a complex process that depends on the type of pattern, gestational age of the fetus, status of the mother, and the presence of indicators of fetal decompensation (Strasburger, 2000). It requires a multidisciplinary team approach, an accurate diagnosis, and an individualized treatment plan for both the woman and her fetus.

Kleinman et al. (2004) state that most referrals for fetal heart irregularities are due to irregularities or "skipped beats." Many have resolved spontaneously prior to diagnosis. In those that have not resolved, a definitive diagnosis should be obtained (Kleinman & Nehgme, 2004). After the diagnosis and the risk-benefit analysis to both mother and fetus are determined, medical treatment can be initiated.

Regardless of the situation, parents should be offered pretreatment counseling. Discussion of treatment options requires openness and cultural sensitivity on the part of the medical and nursing team. Options may range from conservative management, to in-utero pharmacologic treatment, to pregnancy termination, or to planned preterm birth. Table 12-2 describes a selection of medications that may be used in treatment. For example, in cases of SVT or atrial flutter, there is much support for a conservative management scheme in which cases of intermittent fetal tachycardia without evidence of fetal hemodynamic compromise are observed closely, possibly avoiding the need for potentially dangerous pharmacotherapy (Jaeggi & Nii, 2005; Larmay & Strasburger, 2004; Strasburger, 2000).

If needed, medications that have the longest record of safety should be considered as the first-line agents for treating arrhythmic patterns (Joglar & Page, 2001). The risks inherent in antiarrhythmic therapy depend largely on the electrophysiologic mechanisms of the rhythm disturbance and the pattern observed. Use of antiarrhythmic agents also requires knowledge of pharmacology, underlying electrophysiologic mechanisms, and the electrophysiologic and hemodynamic effect of the agents. Treatment for tachyarrhythmias can be difficult and is often associated with significant morbidity and mortality. None of the antiarrhythmic agents is without significant risk to the fetus, the woman, or both, and all have a variety of side effects, including the possibility of producing an arrhythmia in the mother (Kleinman & Nehgme, 2004).

The half-life of these drugs also must be considered when medications are changed or a combined regimen of antiarrhythmic agents is used. Fetal excretion is primarily placental or renal. If the medication metabolites are excreted in the urine, reingestion must be considered (Kleinman & Nehgme).

Individual responses of the woman and her fetus to each agent should be observed during treatment. The decision to treat fetal arrhythmias should be based on an understanding of the natu-

Table 12-2 Drug Therapy

DRUG	INDICATED USE	RECOMMENDED DOSAGE	SIDE EFFECTS	EFFECTIVENESS
Adenosine (Class IV, FDA Class C)	Supraventricular arrhythmias	IV: 100–200 mcg/kg of EFW via rapid IV bolus into umbilical vein; fetal therapy via maternal IV not recommended PO: Not available	Bronchospasm (with asthmatic patients); dyspnea; transient arrhythmias (bradycardia) after cardioversion; known to ↑ AV block	Assists in identifying SVT (reentrant in nature); does not prevent recurrent SVT (Jaeggi & Nii, 2005; Kleinman et al., 2004).
Amiodarone (Class III, FDA Class D)	Supraventricular arrhythmias; ventricular arrhythmias	IV: 5 mg/kg over 20 min; 500–1000 mg over 24 hr, then oral administration PO: Loading dose: 1200–1600 mg divided in two doses for 7–14 days; then 400–800 mg every day for 1–3 wk Maintenance: 200–800 mg/day (Kleinman & Nehgme, 2004; Strasburger, 2000)	Can ↑ digoxin level; maternal-fetal hypo- or hyperthyroidism; corneal microdeposits; prematurity; low birth weight, congenital malformations; photosensitivity; life-threatening pulmonary alveolitis (not found to be dose related); hepatitis; myopathy; neuropathy; nausea; rash; alopecia; tremors; insomnia; nightmares; fetal cretinism; hypotension	Considered "last resort" drug; not recommended for use unless adequate doses of other antiarrhythmic drugs are unsuccessful or not tolerated; adverse reactions require drug discontinuation in about 20% of patients; can be found in breast milk for several weeks after drug administration (Kleinman et al., 2004)
Digoxin (Glycoside, FDA Class C)	Supraventricular arrhythmias; atrial fibrillation (AF) rate control	IV: 1000–1500 mcg/24 hr (loading only) Maintenance: 0.250–1.0 mg/day PO, two divided doses (Kleinman & Nehgme, 2004; Kleinman et al., 2004; Strasburger, 2000)	Toxicity = arrhythmias; nausea and vomiting; anorexia; diarrhea; malaise; fatigue; confusion; facial pain; insomnia; depression; vertigo and colored vision may occur at low serum levels, especially if hypokalemia or hypomagnesemia is present; interacts with other antiarrhythmic agents such as quinidine, verapamil, amiodarone, and propafenone; can also interact with erythromycin; give lower dosage if patient is in renal failure	Contraindicated in ventricular arrhythmias/WPW syndrome; may not be as effective in hydropic fetuses due to poor absorption; requires frequent ECG monitoring to assess toxicity (Kleinman et al., 2004)

Continued

Table 12-2	Drug Therapy—cont'd			
DRUG	**INDICATED USE**	**RECOMMENDED DOSAGE**	**SIDE EFFECTS**	**EFFECTIVENESS**
Disopyramide (Class I-A, FDA Class C)	Supraventricular arrhythmias; ventricular tachyarrhythmias	PO: Loading dose: 300 mg Maintenance: 100–200 mg q6h	Hypotension; negative inotropic effect; torsades de pointes; induction of uterine contractions; vagolytic effects; zero interaction with digoxin; interacts with Class III cardiac agents	Rarely used in children; very limited experience in fetuses; other alternatives are available; may stimulate uterine contractions (Briggs et al., 2005; Kleinman et al., 2004; Vautier-Rit et al., 2000).
Flecainide (Class I-C; FDA Class C)	Supraventricular arrhythmias; ventricular tachyarrhythmias	IV: Not available in United States PO: 100–400 mg/day in divided doses twice a day (Briggs et al., 2005; Kleinman et al., 2004; Strasburger, 2000)	Narrow therapeutic range; lightheadedness, visual disturbances, nausea; may cause arrhythmias, interacts with many antiarrhythmics	Probably safe with structurally normal hearts (Briggs et al., 2005; Kleinman et al., 2004)
Phenytoin (Class I-B, FDA Class D)	Ventricular arrhythmias; arrhythmias due to digoxin toxicity (Briggs et al., 2005)	IV: Not available in United States PO: 100–400 mg twice a day	Hypotension; vertigo; lethargy; dysarthria; mental retardation; gingivitis; macrocytic anemia; lupus; pulmonary infiltrates; growth restriction; fetal hydantoin syndrome	Prolonged QT interval syndrome; better alternative therapies are available; caution advised with breast-feeding (Joglar & Page, 2001)
Procainamide (Class I-A, FDA Class C)	Supraventricular arrhythmias; ventricular tachyarrhythmias	IV: 100 mg bolus over 2 min, up to 25 mg/min to 1 g over first hour Maintenance: 2–6 mg/min PO: 1 g; then up to 500 mg q 3h (Strasburger, et al., 2007; (Kleinman et al., 2004) IV: 600 mg over 20 min PO: 3000–6000 mg/day divided q6h (Strasburger, 2000)	Hypotension with IV; limit oral use to 3–6 months (in patients with lupus), gastrointestinal symptoms; agranulocytosis; interacts with Class III cardiac drugs, causing torsades de pointes; fetal levels may exceed maternal	Long record of safety; oral dose frequency requirement may result in noncompliance. (Briggs et al, 2005); rarely effective; frequency of dosing limits and side effects limit compliance (Kleinman et al., 2004)
Propafenone (Class I-C, FDA Class C)	Supraventricular arrhythmias; ventricular arrhythmias	IV: Not available in United States PO: 150–300 mg three times a day	Increases digoxin level; prolongs QRS complex; negative inotropic effects; proarrhythmias; gastrointestinal side effects common; avoid in patients with coronary artery disease or ventricular dysfunction	Effective in treating arrhythmias associated with WPW syndrome, ventricular premature complexes, and nonsustained ventricular tachycardia (Joglar & Page, 2001); used to treat refractory ventricular tachycardia (Briggs et al., 2005)

Table 12-2	**Drug Therapy—cont'd**			
DRUG	**INDICATED USE**	**RECOMMENDED DOSAGE**	**SIDE EFFECTS**	**EFFECTIVENESS**
Propranolol (Class II, FDA Class C/D)	Supraventricular arrhythmias; ventricular tachyarrhythmias	IV: 1–6 mg slowly PO: 40–160 mg q6h (Kleinman et al., 2004) 80–320 mg/24 hr, divided q6–8h (Strasburger, 2000)	Bronchospasm; central nervous system depression; heart block/↓ inotropic effect; may blunt hypoglycemia in patients with diabetes; may affect glucose tolerance in patients with non-insulin-dependent diabetes; maternal hypotension; contraindicated in sick sinus syndrome and Raynaud's disease; may cause neonatal respiratory depression, apnea, hypoglycemia, or bradycardia	Has been successful in suppressing ectopy in fetuses with reentrant SVT (especially if recurrent) (Briggs et al., 2005; Kleinman et al., 2004); may depress respirations or cause hypoglycemia in neonate; possibly associated with low birth weight (Kleinman et al., 2004)
Quinidine (Class I-A, FDA Class C)	Supraventricular arrhythmias; ventricular arrhythmias	PO: 200–300 mg q6h; 300–600 mg q8–12h if sustained dosage used	Hypotension; gastrointestinal effects; torsades de pointes; ↑ digoxin levels; monitor QRS/QTc intervals; maternal/neonatal thrombocytopenia; idiosyncratic reactions (angioedema/vascular collapse) may occur more commonly; eighth nerve toxicity (Briggs et al., 2005; Joglar & Page, 2001)	Does ↑ mortality; can result in increase in existing atrial arrhythmias/ventricular tachycardia resulting in sudden death (Joglar & Page, 2001)
Sotalol (Class III, FDA Class B/D)	Supraventricular arrhythmias; ventricular tachyarrhythmias; atrial tachycardias	IV: Not available in United States PO: 80–320 mg twice a day (Kleinman, 2004) 40–180 mg twice a day (Strasburger, 2000)	Torsades de pointes with hypokalemia; negative inotropic effect; sinus bradycardia; AV block; arrhythmias more common in renal failure, in females (Kleinman et al., 2004) Fetal death, neurologic sequelae (Briggs et al., 2005)	More successful experience with atrial flutter than with SVT (Kleinman et al., 2004)
Verapamil (Class IV, FDA Class C)	Supraventricular arrhythmias	IV: 5–10 mg over 30–60 sec PO: 80–160 mg three times a day	Calcium channel blocker; negative inotropic agent; ↑ serum digoxin levels; ↓ SA and AV node function; maternal hypotension; contraindicated in sick sinus syndrome with magnesium sulfate therapy, second- or third-degree heart block, shock, congestive heart failure, and with concomitant beta-blocker therapy; fetal bradycardia; heart block; may cause ventricular fibrillation if given to patient in ventricular tachycardia; fatigue, headache; dizziness; skin rash; peripheral edema	IV use for treatment of SVT with cardiac failure is contraindicated in neonates; exercise caution, if used at all, in fetuses (Kleinman et al., 2004)

ral history and precise mechanism of the rhythm disturbances as well as the pharmacology of the specific antiarrhythmic agent. The decision cannot be predicated simply on the basis of presence of arrhythmia or on the frequency of episodes of fetal tachycardia (Kleinman & Nehgme, 2004).

Antiarrhythmic therapy should be initiated on an inpatient basis with close observation of both mother and fetus, including external fetal heart monitoring for 12 to 24 hours (Kleinman & Nehgme, 2004; Larmay & Strasburger, 2004; Strasburger, 2000). Trending FHR patterns may provide additional information regarding changing patterns over the course of time, medication dosages and effectiveness, resolution of hydrops (if present), and other interventions utilized (Strasburger, 2005). Maternal ECG monitoring also is indicated, and some clinicians recommend daily 12-lead ECGs (Kleinman & Nehgme; Strasburger, 2000).

Antiarrhythmic agents are classified according to their predominant effects on cardiac activity. The classes of antiarrhythmic agents are Class IA, IB, IC, II, III, and IV (Table 12-3). For example, Class I agents block the voltage-sensitive sodium channels in the same manner as anesthetics. Class I agents generally cause a decrease in excitability and conduction velocity within the heart and are subdivided into three groups according to their effect on the duration of the action potential. Class II agents, the beta-blocking agents, attenuate adrenergic activity and indirectly block fast sodium channels. Class III agents block potassium channels, prolonging repolarization. Class IV agents block the calcium channels, slowing conduction through the SA and AV nodes (Quintana & Sinert, 2006). Table 12-2 lists the antiarrhythmic medications that may be used to treatment fetal arrhythmias.

Patients taking medications with proarrhythmic effects—that is, medications that can change a normal sinus rhythm pattern to arrhythmic patterns, such as beta-adrenergic sympathomimetics—should discontinue such medications. Patients should also be warned to avoid cocaine. Regardless of the pattern, all neonates will need care using a multidisciplinary team approach involving obstetric, pediatric cardiology, and neonatology personnel until a definitive diagnosis can be established.

Table 12-3	Classification of Antidysrhythmic Drugs	
CLASSIFICATION OF DRUG	MECHANISM OF ACTION	COMMENT
IA	Beta-adrenoreceptor blocker	Blocks cells that are discharging at abnormally high rates (slows phase 0 depolarization)
IB	Na$^+$ channel blocker	Blocks cells that are depolarizing or firing rapidly shortening repolarization (shortens phase 3 repolarization)
IC	Na$^+$ channel blocker	Markedly slows conduction in all cardiac tissue (markedly slows phase 0 depolarization)
II	Beta-adrenoreceptor blocker	Depresses automaticity, prolongs AV conduction, and decreases heart rate and contractility; used to treat supraventricular arrhythmias caused by increased sympathetic nervous system activity; also used for atrial flutter, atrial fibrillation, and AV node reentrant tachycardia (suppresses phase 4 depolarization)
III	K$^+$ channel blocker	Blocks potassium channels diminishing outward potassium current during repolarization (prolongs phase 3 repolarization)
IV	Ca^{2+} channel blocker	Blocks open or inactivated calcium channels, slowing phase 4 spontaneous depolarization and slowing conduction in tissues dependent on calcium current, that is, AV node (shortens action potential)

Source: Joglar & Page (2001); Quintana & Sinert (2006);

PROGNOSIS

The prognosis of a fetus with an arrhythmia depends on a variety of issues, including the associated pathology, the type of pattern, the presence or absence of hydrops, the FHR, and the adequacy of prescribed treatment, including medications. Identifying these variables will help guide the multidisciplinary team to an individualized care plan for both the woman and her fetus. Neonates with arrhythmias should be evaluated by means of a 12-lead ECG to assess ventricular function, especially preexcitation as seen in WPW syndrome, or for junctional reciprocating tachycardia. Should ectopy be found, an echocardiogram is indicated to rule out cardiac structural defects. Neonates with controlled SVT are usually given prophylactic treatment for 6 to 12 months (Larmay & Strasburger, 2004). Neonates with atrial flutter alone and no evidence of WPW syndrome usually require short-term prophylaxis of less than 3 to 6 months if not cardioverted soon after birth (Strasburger, 2000). The prognosis for full-term neonates is excellent; prematurity complicated with hydrops contributes to neonatal morbidity and mortality (Strasburger, 2000).

A fetus with documented complete AV block should be delivered at a tertiary care center where emergency cardiac pacing can be achieved quickly if needed (Strasburger, 2000). For a fetus with isolated complete AV block complicated by hydrops fetalis, a heart rate below 50 bpm, and a mother with a negative maternal anti-SSA antibody status, the prognosis is very poor (Jaeggi et al., 2004). The same is true for fetuses with complete AV block that is associated with structural cardiac disease (Sharland, 2001) or cardiomyopathy (Jaeggi et al.).

SUMMARY

The presumed mechanisms of fetal cardiac failure associated with arrhythmias include the following: (1) decreased ventricular filling time (SVT, atrial fibrillation, and atrial flutter), (2) dissociation between atrial and ventricular depolarization causing loss of the atrial boost mechanism (supraventricular or ventricular arrhythmias), (3) mild impairment of cardiac performance (ventricular arrhythmias), and (4) decrease in cardiac output (third-degree heart block).

When a rhythm abnormality is identified by either electronic monitoring or auscultation, the clinician should communicate the presence of an irregular rhythm to appropriate personnel and document the information appropriately. Multidisciplinary involvement is typically needed after an arrhythmia is recognized. Clinicians caring for these patients should possess knowledge of maternal-fetal physiology; and knowledge of fetal cardiac anatomy and physiology, pathophysiology of the arrhythmic patterns, assessment technology, treatment modalities, and prognoses appropriate to her or his education, training and clinical responsibility. This information will allow the clinician to assess the tracing and participate in the multidisciplinary team that develops a comprehensive individualized care plan and to guide or assist with the interventions necessary to obtain the best outcome possible for the fetus/neonate and the family.

REFERENCES

Bianchi, D., Crombleholme, T., & D'Alton, M. (2000). *Fetology: Diagnosis and management of the fetal patient.* Philadelphia: McGraw-Hill.

Blackburn, S. (2007). *Maternal, fetal, and neonatal physiology: A clinical perspective* (3rd ed., pp. 287–296). St. Louis: Saunders.

Briggs, G. G., Freeman, R. K., & Yaffe, S. J. (2005). *Drugs in pregnancy and lactation: A reference guide to fetal and neonatal risk* (7th ed.). Philadelphia: Lippincott Williams & Wilkins.

Carvalho, J. S., Prefumo, F., Ciardelli, V., Sairam, S., Bhide, A., & Shinebourne, E. A. (2007). Evaluation of fetal arrhythmias from simultaneous pulsed wave Doppler in pulmonary artery and vein. *Heart, 93,* 1448–1453.

Campbell, J. Q., Best, T. H., Eswaran, H., & Lowery, C. L. (2006). Fetal and maternal magnetocardiography during flecainide therapy for supraventricular tachycardia. *Obstetrics and Gynecology, 108,* 767–771.

Cuneo, B. F., & Strasburger, J. F. (2000). Management strategy for fetal tachycardia. *Obstetrics and Gynecology, 96,* 575–581.

Fujioka, S., & Kitaura, Y. (2001). Coxsackie B virus infection in idiopathic dilated cardiomyopathy: Clinical and pharmacological implications. *BioDrugs, 15,* 791–799.

Hamdan, A. H., & Cassady, G. (2006). Hydrops fetalis. (Retrieved February 20, 2007) http://www.emedicine.com/ped/topic1042.htm

Harkness, U., & Crombleholme, T. M. (2005). Twin-twin transfusion syndrome: Where do we go from here? *Seminars in Perinatology, 29,* 296–304.

Huber, A., & Hecher, K. (2004). How can we diagnose and manage twin-twin transfusion syndrome? *Best Practice & Research in Clinical Obstetrics and Gynaecology, 18,* 543–556.

Jaeggi, E. T., Fouron, J. C., Silverman, E. D., Ryan, G., Smallhorn, J., & Hornberger, L. K. (2004). Transplacental fetal treatment improves the outcome of prenatally diagnosed complete atrioventricular block without structural heart disease. *Circulation, 110,* 1542–1548.

Jaeggi, E. T., & Nii, M. (2005). Fetal brady- and tachyarrhythmias: New and accepted diagnostic and treatment methods. *Seminars in Fetal & Neonatal Medicine, 10,* 504–514.

Jain, V., & Fisk, N. M. (2004). The twin-twin transfusion syndrome. *Clinical Obstetrics and Gynecology, 47,* 181–202.

Joglar, J. A., & Page, R. L. (2001). Antiarrhythmic drugs in pregnancy. *Current Opinion in Cardiology, 16,* 40–45.

Kirby, M. L. (2004). Development of the fetal heart. In R. A. Polin, W. W. Fox, & S. H. Abman (Eds.), *Fetal and neonatal physiology* (3rd ed., pp. 613–621). Philadelphia: WB Saunders.

Kleinman, C. S., & Nehgme, R. A. (2004). Cardiac arrhythmias in the human fetus. *Pediatric Cardiology, 25,* 234–251.

Kleinman, C. S., Nehgme, R., & Copel, J. A. (2004). Fetal cardiac arrhythmias: Diagnosis and therapy. In R. K. Creasey & R. Resnik (Eds.), *Maternal-fetal medicine* (5th ed., pp. 465–482). Philadelphia: WB Saunders.

Kumar, S., & O'Brien, A. (2004). Recent developments in fetal medicine. *British Medical Journal, 328,* 1002–1006.

Larmay, H. J., & Strasburger, J. F. (2004). Differential diagnosis and management of the fetus and newborn with an irregular or abnormal heart rate. *Pediatric Clinics of North America, 51,* 1033–1050

Macones, G. A., Hankins, G. D., Spong, C. Y., Hauth, J. D., & Moore, T. (2008). The 2008 National Institute of Child Health Human Development workshop report on electronic fetal monitoring: Update on definitions, interpretations, and research guidelines. *Obstetrics & Gynecology, 112,* 661-666; and *Journal of Obstetric, Gynecologic and Neonatal Nursing, 37,* 510-515.

Menihan, C. A., & Kopel, E. (2008). *Electronic fetal monitoring: Concepts and applications* (2nd ed.). Philadelphia: Lippincott Williams & Wilkins.

Moore, K. L., & Persaud, T. V. N. (2003). *The developing human: Clinically oriented embryology* (7th ed., pp. 329–380). Philadelphia: WB Saunders.

Oudijk, M. A., Michon, M. M., Kleinman, C. S., Kapusta, L., Stoutenbeek, P., Visser, G. H., et al. (2000). Sotalol to treat fetal dysrhythmias. *Circulation, 101,* 2721–2726.

Oudijk, M. A., Ruskamp, J. M., Ambachtsheer, E. B., Ververs, T. F., Stoutenbeek, P., Visser, G. H., et al. (2002). Drug treatment of fetal tachycardia. *Paediatric Drugs, 4,* 49–63.

Oudijk, M. A., Ruskamp, J. M., Ververs, F. F., Ambachtsheer, E. B., Stoutenbeek, P., Visser, G. H., et al. (2003). Treatment of fetal tachycardia with sotalol: Transplacental pharmacokinetics and pharmacodynamics. *Journal of the American College of Cardiology, 42,* 765–770.

Pedra, S. R., Smallhorn, J. F., Ryan, G., Chitayat, D., Taylor, G. P., Khan, R., et al. (2002). Fetal cardiomyopathies: Pathogenic mechanisms, hemodynamic findings and clinical outcomes. *Circulation, 106,* 585–591.

Pickoff, A. S. (2004). Developmental electrophysiology in the fetus and neonate. In R. A. Polin, W. W. Fox, & S. H. Abman (Eds.), *Fetal and neonatal physiology* (3rd ed., pp. 669–690). Philadelphia: WB Saunders.

Quintana, E. C., & Sinert, R. (2006). Toxicity, Antidysrhythmic (Retrieved May 14, 2007). http://www.emedicine.com/emerg/topic45.htm

Rao, A., Sairam, S., & Shehata, H. (2004). Obstetric complications of twin pregnancies. *Best Practice & Research. Clinical Obstetrics and Gynaecology, 18,* 557–576.

Schmolling, J., Renke, K., Richter, O., Pfeiffer, K., Schlebusch, H., & Höller, T. (2000). Digoxin, flecainide, and amiodarone transfer across the placenta and the effects of an elevated umbilical venous pressure on the transfer rate. *Therapeutic Drug Monitor, 22,* 582–588.

Seferovi, P. M., Risti, A. D., Maksimovi, R., Simeunovi, D. S., Risti, G. G., Radovanovi, G., et al. (2006). Cardiac arrhythmias and conduction disturbances in autoimmune rheumatic diseases. *Rheumatology, 45,* iv39–iv42.

Sharland, G. (2001). Fetal cardiology. *Seminars in Neonatology, 6,* 3–15.

Simpson, K. R. (2008). Fetal assessment during labor. In K. R. Simpson & P. A. Creehan (Eds.), *Perinatal nursing* (3rd ed., pp. 399–442). Philadelphia: Lippincott Williams and Wilkins.

Singh, G. K. (2004). Management of fetal tachycardia. *Current Treatment Options in Cardiovascular Medicine, 6,* 399-406.

Sivasankaran, S., Sharland, G. K., & Simpson, J. M. (2005). Dilated cardiomyopathy presenting during fetal life. *Cardiology in the Young, 15,* 409–416.

Strasburger, J. F. (2000). Fetal arrhythmias. *Progress in Pediatric Cardiology, 11,* 1–17.

Strasburger, J. F. (2005). Prenatal diagnosis of fetal arrhythmias. *Clinics in Perinatology, 32,* 891–912.

Strasburger, J. F., Cheulkar, B., & Wichman, H. J. (2007). Perinatal arrhythmias: Diagnosis and management. *Clinics in Perinatology, 34,* 627-652.

Tanel, R. E., & Rhodes, L. A. (2001). Fetal and neonatal arrhythmias. *Clinics in Perinatology, 28,* 187–207.

Trines, J., & Hornberger, L. K. (2004). Evolution of heart disease in utero. *Pediatric Cardiology, 25,* 287–298.

Tulzer, G. (2000). Fetal cardiology. *Current Opinion in Pediatrics, 12,* 492–496.

Vautier-Rit, S., Dufour, P., Vaksmann, G., Subtil, D., Vaast, P., Valat, A. S., et al. (2000). Fetal arrhythmias: Diagnosis, prognosis, treatment, apropos of 33 cases. *Gynecologic & Obstetric Fertility, 28,* 729–737.

Vlagsma, R., Hallensleben, E., & Meijboom, E. J. (2001). Supraventricular tachycardia and premature atrial contractions in fetus. *Nederlands Tijdschrift Voor Geneeskunde, 145,* 295–299.

Wee, L. Y., & Fisk, N. M. (2002). The twin-twin transfusion syndrome. *Seminars in Neonatology, 7,* 187–202.

Wren, C. (2006). Cardiac arrhythmias in the fetus and newborn. *Seminars in Fetal and Neonatal Medicine, 11,* 182–190.

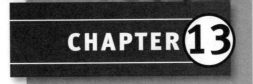

CHAPTER 13

Case Study Exercises

Rebecca L. Cypher

This chapter provides advanced case study exercises that are an adjunct to those presented in Chapter 10 as well as the Intermediate and Advanced Fetal Monitoring courses. The goal of this chapter is to provide participants with a series of adaptations from actual case studies that will promote and support critical thinking analysis of EFM tracings that keep within the framework of Association of Women's Health, Obstetric and Neonatal Nurses (AWHONN) fetal monitoring courses.

A practice case answer sheet is provided to facilitate analysis of the case studies and EFM tracings. For each case study exercise, readers are encouraged to (1) review the brief history and data provided, (2) analyze the EFM tracing, and (3) complete the practice case answer sheet. Answer keys for each exercise are provided at the end of each scenario. Readers should review their

work and identify areas of strength and those areas requiring more practice or review related to electronic FHR monitoring interpretation.

Objectives

For each case study exercise, the participant will be able to do the following:

- Interpret the fetal heart rate (FHR) baseline and variability using National Institute of Child Health and Human Development terminology.
- Identify periodic and episodic FHR patterns to include accelerations, late decelerations, variable decelerations, early decelerations, and prolonged decelerations.
- Determine the frequency, duration, intensity, and resting tone for the contraction pattern.
- Describe the appropriate interventions for each case study.

PRACTICE CASE ANSWER SHEET
Case Study Exercise: _____

1. Baseline FHR:

2. Variability   a. Absent (undetectable)   _____
                             b. Minimal (>0 but ≤ 5 bpm)   _____
                             c. Moderate (6–25 bpm)   _____
                             d. Marked (>25 bpm)   _____
                             e. Unable to determine   _____

3. Contractions   Frequency: _____
                             Duration: _____
                             Intensity: _____
                             Resting tonus: _____

4. Accelerations and decelerations. When present, circle P if periodic or E if episodic.

Accelerations	P	E
Early decelerations	P	
Variable decelerations	P	E
Late decelerations	P	
Prolonged decelerations	P	E
None present		

5. Interpretation   Category I   _____
                             Category II   _____
                             Category III   _____

6. List possible underlying physiologic mechanisms or rationales for observed patterns.

7. List in order of priority the physiologic goal(s) for observed patterns.

8. List actions and interventions indicated based on overall interpretation (physiologic based, instrumentation based, and further assessments).

Case Study Exercise A: Mary

Age:	24 years old
Gravida/Para:	G3 P1011
Gestational Age:	40-1/7 weeks
Medical History:	Tuberculosis at age 19—treated with INH, negative chest x-ray
Surgical History:	Unremarkable
Psychosocial History:	Migrant worker; single parent; father of baby not involved
Past Obstetric History:	Normal spontaneous vaginal birth at 39 2/7 weeks
	Spontaneous abortion at 9 weeks requiring dilation and curettage
Current Obstetric History:	Normal prenatal laboratory results
	Rh negative: received RhoGAM at 28 weeks
	2nd trimester ultrasound consistent with last menstrual period (LMP), normal anatomy
	Five prenatal visits in community clinic

Mary presented to obstetric triage for decreased fetal movement for 4 days. Her membranes were intact. Vaginal examination (VE) revealed a cervix that was 2 cm dilated, 75% effaced, and a fetal vertex that was −2 station. Her vital signs were as follows: oral temperature: 97.8° F (36.5° C); blood pressure: 110/68 mm Hg; pulse: 92 bpm; respiration: 20 breaths per minute. This tracing occurred within the first 15 minutes of monitor placement.

Figure 13-1   Mary: Triage Tracing Using Ultrasound and Tocodynamometer

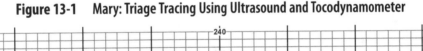
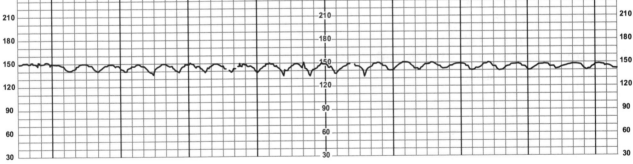
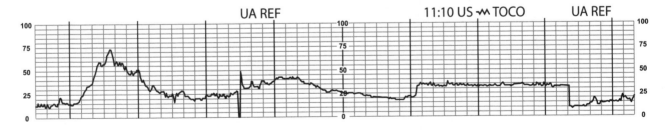

PRACTICE CASE ANSWER SHEET
Case Study Exercise A: Mary

1. Baseline FHR: **145 bpm**

2. Variability

Absent (undetectable)	_____
Minimal (>0 but ≤ 5 bpm)	_____
Moderate (6–25 bpm)	_____
Marked (>25 bpm)	_____
Unable to determine	_____ (Sinusoidal)

3. Contractions

Frequency:	**Irregular**
Duration:	**110–130 seconds**
Intensity:	**Palpate**
Resting tonus:	**Palpate**

4. Accelerations and decelerations. When present, circle P if periodic or E if episodic.

Accelerations	P	E
Early decelerations	P	
Variable decelerations	P	E
Late decelerations	P	
Prolonged decelerations	P	E
None present		

5. Interpretation

Category I	_____
Category II	_____
Category III	_____

6. List possible underlying physiologic mechanisms or rationales for observed patterns.
   - **Severe fetal anemia**
   - **Rh isoimmunization**
   - **Abruptio placentae**
   - **Fetal maternal hemorrhage**
   - **Narcotic or analgesic administration or ingestion**
   - **Fetal thumb sucking**
   - **Unknown etiology**

7. List in order of priority the physiologic goal(s) for observed patterns.
   - **Maximize oxygenation.**
   - **Maximize uteroplacental blood flow.**
   - **Reduce uterine activity.**

8. List interventions to achieve the physiologic goals and actions needed (physiologic based, instrumentation based, and further assessments).
   - **Administer maternal supplemental oxygen at 10 Liters/minute via a tight non-rebreather face mask.**
   - **Change maternal position to maximize uterine blood flow.**
   - **Hydrate with intravenous (IV) fluids.**
   - **Notify provider for immediate bedside evaluation.**
   - **Prepare for possible emergent birth if FHR pattern cannot be improved.**
   - **Alert neonatal team for possible emergent birth.**
   - **Interview the woman about fetal activity patterns prior to admission.**
   - **Question woman about recent trauma, abuse (e.g., abdominal trauma), and medication use (legal and illegal substances).**
   - **Review prenatal records for Rh status and RhoGAM® administration.**
   - **Consider fetal surveillance techniques such as biophysical profile.**
   - **Evaluate FHR responses to interventions.**
   - **Consider Kleihauer-Betke test and drug screen profile.**
   - **Palpate uterus to validate uterine monitoring data.**
   - **Keep provider notified of FHR pattern (undulating tracing) and evaluate maternal-fetal response to interventions.**

Case Study Exercise: _____

1. Baseline FHR:

2. Variability   a. Absent (undetectable)   _____
                        b. Minimal ($>$0 but $\leq$ 5 bpm)   _____
                        c. Moderate (6–25 bpm)   _____
                        d. Marked ($>$25 bpm)   _____
                        e. Unable to determine   _____

3. Contractions   Frequency: _____
                        Duration: _____
                        Intensity: _____
                        Resting tonus: _____

4. Accelerations and decelerations. When present, circle P if periodic or E if episodic.

                        Accelerations   P   E
                        Early decelerations   P
                        Variable decelerations   P   E
                        Late decelerations   P
                        Prolonged decelerations   P   E
                        None present

5. Interpretation   Category I   _____
                        Category II   _____
                        Category III   _____

6. List possible underlying physiologic mechanisms or rationales for observed patterns.

7. List in order of priority the physiologic goal(s) for observed patterns.

8. List actions and interventions indicated based on overall interpretation (physiologic based, instrumentation based, and further assessments).

Case Study Exercise B: Eleanor

Age:	28
Gravida/Para:	G3 P1011
Gestational Age:	41-4/7 weeks
Medical History:	Unremarkable
Surgical History:	Cesarean section
Psychosocial History:	Unremarkable
Past Obstetric History:	Previous low transverse cesarean section for arrest of dilation at 6 cm
	Spontaneous abortion at 6 weeks
Current Obstetric History:	Normal prenatal laboratory results
	2nd trimester ultrasound consistent with LMP, normal anatomy

Eleanor presented to labor and delivery at 1330 with spontaneous rupture of membranes that occurred at 1100. The fluid was meconium stained. The FHR was normal, with a baseline of 140, moderate variability, and spontaneous accelerations. She was having contractions every 2 to 4 minutes, lasting 60 to 90 seconds, and moderate on palpation. A VE on admission revealed a cervix that was 2 cm dilated, 50% effaced, and a fetal vertex that was −2 station. Her vital signs were as follows: oral temperature: 97.8° F (36.5° C); blood pressure: 112/58 mm Hg; pulse: 86 bpm; respiration 22 breaths per minute. Eleanor requested an epidural shortly after admission because of the increasing intensity of contractions. There was arrest of dilation at 6 cm. Internal monitors were placed at 1640, and an oxytocin infusion was started due to inadequate Montevideo units (140–180).

The FHR gradually changed to a baseline of 135 bpm, minimal variability, and recurrent variable decelerations with an occasional late deceleration. The nurse performed intrauterine resuscitation maneuvers. The physician reviewed the FHR tracing but asked that the oxytocin infusion continue at the current rate of 9 mU/minute. The nurse voiced her concern but followed the order as directed.

At 2045, the cervix was 10 cm dilated, 100% effaced, and vertex at +1 station in the occiput posterior position. At 2100, the IUPC was dislodged, and the tocodynamometer was reapplied. The physician instructed the patient to start pushing. The nurse again expressed her concern about the FHR tracing but was told by the physician that he would find another nurse to care for the patient if she refused to push with the patient.

Figure 13-2   Eleanor: Labor and Delivery at 2205 Using Fetal Spiral Electrode and Tocodynamometer

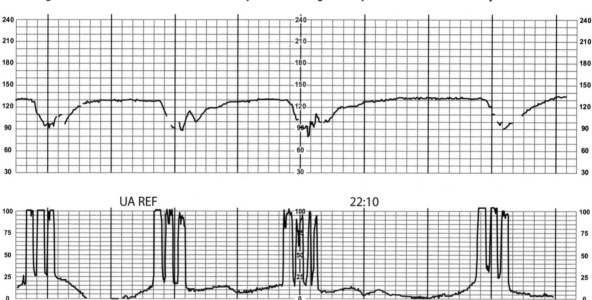

PRACTICE CASE ANSWER SHEET
Case Study Exercise B: Eleanor

1. Baseline FHR: **130 bpm**

2. Variability   **Absent (undetectable)**   (first five minutes of tracing)
        Minimal (>0 but ≤5 bpm)   (last three minutes of tracing)
        Moderate (6–25 bpm)   _____
        Marked (>25 bpm)   _____

3. Contractions   Frequency: **q 2 to 3 minutes**
        Duration: **50–60 seconds**
        Intensity: **Palpate**
        Resting tone: **Palpate**

4. Accelerations and decelerations. When present, circle P if periodic or E if episodic.

Accelerations	P	E
Early decelerations	P	
Variable decelerations	**P**	**E**
Late decelerations	P	
Prolonged decelerations	E	
None present		

5. Interpretation   Category I   _____
        Category II   _____
        Category III

        _____ This tracing has criteria that could be interpreted as category II or category III. It is an example of the need for clinical judgment and decision making based on the overall clinical picture: the decision to interpret as indeterminate or abnormal will depend on the preponderance of minimal versus absent variability in a larger segment of tracing.

6. List possible underlying physiologic mechanisms or rationales for observed patterns.
   • **Decreased umbilical cord perfusion**
   • **Umbilical cord compression**
       o **Knot in cord**
       o **Short cord**
       o **Decreased Wharton's jelly**
       o **Thin cord**
   • **Strong vagal stimulation resulting from head compression**
   • **Decreasing fetal oxygen reserves related to placental changes**
   • **Umbilical cord prolapse (occult)**
   • **Decreased amniotic fluid (oligohydramnios)**

7. List in order of priority the physiologic goal(s) for observed patterns.
- **Maximize umbilical circulation.**
- **Maximize oxygenation.**
- **Reduce uterine activity.**
- **Maximize placental blood flow.**

8. List actions and interventions indicated based on overall interpretation (physiologic based, instrumentation based, and further assessments).
- **Discontinue oxytocin.**
- **Push every 2nd or 3rd contraction.**
- **Perform VE to assess fetal descent, presentation for most expeditious route of birth, and possibility of cord prolapse.**
- **Change maternal position to maximize uterine blood flow and optimize oxygenation.**
- **Initiate chain of command or authority.**
- **Continue to hydrate with IV fluids to increase maternal blood volume and maximize uterine blood flow.**
- **Continue to administer maternal supplemental oxygen at 10 Liters/minute via a tight non-rebreather face mask.**
- **Prepare for possible expedited birth.**
- **Notify neonatal team for possible resuscitation.**
- **Keep provider notified of FHR pattern and evaluate maternal-fetal response to interventions.**
- **Consider fetal scalp stimulation when FHR is at baseline.**
- **Validate uterine monitoring data.**
- **Continue assessments and interventions based upon clinical findings and facility protocols**
- **Keep family informed of clinical situation.**

Case Study Exercise: _____

1. Baseline FHR:

2. Variability   a. Absent (undetectable)   _____
     b. Minimal (>0 but ≤5 bpm)   _____
     c. Moderate (6–25 bpm)   _____
     d. Marked (>25 bpm)   _____
     e. Unable to determine   _____

3. Contractions   Frequency: _____
     Duration: _____
     Intensity: _____
     Resting tonus: _____

4. Accelerations and decelerations. When present, circle P if periodic or E if episodic.

Accelerations	P	E
Early decelerations	P	
Variable decelerations	P	E
Late decelerations	P	
Prolonged decelerations	P	E
None present		

5. Interpretation   Category I   _____
     Category II   _____
     Category III   _____

6. List possible underlying physiologic mechanisms or rationales for observed patterns.

7. List in order of priority the physiologic goal(s) for observed patterns.

8. List actions and interventions indicated based on overall interpretation (physiologic based, instrumentation based, and further assessments).

Case Study Exercise C: Nancy

Age:	32 years old
Gravida/Para:	G3 P2002
Gestational Age:	38-5/7 weeks
Medical History:	Unremarkable
Surgical History:	Unremarkable
Psychosocial History:	Single; father of baby involved
Past Obstetric History:	Normal spontaneous vaginal birth at 39-6/7 weeks
	Normal spontaneous vaginal birth at 38-1/7 weeks
Current Obstetric History:	Normal prenatal laboratory results

* Rh negative
* Group B streptococcus (GBS) positive

2nd trimester ultrasound consistent with LMP, normal anatomy

Nancy presented to obstetric triage at 0400 with complaint of leaking small amounts of clear fluid since 0115. She also had increasing frequency and intensity of contractions prior to admission. She denied headache, blurred vision, or epigastric pain. A VE at admission showed a cervix that was 2 cm dilated, 50% effaced, and a fetal vertex that was +1 station. Her vital signs were as follows: temperature oral: 97.8° F (36.5° C); blood pressure: 126/74 mm Hg; pulse: 98 bpm; respiration: 24 breaths per minute. Oxytocin augmentation was started at 0830 related to arrest of dilation at 2 cm despite regular, painful contractions. The patient declined an epidural and received 2 mg Stadol and 12.5 mg Phenergan IV for pain relief at 0845. The patient received relief rating her pain 2–3 out of 10.

A seizure was witnessed at 1040 and the patient became unresponsive. The patient was hypotensive with a palpable pulse. An anesthesiologist was called to the bedside to assist with airway and fluid management. The charge nurse called the primary care provider to the bedside stat. Eclampsia was the presumptive diagnosis, and the patient received a 4 gram magnesium sulfate loading dose. The subsequent diagnosis, after delivery, was anaphylactoid syndrome of pregnancy, commonly referred to as an amniotic fluid embolism.

FIGURE 13-3   Nancy: Labor and Delivery Tracing Using Fetal Spiral Electrode and Tocodynamometer at 1050

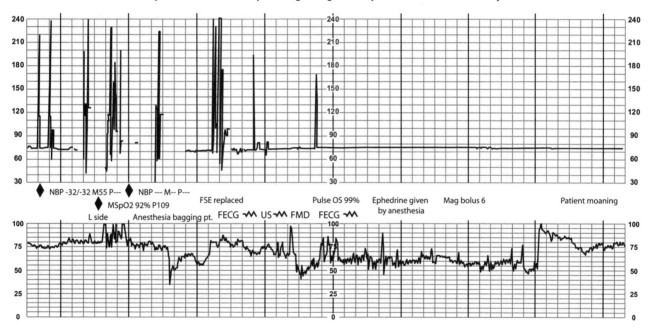

PRACTICE CASE ANSWER SHEET

Case Study Exercise C: Nancy

1. Baseline FHR: **75 bpm**

2. Variability   **Absent (undetectable)**   _____
   Minimal (>0 but ≤5 bpm)   _____
   Moderate (6–25 bpm)   _____
   Marked (>25 bpm)   _____
   Unable to determine   _____

3. Contractions   Frequency: **Unable to assess**
   Duration: **Unable to assess**
   Intensity: **Unable to assess**
   Resting tone: **Need to palpate**

4. Accelerations and decelerations. When present, circle P if periodic or E if episodic.

   Accelerations   P   E
   Early decelerations   P
   Variable decelerations   P   E
   Late decelerations   P
   Prolonged decelerations   P   E (Presumed bradycardia)
   None present

5. Interpretation   Category I   _____
   Category II   _____
   Category III   _____

6. List possible underlying physiologic mechanisms or rationales for observed patterns.
   • **Decreased uteroplacental perfusion related to maternal hypotension**
   • **Decreased uteroplacental perfusion during maternal seizure**
   • **Hypoxia secondary to maternal seizure**

7. List in order of priority the physiologic goal(s) for observed patterns.
   • **Maximize oxygenation.**
   • **Maximize placental blood flow.**

8. List actions and interventions indicated based on overall interpretation (physiologic based, instrumentation based, and further assessments).
   • **Maintain maternal airway and resuscitate.**
   • **Change maternal position with lateral tilt to maximize uterine blood flow as well assist with CPR.**
   • **Discontinue oxytocin.**
   • **Prepare for perimortem cesarean if unable to resuscitate mother within 5 minutes.**

- **Assess for alternative causes of FHR bradycardia (i.e., uterine rupture)**
- **Maintain IV access for fluid administration to increase maternal blood volume and maximize uterine blood flow.**
- **Prepare and administer magnesium sulfate bolus for seizure prophylaxis as ordered by provider.**
- **Prepare for emergent birth after Nancy is stabilized.**
- **Alert neonatal team to prepare for emergent birth and resuscitation.**
- **Have ephedrine 5–10 mg IV push ready to treat hypotension, if necessary.**
- **Differentiate FHR from maternal pulse by manual palpation of maternal pulse, auscultation of FHR, or ultrasound of FHR.**
- **Use pulse oximeter to verify maternal oxygenation during ventilation.**
- **Evaluate FHR responses to interventions.**
- **Palpate uterus to validate uterine monitoring data.**
- **Continue assessments and interventions based upon clinical findings and facility protocols**
- **Keep family informed of clinical situation.**

Case Study Exercise: _____

1. Baseline FHR:

2. Variability
   a. Absent (undetectable) _____
   b. Minimal (>0 but ≤ 5 bpm) _____
   c. Moderate (6–25 bpm) _____
   d. Marked (>25 bpm) _____
   e. Unable to determine _____

3. Contractions
   Frequency: _____
   Duration: _____
   Intensity: _____
   Resting tonus: _____

4. Accelerations and decelerations. When present, circle P if periodic or E if episodic.

Accelerations	P	E
Early decelerations	P	
Variable decelerations	P	E
Late decelerations	P	
Prolonged decelerations	P	E
None present		

5. Interpretation
   Category I _____
   Category II _____
   Category III _____

6. List possible underlying physiologic mechanisms or rationales for observed patterns.

7. List in order of priority the physiologic goal(s) for observed patterns.

8. List actions and interventions indicated based on overall interpretation (physiologic based, instrumentation based, and further assessments).

Case Study Exercise D: Ruth

Age:	41 years old
Gravida/Para:	G1 P0
Gestational Age:	39-1/7 weeks
Medical History:	Chronic hypertension controlled on Aldomet twice a day
Surgical History:	None
Psychosocial History:	Married
Past Obstetric History:	In vitro fertilization pregnancy using donor egg and sperm
Current Obstetric History:	Normal prenatal lab
	1st trimester screening normal
	2nd trimester ultrasound normal anatomy, declined amniocentesis
	Blood pressure ranges prenatally: 130–160s/80–90s mm Hg

Ruth presented for labor induction at 0100 because of chronic hypertension. Her cervix was closed and 50% effaced on admission. A Foley bulb was placed for mechanical dilation of the cervix with a low-dose oxytocin infusion of 2 mU/minute. The Foley bulb came out spontaneously at 0720. Her cervix was 3–4 cm, 50% effaced, and the fetal vertex was at −3 station. The FHR baseline was 145 bpm with moderate variability and accelerations. Ruth progressed slowly to 6 cm, 90% effaced, and 0 station with oxytocin. Amniotomy was performed at 1430 and a large amount of clear fluid was observed. Blood pressures during the labor were 130–150s/80s mm Hg.

Ruth requested an epidural at 1545. Shortly after the epidural was placed, Ruth became hypotensive, with blood pressure ranges of 64–98/41–56 mm Hg. The FHR baseline was 155 bpm with moderate variability. She became lightheaded and nauseated. A 5-mg dose of ephedrine was given IV push by the anesthesiologist. An increasing amount of bloody vaginal fluid was noted.

FIGURE 13-4A   Ruth: Labor and Delivery Tracing Using Fetal Spiral Electrode and Intrauterine Pressure Catheter at 1530

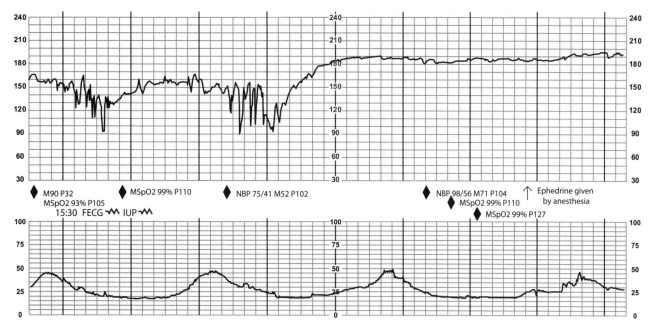

PRACTICE CASE ANSWER SHEET
Case Study Exercise D1: Ruth

1. Baseline FHR: **155 bpm initially (presumed to be stable before this segment)**
   185 bpm post decelerations

2. Variability

Absent (undetectable)	_____
Minimal (>0 but ≤5 bpm)	_____
Moderate (6–25 bpm)	_____
Marked (>25 bpm)	_____
Unable to determine	_____

3. Contractions

Frequency:	**2½–3 minutes**
Duration:	**90–110 seconds**
Intensity:	**45–55 mm Hg**
Resting tone:	**15–20 mm Hg**

4. Accelerations and decelerations. When present, circle P if periodic or E if episodic.

Accelerations	P	E
Early decelerations	P	
Variable decelerations	P	E
Late decelerations	**P**	
Prolonged decelerations	P	E
None present		

5. Interpretation

Category I	_____
Category II	_____
Category III	_____

6. List possible underlying physiologic mechanisms or rationales for observed patterns.
   - **Decreased uteroplacental perfusion related to abrupt decrease in maternal blood pressure following epidural placement**
   - **Possible placental abruption related to rapid decrease in blood pressure and increasing amount of blood-tinged vaginal fluid**
   - **Fetal tachycardia as a compensatory effort following episode of suspected maternal and fetal hypoxemia**
   - **Possible elevation in maternal temperature**
   - **Endogenous catecholamine response**

7. List in order of priority the physiologic goal(s) for observed patterns.
   - **Maximize placental blood flow.**
   - **Maximize oxygenation.**
   - **Reduce uterine activity.**

8. List actions and interventions indicated based on overall interpretation (physiologic based, instrumentation based, and further assessments).

- **Change maternal position to maximize uterine blood flow and optimize oxygenation.**
- **Hydrate with IV fluids to increase maternal blood volume and maximize uterine blood flow.**
- **Administer maternal supplemental oxygen at 10 Liters/minute via a tight non-rebreather face mask.**
- **Evaluate FHR responses to interventions.**
- **Check maternal temperature.**
- **Notify primary care provider of changing maternal-fetal status.**
- **Provide support to decrease maternal anxiety and catecholamine response.**
- **Prepare for a possible emergent birth.**
- **Alert neonatal team for possible emergent birth.**
- **Continue assessments and interventions based upon clinical findings and facility protocols.**
- **Keep family informed of clinical situation.**

PRACTICE CASE ANSWER SHEET
Case Study Exercise: _____

1. Baseline FHR:

2. Variability   a. Absent (undetectable)   _____
                          b. Minimal ($>$0 but $\leq$ 5 bpm)   _____
                          c. Moderate (6–25 bpm)   _____
                          d. Marked ($>$25 bpm)   _____
                          e. Unable to determine   _____

3. Contractions   Frequency: _____
                          Duration: _____
                          Intensity: _____
                          Resting tonus: _____

4. Accelerations and decelerations. When present, circle P if periodic or E if episodic.

Accelerations	P	E	
Early decelerations	P		
Variable decelerations	P	E	
Late decelerations	P		
Prolonged decelerations	P	E	
None present			

5. Interpretation   Category I   _____
                          Category II   _____
                          Category III   _____

6. List possible underlying physiologic mechanisms or rationales for observed patterns.

7. List in order of priority the physiologic goal(s) for observed patterns.

8. List actions and interventions indicated based on overall interpretation (physiologic based, instrumentation based, and further assessments).

Ruth responded to the ephedrine dose with blood pressures returning to the pre-epidural range, and her temperature was 99.0 F (.37.2 C) A VE was performed because of the increased amount of bleeding and fetal tachycardia. She was 10 cm dilated, 100% effaced, and +2 station. The IUPC was removed and a tocodynamometer applied. The patient was instructed to start pushing with every other contraction. The FHR tracing remained indeterminate, and the patient was moved to the operating room for operative vaginal delivery versus cesarean section. Figure 13-4B is the FHR tracing before the patient was moved to the operating room.

FIGURE 13-4B   Ruth: Labor and Delivery Tracing Using Fetal Spiral Electrode and Tocodynamometer

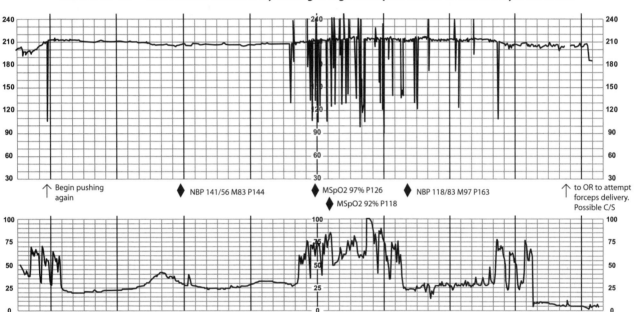

PRACTICE CASE ANSWER SHEET
Case Study Exercise D2: Ruth

1. Baseline FHR: **210 bpm**

2. Variability   Absent (undetectable)   _____
   Minimal (>0 but ≤5 bpm)   _____
   Moderate (6–25 bpm)   _____
   Marked (>25 bpm)   _____
   Unable to determine   _____

3. Contractions   Frequency: **Unable to assess**
   Duration: **Unable to assess**
   Intensity: **Unable to assess**
   Resting tone: **Need to palpate**

4. Accelerations and decelerations. When present, circle P if periodic or E if episodic.

Accelerations	P	E
Early decelerations	P	
Variable decelerations	P	E
Late decelerations	P	
Prolonged decelerations	E	
None present		

5. Interpretation   Category I   _____
   Category II   _____
   Category III   _____

6. List possible underlying physiologic mechanisms or rationales for observed patterns.
   - **Fetal response to ephedrine**
   - **Decreased uteroplacental perfusion related to maternal hypotension**
   - **Possible placental abruption related to increased amount of blood-tinged vaginal fluid**
   - **Elevation in maternal temperature**

7. List in order of priority the physiologic goal(s) for observed patterns.
   - **Maximize placental blood flow.**
   - **Maximize oxygenation.**
   - **Reduce uterine activity.**

8. List actions and interventions indicated based on overall interpretation (physiologic based, instrumentation based, and further assessments).
   - **Change maternal position to maximize uterine blood flow.**
   - **Continue IV fluid maintenance.**
   - **Continue maternal supplemental oxygen at 10 Liters/minute via a tight non-rebreather face mask.**
   - **Evaluate FHR responses to interventions.**
   - **Prepare to expedite birth.**
   - **Alert neonatal team about imminent birth.**
   - **Continue assessments and interventions based upon clinical findings and facility protocols.**
   - **Keep family informed of clinical situation.**

Glossary of Key Terms

Abrupt—Timing from onset to nadir or peak of FHR change is < 30 seconds. Refers to characteristics of periodic or episodic FHR changes.

Acceleration—An abrupt transitory increase in the fetal heart rate from the baseline rate; associated with sympathetic nervous stimulation. When using EFM to assess FHR data in the term fetus, an acceleration is a visually apparent abrupt increase in FHR peaking at least 15 beats per minute above the FHR baseline, lasting at least 15 seconds from onset to return to baseline. In the fetus under 32 completed weeks gestation an acceleration increases at least 10 beats per minute above baseline and lasts at least 10 seconds from onset to return to baseline.

Acidemia—An abnormal excess hydrogen ion concentration in the blood due to accumulation of acid or consumption of base.

Acidosis—An abnormal excess hydrogen ion concentration in tissues due to accumulation of acid or consumption of base.

Adrenergic response—Activated by, characteristic of, or secreting epinephrine or substances with similar activity. The term is applied to nerve fibers transmitting norepinephrine at a synapse when a nerve impulse passes (i.e., sympathetic fibers).

Aerobic metabolism—Growing, living, or occurring in the presence of oxygen; requiring oxygen for respiration. Specifically, the chemical process of using oxygen to produce energy from carbohydrates (sugars). This process is also called aerobic respiration, oxidative metabolism, and cellular respiration.

Alkalosis—An abnormal deficit of hydrogen ion in the tissues, resulting in an increase in pH value (decreased hydrogen ion concentration) above normal.

Amnioinfusion—Instillation of fluid into the uterus through an intrauterine catheter. Used to increase amniotic fluid volume in situations of oligohydramnios or umbilical cord compression with associated variable decelerations.

Amniotic Fluid Index (AFI)—The amount of amniotic fluid measured by ultrasonography in centimeters. AFI is expressed as the sum of the measurements of the deepest amniotic fluid pocket in all four abdominal quadrants.

Amplitude—The distance between high and low points of the FHR tracing oscillations. Describes the range of variation in fetal heart rate changes from peak to trough.

Anaerobic metabolism—Chemical processes of energy production from carbohydrates that take place in the absence of oxygen.

Antenatal—Before birth; used synonymously with prenatal.

Antepartum—The period of pregnancy occurring before labor or childbirth.

Antiarrhythmic therapy—Medication regimens used to treat fetal arrhythmias.

Arrhythmia—Any deviation from a normal heart rate; a heart rate without rhythm. Describes FHRs that are too fast (> 160 bpm), too slow (< 110 bpm), sporadic, or irregular. An arrhythmia may be associated with disordered impulse formation, disordered impulse conduction, or a combination of both. The term is sometimes used interchangeably with dysrhythmia.

Artifact—Inaccurate variation or absence of FHR on the fetal monitor tracing due to mechanical or technical limitations or electrical interference of the monitoring system.

Aspartate Aminotransferase (AST)—An enzyme that contributes to protein metabolism. This enzyme is present in the liver and is important in the biosynthesis of amino acids as it catalyzes the reversible transfer of an amino group between glutamic and aspartic acid. The former term was SGOT (serum glutamic-oxaloacetic transaminase). When cell damage occurs, especially in the liver (as seen with severe preeclampsia, HELLP syndrome, or trauma), AST is released into the tissues and bloodstream and AST levels are increased.

Asphyxia—Decrease in oxygen in body tissue (hypoxia), increase in CO_2 level (hypercapnia), and decrease in pH (metabolic and/or respiratory acidosis) with buildup of lactic acid in the tissue. In order to make a diagnosis of asphyxia in the neonate there must be evidence of all four of the following findings: arterial pH < 7.00, 5-minute Apgar score of 3 or below, neonatal neurologic sequelae, and multi-organ system dysfunction (AAP/ACOG, 2003).

Atrial flutter—An extremely rapid tachyarrythmia resulting from reentrant electrical conduction. The atrial rate may range from 300–500 bpm in the fetus and 300–360 bpm in the neonate. The AV node slows or blocks transmission of some of the atrial electrical impulses, resulting in a variable ventricular response. The ventricular rate usually ranges 190-240 bpm. The relationship between atrial and ventricular impulses may be fixed (2:1 or 3:1 AV block) and regular, or variable and irregular (e.g., varying degrees of AV block).

Atrial fibrillation—Tachycardiac atrial FHR rarely identified in the fetus. Often accompanied by a variable degree of AV block that will cause the ventricular rate to vary from 60 to 200 bpm.

Atrioventricular (AV) arrhythmias—Arrythmias resulting from a defect in the AV junction that disrupts or changes conduction of impulses through the AV node. AV arrhythmias consist of second- and third-degree AV block.

Auscultation—An auditory assessment made by listening for sounds within the body, such as fetal heart sounds. Fetal heart sounds are auscultated to determine rate and rhythm. Technically, "true" auscultation of fetal heart sounds is performed with a fetoscope, or stethoscope (e.g. Pinard), but this term also includes the use of a hand-held Doppler ultrasound device to assess the FHR through detection of heart motion by ultrasound.

Autocorrelation—Computerized comparison of consecutive points of waveforms generated by the electronic fetal monitor. Comparison is based on ultrasound waves reflected from the moving fetal heart valves. Current EFM terminology and practices assume the use of this technology in generating EFM data.

Automaticity—The inherent ability of cardiac muscle cells to depolarize spontaneously. Exhibited most strongly by the SA node, the AV node, the bundle of HIS, and the Purkinje fibers, but can be expressed by any cardiac muscle cell.

Baroreceptors—Pressure-sensitive stretch receptors in carotid sinus and aortic arch that detect changes in blood pressure. Stimulation of fetal baroreceptors alters the FHR by stimulating the autonomic nervous system to increase or decrease the FHR via the sympathetic or parasympathetic branch.

Base deficit—Measures the amount of base buffer reserves below normal levels. A large positive base deficit (e.g., > 12 mEq/liter) indicates that base buffers have been used to buffer acids, that sufficient base reserves are not present, and that metabolic acidosis is present.

Base excess—Measures the amount of base buffer reserves above normal levels. A large negative base excess [e.g., < -12 mEq/liter (-13, -14, etc.)] indicates that base buffers have been used to buffer acids, that sufficient base reserves are not present, and that metabolic acidosis is present.

Baseline fetal heart rate—Approximate mean FHR rounded to increments of 5 beats per minute (bpm) during a 10-minute period, excluding accelerations and decelerations and periods of marked FHR variability (more than 25 bpm). There must be at least 2 minutes of identifiable baseline segments (not necessarily contiguous) in any 10-minute period, or the baseline for that period is indeterminate.

Baseline fetal heart rate variability—Fluctuations in the baseline FHR that are irregular in amplitude and frequency. The fluctuations are visually quantitated as the amplitude of the peak-to-trough in bpm. Variability is a characteristic of the baseline: it is determined in a 10-minute period excluding accelerations and decelerations, and quantified as **absent** (visually undetectable), **minimal** (visually detectable but ≤5 bpm), **moderate** (6-25 bpm), or **marked** (> 25 bpm).

Beta-adrenergic receptors—Cellular binding sites sensitive to epinephrine and norepinephrine. Myometrial smooth muscle beta-2 receptors are highly sensitive to epinephrine and have a high affinity to bind with terbutaline.

Betamimetic drugs—Medications that mimic stimulation of the sympathetic nervous system. Specifically in myometrial cells they have a relaxant or depressant effect on uterine contractility. (Sometimes referred to as sympathomimetic or betasympathomimetic.)

Biophysical Profile (BPP)—An antenatal assessment of fetal well-being that combines NST results with multiple physiologic parameters observed with real-time ultrasound. The BPP includes the assessment of five parameters: fetal breathing movement, gross body movement, fetal tone, amniotic fluid volume, and fetal heart rate reactivity (NST).

Bishop score—A method for determining cervical readiness for induction of labor by scoring 5 components: cervical dilation, effacement, consistency, position, and station of the presenting part. Higher scores (≥6) are associated with successful induction of labor.

Bradyarrhythmia—A slow heart rate rhythm usually occurring when FHR is below 90 beats per minute (e.g., sinus bradycardia or heart block).

Bradycardia—Baseline FHR below 110 beats per minute for a period of 10 minutes or more.

Cardiotocography—The monitoring of the fetal heart rate and uterine activity during labor and birth. Also referred to as cardiotokography.

Category I FHR patterns—FHR tracings demonstrating normal baseline rate, moderate variability, and the absence of late or variable decelerations. Accelerations and early decelerations may or may not be present. Tracings with these features are strongly predictive of normal fetal acid base status at the time of observation.

Catgory II FHR patterns—Tracings which cannot be classified as either category I or category III patterns. These tracings are not predictive of abnormal acid-base status, but there is not enough evidence to classify them in category I or III.

Category III FHR patterns—Tracings exhibiting a sinusoidal pattern or exhibiting absent variability in conjunction with bradycardia or recurrent late or variable decelerations. These tracings are predictive of abnormal fetal acid base status at the time of observation.

Chain of command or authority—Definition of the lines of authority and responsibility for clinical problem resolution within an organization. Describes the persons to contact and the order in which to contact them when differences of opinion about clinical management of patients cannot be resolved directly between providers.

Chemoreceptor—Sensory nerve endings or cells stimulated by increased or decreased blood concentrations of a chemical substance. Sensitive to change in oxygen, carbon dioxide, and pH levels in the blood. Chemoreceptors are located in the aortic and carotid bodies and in the medulla.

Compensatory response to hypoxemia—Describes the ability of the fetus to adjust to low blood oxygen levels by drawing on fetal reserves and mobilizing physiologic responses to maintain central oxygenation. The presence of moderate variability implies adequate physiologic compensation and fetal reserves.

Competence validation—Process of documenting the verification of individual's knowledge and skills according to predetermined criteria.

Computer Analysis (CA)—The use of artificial intelligence (AI) to objectively analyze FHR signals according to predetermined algorithms. CA can also alert care providers, interpret patterns and offer management options.

Conductivity—The capacity of the cardiac cells to conduct a current through the cells.

Conflict management—Process of managing professional disagreements through effective interpersonal communication and/or within the mechanisms of institutional policies, procedures, and protocols. May involve implementing the chain of command or authority.

Contraction Stress Test (CST)—Assessment of the FHR response to uterine activity typically conducted in the antenatal period. A CST may be assessed when there are at least 3 contractions of at least 40 seconds duration in 10 minutes. Contractions may be spontaneous, induced by oxytocin administration, or induced with endogenous oxytocin via nipple or breast stimulation. The presence of late decelerations in response to these contractions (a positive CST) may be an indicator of fetal compromise.

Deceleration—A transitory decrease in the FHR from the baseline rate.

Digyzotic—Pertaining to or derived from two separate zygotes (fertilized ova), as in twin gestation occurring from two fertilized ova. Results in fraternal twins.

Doppler—An instrument that emits ultrasound waves and receives a return signal. In the context of FHR monitoring, a Doppler usually refers to a hand-held ultrasound device used to detect the FHR. It converts the sound waves reflected from the motion of the heart valves into a fetal heart rate.

Doppler velocimetry—Use of specialized ultrasonography to measure the blood flow velocity in the uterine artery, umbilical arteries and fetal middle cerebral artery. Also referred to as Doppler flow.

Early deceleration—Early decelerations are visually apparent gradual decreases in the FHR. The onset, nadir, and recovery of early decelerations generally occur coincident with the onset, peak, and recovery of uterine contractions. Early decelerations are typically symmetrical in shape

Electronic fetal monitoring—An auditory and visual assessment of the FHR and uterine activity with data generated by fetal monitor technology. The data generated includes an auditory FHR signal, a digital or graphic display of FHR and UA data, and a permanent record on paper or computerized storage.

Episodic changes—Accelerations or decelerations of the FHR which are not associated with uterine contractions.

Excitability—The readiness of the cardiac cells to respond to a stimulus or irritation.

External fetal monitoring—Collection and assessment of FHR and UA data using an ultrasound transducer to monitor the fetal heart rate and a tocodynamometer to monitor uterine contractions.

Extrinsic influences—Factors outside the fetus that may affect fetal oxygenation and FHR characteristics (e.g., maternal, placental, or umbilical cord factors).

False negative—When an assessment incorrectly identifies a compromised fetus as healthy.

False positive—When an assessment incorrectly identifies a healthy fetus as compromised.

Favorable physiologic response—An FHR response predictive of a fetus that is able to respond appropriately to the environment and maintain fetal reserves.

Fetal attitude—The relationship of the fetal parts to each other, especially the referring to the position of the fetal head in relation to the fetal body when the vertex is presenting. The vertex may be flexed, deflexed, or extended.

Fetal lie—The relationship of the fetal body to the maternal body. Fetal lie may be longitudinal (fetal body is parallel to maternal spine), transverse (fetal body is perpendicular to maternal spine), or oblique (fetal body is at an angle between longitudinal and transverse lie).

Fetal presentation—The lowest part of the fetus that comes out of the uterus first. Most often the presentation is vertex (occiput first), but it can also be breech (buttocks or feet first), shoulder (shoulder first), face or brow (face or brow first) or compound (hand with head or foot with buttocks).

Fetal scalp blood sampling—The collection of small sample of blood from the fetal scalp via a capillary tube that is analyzed for pH level by a blood gas machine. An invasive method of assessing pH level of the fetus. Requires ruptured membranes and lancing the fetal scalp.

Fetal scalp stimulation—An indirect method of assessing acid-base status of the fetus by rubbing the fetal head to elicit an acceleration. Can be performed with or without ruptured membranes. Scalp stimulation is performed during a period of baseline FHR. It is not a resuscitative measure, and should not be performed during decelerations.

Fetal surveillance—Assessment of fetal well-being via indirect methods such as auscultation, electronic fetal monitoring, and antepartum testing.

Fetal reserve—The ability to maintain tissue oxygenation and essential physiologic function in response to decreased availability of oxygen or other physiologic stressors. This term is also used to refer to the excess amount of oxygen available to the fetus beyond that normally required for metabolism.

Fetoscope—Stethoscope adapted for auscultation of the FHR (also known as DeLee fetoscope).

First-generation monitor—An electronic fetal monitor that uses a refractory window and peak-to-peak comparison of fetal heart waveforms generated by an external ultrasound transducer. FHR was calculated by averaging peaks. Current EFM terminology and practices assume the use of autocorrelation techniques which are not available in first-generation monitors.

Funic souffle (bruit)—A soft "blowing" sound heard on auscultation over the umbilical cord. The rate is synchronous with the FHR.

Gradual—Timing from onset to nadir or peak of FHR change is ≥30 seconds. Refers to characteristics of periodic and episodic changes in the FHR.

Heart block—An AV conduction defect in which the electrical impulses in the heart are not conducted normally from the atrium to the ventricles via atrioventricular (AV) nodes. Results in bradycardia.

Hydrops fetalis—Generalized edema in the abdomen, scalp, liver and spleen of the fetus. Hydrops is a serious and often life threatening condition resulting from cardiac pump failure. Hydrops may result from immune disorders such as Rh incompatibility or non-immune causes such as cardiac malformations, cardiac arrhythmias, anemia, or twin-to-twin transfusion syndrome.

Hydrostatic pressure—The pressure exerted by a fluid in a closed system, such as pressure created by amniotic fluid in the uterus. An intrauterine pressure catheter (IUPC) measures hydrostatic pressure in the uterus during and between uterine contractions.

Hyperstimulation—A retired term for excessive uterine activity.

Hypoxemia—Low levels of oxygen in the blood.

Hypoxia—Low levels of oxygen in the tissue, oxygen levels inadequate to meet metabolic needs of the tissue.

Indeterminate—Not definitely or precisely determined or fixed; not leading to a definite end or result. Category II FHR patterns are indeterminate: they are not predictive of abnormal fetal acid-base status, yet there is not adequate evidence at present to classify these as Category I or Category III. Category II FHR tracings require evaluation and continued surveillance and re-evaluation, taking into account the entire associated clinical circumstances.

Intermittent auscultation—Auditory assessment of the FHR at intervals either by fetoscope or hand-held Doppler.

Intermittent decelerations—Occur with fewer than 50% of contractions in a 20-minute period.

Internal fetal monitoring—An invasive assessment of the FHR or uterine contractions or both. A fetal spiral electrode provides auditory and visual fetal heart ECG data. An intrauterine pressure catheter provides visual intrauterine pressure measurements during and between contractions.

Intrapartum—The period of pregnancy that includes labor and birth.

Intrauterine Pressure Catheter (IUPC)—A catheter used to directly measure intrauterine pressure during and between uterine contractions. The catheter may be fluid filled or sensor tipped.

Intrinsic factors—Internal fetal regulatory mechanisms that control the heart rate, including sympathetic, parasympathetic, and central nervous systems, baroreceptor, chemoreceptor, and hormonal responses.

Kleihauer-Betke test—A blood analysis to detect the presence and relative amount of fetal hemoglobin in the maternal blood specimen. When a blood specimen is stained on a slide, cells characterized with fetal hemoglobin can be viewed and counted to determine the ratio of fetal blood cells to maternal blood cells. Used to detect and/or estimate the severity of feto-maternal hemorrhage.

Late deceleration—Late decelerations are visually apparent gradual decreases in the FHR that are associated with uterine contractions. Late decelerations are delayed in timing, meaning the deceleration reaches its nadir (lowest point) after the peak of the contraction. In most cases the onset, nadir, and recovery of the deceleration occur after the respective onset, peak, and resolution of the contraction as well. Late decelerations are typically symmetrical in shape.

Leopold's maneuvers—A systematic method of abdominal palpation to assess fetal position, attitude, and lie.

Long-term variability—The frequency of oscillations (cycles) in the FHR over 1 minute. In current practice, FHR variability is visually assessed as a unit and no distinction is made between short-term and long-term variation in the heart rate.

Medulla oblongata—The lower portion of the brain stem; the relay center for the parasympathetic and sympathetic nervous system.

Meta-analysis—A research strategy used to analyze findings from multiple studies. The process includes: defining the hypotheses, standardized terminology, independent and dependent variables, and the instruments; defining key words for literature review; defining study inclusion and exclusion criteria; and performing analysis using specialized statistical techniques.

Metabolic acidosis—Decrease in blood pH due to an increase in hydrogen ion concentration, decrease in PO_2, and consumption of buffer bases (expressed as an increased base deficit or base excess). The PCO_2 may be normal.

Metabolic alkalosis—Increase in blood pH due to a decreased hydrogen ion concentration and associated with decreased PCO_2.

Mixed acidosis—Combination of metabolic and respiratory acidosis, reflected as a decrease in pH, decrease in PO_2, an increase in PCO_2 levels, and an increase in base deficit or excess.

Modified biophysical profile—Antepartum test for fetal wellbeing consisting of an NST and an amniotic fluid index.

Monozygotic—Pertaining to or derived from a single zygote (fertilized ovum), as in twin gestation occurring from a single fertilized ovum. Results in identical twins.

Montevideo units—Total pressure in mm Hg for all uterine contractions within a 10-minute time frame. Calculated by measuring the peak intensity or amplitude (in mm Hg) for each contraction occurring in a 10-minute period and adding the numbers together. Contraction amplitude is the difference between the resting tone and the peak of the contraction (in mm Hg). It is important to note that these calculations are dependent on the accuracy of IUPC data.

Nadir—The lowest FHR value in a deceleration. With electronic monitoring, it is visually the lowest point in the deceleration curve.

Neurohormonal response—A physiologic response involving both neural and hormonal mechanisms.

Nonhypoxic reflex response—Refers to a FHR response to an event not associated with decreased PO_2. Fetus quickly responds to change caused by an event (e.g., baroreceptor and vagal response affecting fetal blood pressure because of brief compression of the umbilical cord).

Nonreassuring fetal heart rate pattern—"Nonreassuring fetal status describes the clinician's interpretation of data regarding fetal status (ie, the clinician is not reassured by the findings). This term acknowledges the imprecision inherent in the interpretation of the data. Therefore, the diagnosis of nonreassuring fetal status can be consistent with the delivery of a vigorous neonate" (ACOG, 2005). This term is no longer recommended for interpretation of fetal heart monitoring data, but is used in multiple studies to refer to various FHR characteristics which might now be classified as category II or III patterns.

Nonstress Test (NST)—Antepartum fetal assessment test used to assess fetal wellbeing. The FHR is monitored for 2 accelerations (in a term fetus, FHR increases at least 15 bpm above baseline lasting for 15 seconds from the time the FHR leaves the baseline to the time it returns to the baseline) in 20 minutes. In a fetus under 32 weeks gestation accelerations are increases of at least 10 bpm for 10 bpm duration. The presence of accelerations indicates adequate fetal oxygenation.

Oxytocic—Having the effect of stimulating the uterus to contract.

Para (P)—Number of pregnancies that have resulted in birth. The TPAL method of describing gravidity (the number of pregnancies, including the present pregnancy) refers to the number of term births (T), preterm births (P), abortions (A), and living children (L) (e.g., gravida 3, para 1102).

Parasympathetic nervous system—Part of autonomic nervous system. Includes the vagus nerve which decreases the heart rate when stimulated.

Perinatal—Occurring during, or pertaining to, the periods before, during, or after the time of birth up to 28 days after delivery

Periodic changes—Accelerations or decelerations of the FHR that are associated with uterine contractions.

Phonocardiography—The graphic representation of heart sounds and murmurs, and includes pulse tracings (carotid, apex, and jugular pulse).

Piezoelectric effect—The crystals in the ultrasound transducer generate sound waves that are reflected back from moving structures. A shift in frequency of the waveforms reflected is used to identify the FHR.

Postterm or postdates pregnancy—Pregnancy lasting beyond 42 completed weeks of gestation.

Premature Atrial Contraction (PAC)—Characterized by the early discharge of an atrial focus, as seen by a premature P wave followed by a narrow, normal-appearing QRS complex. Can be either conducted (i.e., PAC followed by a ventricular contraction, then a compensatory pause followed by normal sinus rhythm) or nonconducted (i.e., PAC followed by compensatory pause). Often followed by an incomplete compensatory pause, produced by the incomplete depolarization of the fetal heart.

Premature Rupture of Membranes (PROM)—Rupture of membranes that occurs after 37 completed weeks of gestation, without signs and symptoms of labor.

Preterm PROM (PPROM)—Rupture of membranes that occurs prior to 37 completed weeks of gestation, without signs and symptoms of labor.

Premature Ventricular Contraction (PVC)—Premature depolarization in the heart with resultant irregularity in the heart rate and rhythm. PVCs will show no P wave, and the premature QRS is bizarre and wide, with the T wave usually directed opposite to the polarity of the QRS complex. The full compensatory pause may or may not be present.

Prolonged deceleration—Prolonged decelerations are visually apparent decreases in the FHR that drop at least 15 bpm below baseline and last at least 2 minutes but less than 10 minutes from their onset to the return to baseline.

Pseudosinusoidal pattern—A sinusoidal-appearing, undulating FHR pattern of short duration which is both preceded and followed by an FHR with normal characteristics.

Pulse oximetry—An additional method of assessing the fetal status during labor with internal oxygen saturation monitor. The monitor is placed on the fetal cheek via a vaginal exam. An SpO_2 result of 30% or more is considered reassuring and means the fetus is adequately oxygenated. Also referred to as fetal pulse oximetry or fetal oxygen saturation monitoring. While used in some research settings, this technology is not in use in general clinical practice in the United States.

Reassuring—A descriptive term reflecting the clinician's conclusion that he or she can be reasonably assured of fetal wellbeing at the present time, based on available assessment data. This term is no longer recommended for use in describing interpretation of EFM data, but is used at times to refer to the clinician's interpretation of antepartum testing results (e.g. an 8/10 or 10/10 biophysical profile score). The term is used in multiple research reports to refer to various FHR characteristics which might now be classified as category I FHR patterns.

Recurrent decelerations—Occurring with at least 50% of the contractions in a 20-minute period.

Refractory window—An inhibitory period in which the electronic ultrasound transducer does not attempt to count the incoming signal. Mechanism in first-generation fetal monitors.

Respiratory acidosis—A decrease in pH due to increased CO_2 and carbonic acid in the blood., Base deficit or excess may be within normal range. If pulmonary or placental exchange is increased, the amount of CO_2 in the extracellular tissue may decrease.

Respiratory alkalosis—An increase in pH due to decreased hydrogen ion concentration and a decrease in PCO_2 (often associated with hyperventilation).

Rhythm—Regularity or irregularity of the baseline FHR.

Second generation monitor—An electronic ultrasound fetal monitor that uses multiple comparison points in the waveforms generated by the external ultrasound transducer. Rate calculated by autocorrelation. Current EFM terminology and practice assume the use of this technique in the generation of FHR data.

Short-term variability—Changes in the FHR from one beat to the next. Measures the R-to-R intervals of subsequent fetal cardiac cycles (QRS). Historically, short-term variability and long-term variability were assessed independently of each other and an internal electrode was necessary for assessment of short term variability. In current clinical practice FHR variability is visually assessed as a unit by peak-to-trough amplitude fluctuations regardless of electronic monitoring method. No distinction is made between short term and long term FHR variation.

Sinusoidal pattern—A sinusoidal fetal heart rate pattern is a visually apparent undulating smooth sine wave-like pattern in FHR baseline with a cycle frequency of 3-5 per minute which persists for at least 20 minutes. There is an absence of accelerations and no response to uterine contractions, fetal movement, or stimulation.

Solid sensor-tipped IUPC—An intrauterine pressure catheter that has a microprocessor transducer at the catheter tip which measures the intrauterine pressure directly.

Specificity—The probability that a test will be negative when the infection or specific condition being tested for is not present.

Spiral electrode—An internal device for recording the FHR that is applied directly to the fetal presenting part and receives signals from the electrocardiac impulses of the fetal heart. Used to directly determine FHR based on changes in the R-to-R intervals in successive QRS complexes.

Strain gauge—A pressure transducer that electronically converts uterine pressure changes exerted on a diaphragm into mm Hg. Component of closed pressure system using a fluid-filled intrauterine catheter.

Supraventricular arrhythmias—Rhythm disturbances that originate above the ventricles, i.e., in the atria.

Supraventricular tachycardia—A sustained, rapid, regular atrial arrhythmia resulting from reentrant electrical conduction in the atria or the establishment of an irritable ectopic focus taking on the role of pacemaker. The rate may range from 210-320 bpm, but SVT rates are typically between 240 and 260 bpm. May be intermittent or sustained. Supraventricular tachycardia is often characterized by a fixed R-to-R interval with P waves preceding each QRS complex, as identified by ECG.

Sympathetic nervous system—A part of the autonomic nervous system. Stimulation results in FHR increase.

Tachycardia—Baseline FHR above 160 beats per minute for a period of ten minutes or more.

Tachysystole—Greater than 5 contractions in 10 minutes, averaged over 30 minutes. Uterine activity is quantified as the number of contractions in 10 minutes over an average of 30 minutes, and tachysystole is further qualified by the presence or absence of associated FHR decelerations.

Tocodynamometer (tocotransducer)—The transducer on an electronic fetal monitor that externally detects abdominal pressure or contour changes resulting from uterine contractions and transmits this information to the monitor to be displayed in graphic form.

Tocolytic—A medication that diminishes or stops uterine activity by altering smooth muscle activity.

Tonus—Intensity of uterine tone or intrauterine pressure between uterine contractions.

Ultrasound transducer—An external monitor that detects movement of the fetal heart valves opening and closing through transmission of a sound wave and Doppler shift. Monitor processor converts reflected sound waves into an electronic signal corresponding to the FHR.

Uterine bruit—The sound heard when listening to the blood flow in the maternal uterine vessels (also known as uterine souffle). Synchronous with maternal pulse.

Variable deceleration—Visually apparent, abrupt (onset to nadir < 30 seconds) decrease in the FHR below baseline. The decrease is calculated from onset to the beginning of the nadir of the deceleration. The FHR decreases ≥ 15 bpm, lasting ≥ 15 sec and < 2 minutes in duration. May occur with or without relationship to uterine contractions. When variable decelerations are associated with uterine contractions, their onset, depth, and duration typically vary with successive uterine contractions.

Ventricular arrhythmias—Rhythm disturbances originating from the ventricles, as a result of premature electrical discharge below the AV junction.

Vibroacoustic Stimulation (VAS)—A method of assessing fetal well-being in the antepartum and intrapartum periods using sound from an artificial larynx to elicit an acceleration. May also be referred to as fetal acoustic stimulation or simply acoustic stimulation.

REFERENCES

American College of Obstetricians and Gynecologists. (2005). *Inappropriate use of the terms fetal distress and birth asphyxia* (ACOG Committee Opinion No. 326). Washington, DC: Author.

American College of Obstetricians and Gynecologists and American Academy of Pediatrics. (2003). *Neonatal encephalopathy and cerebral palsy: Defining the pathogenesis and pathophysiology.* Washington, DC: Author.

Index

Note: Page numbers followed by *b* indicate boxes;
f indicates figures; *t* indicates tables.